CHALLENGES IN

Rheumatoid Arthritis

EDITED BY

Howard A. Bird
MD, FRCP
Professor of Pharmacological Rheumatology
University of Leeds
Research School of Medicine
Chapel Allerton Hospital
Leeds

Michael L. Snaith
MD, FRCP
Rheumatology Section
Division of Molecular and Genetic Medicine
The Medical School
The University of Sheffield
Sheffield

Blackwell
Science

© 1999 by
Blackwell Science Ltd
Editorial Offices:
Osney Mead, Oxford OX2 0EL
25 John Street, London WC1N 2BL
23 Ainslie Place, Edinburgh EH3 6AJ
350 Main Street, Malden
  MA 02148 5018, USA
54 University Street, Carlton
  Victoria 3053, Australia
10, rue Casimir Delavigne
  75006 Paris, France

Other Editorial Offices:
Blackwell Wissenschafts-Verlag GmbH
Kurfürstendamm 57
10707 Berlin, Germany

Blackwell Science KK
MG Kodenmacho Building
7–10 Kodenmacho Nihombashi
Chuo-ku, Tokyo 104, Japan

First published 1999

Set by Graphicraft Limited,
Hong Kong
Printed and bound in Great Britain
by MPG Books Ltd, Bodmin, Cornwall

A catalogue record for this title is
available from the British Library
and the Library of Congress

ISBN 0-632-04939-1

For further information on
Blackwell Science, visit our website:
www.blackwell-science.com

DISTRIBUTORS

Marston Book Services Ltd
PO Box 269
Abingdon, Oxon OX14 4YN
(*Orders*: Tel: 01235 465500
      Fax: 01235 465555)

USA
Blackwell Science, Inc.
Commerce Place
350 Main Street
Malden, MA 02148 5018
(*Orders*: Tel: 800 759 6102
         781 388 8250
      Fax: 781 388 8255)

Canada
Login Brothers Book Company
324 Saulteaux Crescent
Winnipeg, Manitoba R3J 3T2
(*Orders*: Tel: 204 837-2987)

Australia
Blackwell Science Pty Ltd
54 University Street
Carlton, Victoria 3053
(*Orders*: Tel: 3 9347 0300
      Fax: 3 9347 5001)

CHALLENGES IN
Rheumatoid Arthritis

Contents

List of contributors

EDITORS

Howard A. Bird MD, FRCP, *Professor of Pharmacological Rheumatology, University of Leeds, Research School of Medicine, Chapel Allerton Hospital, Chapeltown Road, Leeds, LS7 4SA, UK*

Michael L. Snaith MD, FRCP, *Rheumatology Section, Division of Molecular and Genetic Medicine, The Medical School, The University of Sheffield, Beech Hill Road, Sheffield, S10 2RZ, UK*

CONTRIBUTORS

Khalid Ahmed MB BS, PhD, MRCP, *Senior Registrar, Rheumatology Department, Leeds General Infirmary, Great George Street, Leeds, LS9 3EX, UK*

Arne N. Akbar PhD, MRCPath, *Department of Clinical Immunology, The Royal Free Hospital, Pond Street, London, NW3 2QG, UK*

Stephen Brady BMed, FRACP, *Director of Medicine, Mount Isa Base Hospital, Camooweal Street, Mount Isa, Queensland 4825, Australia*

Ferdinand C. Breedveld MD, PhD, *Professor of Rheumatology, Department of Rheumatology, C4R, Leiden University Medical Centre, PO Box 9600, 2300-RC Leiden, The Netherlands*

Peter M. Brooks MB BS, MD, FRACP, FAFRM, FAFPHM, MD (Lund) Hon. Causa, *Executive Dean, Health Sciences, University of Queensland, Brisbane 4029, Australia*

W. Paul Butt MD, FRCR, FRCPC, *Consultant Radiologist, Department of Clinical Radiology, Chancellor's Wing, St James University Hospital, Leeds, LS9 7TF, UK*

Margaret Byron MD, FRCP, *Consultant and Honorary Senior Lecturer in Rheumatology, Rheumatology Unit, University of Bristol, Division of Medicine, Bristol Royal Infirmary, Bristol, BS2 8HW, UK*

Hilary A. Capell MB BCh, BA, MD, FRCP, *Consultant Rheumatologist, Centre for Rheumatic Disease, Wards 14/15, Royal Infirmary, Glasgow, G4 0SF, UK*

Kaushik Chaudhuri MRCP (UK), *Department of Rheumatology, Walsgrave Hospital, Clifford Bridge Road, Walsgrave, Coventry, CV2 2DX, UK*

Anthony K. Clarke FRCP, *Consultant in Rheumatology and Rehabilitation, Royal National Hospital for Rheumatic Diseases, Upper Borough Walls, Bath, Somerset, BA1 1RL, UK*

Andrew Cope PhD, MRCP, *Wellcome Trust Clinical Research Fellow in Rheumatology, Kennedy Institute of Rheumatology, 1 Aspenlea Road, Hammersmith, London, W6 8LH, UK*

Richard O. Day MD, FRACP, *Professor and Director of Clinical Pharmacology, St Vincent's Hospital, Victoria Street, Darlinghurst, NSW 2010, Australia*

Jo C.W. Edwards MD, FRCP, *Professor of Connective Tissue Medicine, University College London Centre for Rheumatology, Arthur Stanley House, 45–50 Tottenham Street, London, W1P 9PG, UK*

Paul Emery MA, MD, FRCP, ARC, *Professor of Rheumatology, Clinical Director, Rheumatology Department, Leeds General Infirmary, Great George Street, Leeds, LS9 3EX, UK*

Christopher H. Evans PhD, DSc, FRCPath, *Henry Mankin Professor of Orthopaedic Surgery, University of Pittsburgh School of Medicine, Department of Orthopaedic Surgery, Ferguson Laboratory, 200 Lothrop Street, Room C313 Presbyterian-University Hospital, Pittsburgh, PA 15213, USA*

Juliane Franz MD, *WHO Collaborating Center for Molecular Biology and Novel Therapeutic Strategies for Rheumatic Diseases, Department of Rheumatology, University Hospital, Gloriastrasse 25, CH-8091 Zurich, Switzerland*

Renate E. Gay MD, *WHO Collaborating Center for Molecular Biology and Novel Therapeutic Strategies for Rheumatic Diseases, Department of Rheumatology, University Hospital, Gloriastrasse 25, CH-8091 Zurich, Switzerland*

Steffen Gay MD, *Professor of Experimental Rheumatology, WHO Collaborating Center for Molecular Biology and Novel Therapeutic Strategies for Rheumatic Diseases, Department of Rheumatology, University Hospital, Gloriastrasse 25, CH-8091 Zurich, Switzerland*

Anke M. van Gestel MSc, *Health Scientist, University Hospital Nijmegen, Department of Rheumatology, Geert Grooteplein 8, 6525 GA Nijmegen, The Netherlands*

Garry G. Graham PhD, *Honorary Visiting Professor, School of Physiology and Pharmacology, University of New South Wales, Sydney 2052, Australia*

Anthony P. Hollander PhD, *Lecturer, Human Metabolism & Clinical Biochemistry in the Division of Biochemical & Musculoskeletal Medicine, University of Sheffield Medical School, Beech Hill Road, Sheffield, S10 2RX, UK*

John D. Isaacs PhD, FRCP, *Senior Lecturer in Rheumatology, University of Leeds, Molecular Medicine Unit, Clinical Sciences Building, St James's University Hospital, Leeds, LS9 7TF, UK*

John R. Kirwan MD, FRCP, *Consultant and Reader in Rheumatology, Head of Rheumatology Unit, University of Bristol Division of Medicine, Bristol Royal Infirmary, Bristol, BS2 8HW, UK*

Matthew H. Liang MD, MPH, *Professor of Medicine, Division of Rheumatology, Immunology and Allergy, Brigham and Women's Hospital, Robert B Brigham Multipurpose Arthritis and Muscolosketetal Diseases Center, 75 Francis Street, Boston, MA 02115, USA*

Lisa A. Mandl MD, FRCP, *Fellow, Division of Rheumatology, Immunology and Allergy Brigham and Women's Hospital, Robert B Brigham Multipurpose Arthritis and Muscolosketetal Diseases Center, 75 Francis Street, Boston MA 02115, USA*

Michael F.R. Martin MA, MRCP, FRCP, *Consultant Rheumatologist, St James's University Hospital, Beckett Street, Leeds, LS9 7TF, UK*

Thomas Pap MD, *WHO Collaborating Center for Molecular Biology and Novel Therapeutic Strategies for Rheumatic Diseases, Department of Rheumatology, University Hospital, Gloriastrasse 25, CH-8091 Zurich, Switzerland*

Piet L.C.M. van Riel MD, PhD, *Professor of Rheumatology, University Hospital Nijmegen, Department of Rheumatology, Geert Grooteplein 8, 6525 GA Nijmegen, The Netherlands*

Paul D. Robbins PhD, *Associate Professor, Department of Molecular Genetics and Biochemistry, University of Pittsburgh School of Medicine, Presbyterian-University Hospital, Pittsburgh, PA 15213, USA*

Michael Salmon PhD, MRCPath, *Division of Immunity and Infection, The Medical School, Vincent Drive, Birmingham, B15 2TT, UK*

Ian Stockley MD, FRCS, *Consultant Orthopaedic Surgeon, Northern General Hospital, Herries Road, Sheffield, S5 7AU, UK*

Paul P. Tak MD, PhD, *Associate Professor, Department of Rheumatology, C4R Leiden University Medical Centre, PO Box 9600, 2300-RC Leiden, The Netherlands*

Alan Tyndall FRACP, FMH, *Professor and Head, University Department of Rheumatology, Felix Platter-Spital, Burgfelderstrasse 101, 4012 Basel, Switzerland*

A. Gerry Wilson PhD, MRCP, *Senior Lecturer in Molecular Medicine and Rheumatology, The University of Sheffield, Royal Hallamshire Hospital, Sheffield, S10 2JX, UK*

Frank A. Wollheim MD, PhD, FRCP, *Professor of Rheumatology, Department of Rheumatology, Lund University Hospital, S-221 85 Lund, Sweden*

Preface

Rheumatoid arthritis, the most common and arguably the most severe of the various inflammatory polyarthritides encountered world-wide, continues to intrigue. Many challenges remain, not least because its cause remains a secret. Even in terms of management there are controversies over the clinical effectiveness of the various programmes for disease control which are emerging and which are evaluated, for example, by using improved techniques for imaging. This is the second volume in a series devoted to common diseases that still provoke controversy. It may not answer all such questions but seeks to air the various arguments that need to be considered before the clinician can present a treatment option to the patient.

It seems unlikely that the cause in rheumatoid synovitis will prove to be singular. The first section of this volume, directed at this, brings together experts who were invited to provide a critical review of the evidence in those expanding fields that, in the last few years, have seemed most relevant to pathogenesis.

Discussion of pathogenesis leads automatically to disease progression and management. The second section airs the continued debate on how we can assess prognosis for groups of patients and how we can best distinguish between the undoubted variations in disease progression that is observed between different individuals. Outcome measures, histology, arthroscopy and the most recent advances in imaging are all discussed.

This leads to the most relevant and safest treatment. These sections are unashamedly devoted to medication, not just because of the vast investment currently being placed in this area by industry but also because the therapeutic/toxicity ratio for drugs, old and new, is often disappointingly small, providing additional fuel for the controversy on how aggressively rheumatoid arthritis should be treated.

The final section, loosely entitled 'benefits and risks', is perhaps the most speculative, tying up some loose ends and raising what we suggest will become the challenges of the future. The success of joint replacement is undoubted, although controversy still remains as to the timing and nature of surgical intervention. The increasing contribution of paramedicals, particularly physiotherapists and occupational therapists, is now being validated more rigorously. More thorny issues also receive attention, such as whether prognosis is changing, whether there will be a role for gene therapy and how all of this can be resourced from the limited funds available. The editors were relieved that these tasks could be delegated so they did not themselves have to provide the answers.

In general, a single author was invited to argue all aspects of each topic. Where the difference between physicians or scientists was more manifest, authors likely to hold opposing views were invited to contribute adjacent chapters.

It will be appreciated that the book provided a considerable challenge in design to the two editors. We both remain grateful to all authors who have contributed so ably in their respective fields and hope that readers will gain as much from it as we have in putting it together. More importantly, we hope that patients will ultimately gain from more rational decisions based upon appropriate consideration, by their medical attendant, of the controversies we have aired.

Howard A. Bird
Michael L. Snaith

Note added in proof

Whilst this book was in production an important international agreement on the nomenclature of drugs was announced by the Medicines Control Agency. This announcement was made too late to be implemented in this book.

Part 1: Pathogenesis of Rheumatoid Synovitis

1: Is rheumatoid factor relevant?

J.C.W. Edwards

Introduction

Rheumatoid factor (RF) has been out of fashion.

Rheumatoid arthritis (RA) is often described as an immune-complex disease. Immune complexes present in the serum and synovial fluid of patients contain RFs (autoantibodies to IgG Fc) [1]. A collation of conventional immunological dogma [2] suggests that RA is consistent with the predicted outcome of RF production (Fig. 1.1). Why then, has there been almost no recent interest in the potential pathogenic role of RF?

Between 1960 and 1980 a programme of analytical chemistry initiated by Henry Kunkel in the USA, and developed by Roitt and Natvig in Europe, promised to define the role of RF, and, in particular, IgG RF, in RA [1]. Then interest subsided. In the absence of a reason why persistent RF production should be a primary event, it became fashionable to see RF production as secondary to some deeper, more meaningful, immune disturbance. Nobody could explain why RFs should end up in joints, and interest was directed at articular or arthrotropic antigens and T-cell responses.

Current controversy over the identity of the villain in RA embraces competing claims for the T cell [3], the macrophage [4] and the synovial fibroblast [5]. Defects in the function of each of these cell types have been invoked to explain specific aspects of joint pathology. However, a viable theoretical model for the pathogenesis of RA must explain every genetic, demographic, clinical, pathological and serological feature of the disease; summarized in Table 1.1. Without a specific role for RFs and immune complexes this proves very difficult. In particular, it is difficult to see how RF production can be secondary to an inflammatory reaction in a joint when elevated RF levels frequently precede clinical disease [6]. Perhaps we have thrown the baby out with the bath water. The object of this chapter is to review, in the context of all aspects of RA, the arguments for and against reinstating a central role for RF in rheumatoid pathogenesis.

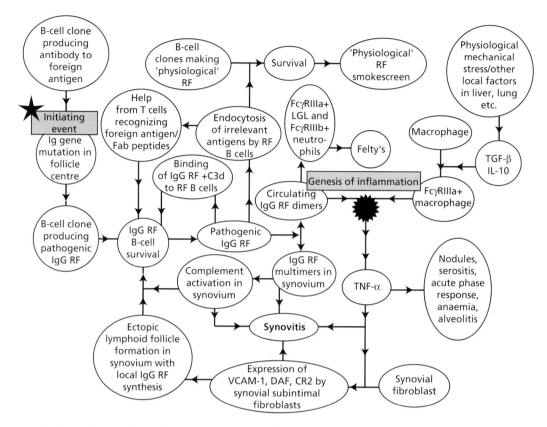

Fig. 1.1 Flow diagram of how RF may be involved in RA pathogenesis.

The prima facie case for RFs in RA pathogenesis

The circumstantial evidence for the involvement of autoantibodies in RA is impressive. RA overlaps or associates with a range of disorders, most obviously systemic lupus, Sjögren's syndrome and autoimmune thyroid disease, in many of which a pathogenic role for autoantibodies seems very likely. These conditions show a female preponderance, perhaps reflecting the tendency for antibody responses to be greater in females [7]. Moreover, RA is distinct from seronegative arthropathies, which lack autoantibodies, may show male preponderance and which have links with pathology in specific T-cell trafficking domains; the skin in psoriasis, the gut in Crohn's disease and mucosae in Reiter's syndrome.

Serum autoantibodies, and most consistently RFs, are present in 75–80% of cases of RA [8]. Immune complexes are found in the circulation and in joints, with evidence of complement activation in the latter [9]. Analysis of these complexes has failed to identify antigens other than IgG itself [10]. The complexes found in the serum (Fig. 1.2) include

Table 1.1 Features of rheumatoid arthritis.

Female preponderance
Association with HLA-DR4
Onset at any time in adult life with peak in midlife
Absence of epidemics or temporal relationship to external factors
Fluctuating but persistent course
Widespread synovitis, chiefly MCP, PIP, wrist, knee joints
Tendon sheath and bursal involvement
Suppression of erythropoiesis
Acute-phase response, raised serum levels of hepatic enzymes
Bone erosion, usually, but not always, contiguous with synovium
Subcutaneous nodules at sites of stress
Mononeuropathies at sites of stress (median, ulnar, lateral popliteal)
Alveolitis, pericarditis, pleurisy, lung nodules
Sicca syndrome
Circulating rheumatoid factors and immune complexes
A range of other autoantibodies to, e.g., nuclear antigens and keratin
Complement consumption in joints but not in the circulation
Marked increase in synovial intimal macrophage size and number
Lymphocyte accumulation with follicle formation in synovium
No significant central nervous system, gut or glomerular involvement
Amyloidosis
Nailford microinfarcts

Rarely
Splenomegaly, neutropenia and lymphadenopathy
Large granular lymphocyte pseudoleukaemia
Nodular hyperplasia of the liver
Major vasculitis, diffuse peripheral neuropathy

MCP, metacarpophalangeal; PIP, proximal interphalangeal.

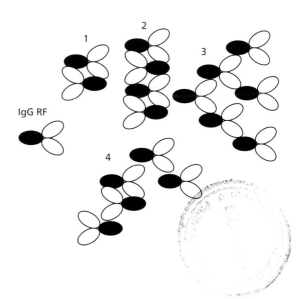

Fig. 1.2 Possible modes of self-association of IgG RF. Dimers (1) are found in serum in RA. Larger complexes, of which 3–5 are possible structures, are found in synovial fluid. Structure 2 requires the Fc antigenic epitope to be divalent. Structure 3 can interact with B-cell surface Ig most readily.

IgG RF dimers, which do not fix complement well [11], are small enough to reach the extravascular space and have the ability to activate cells resident in connective tissue [12]. The larger RF complexes found in joints fix complement [9].

The chief argument against a pathogenic role for autoantibodies in RA is the inconsistent correlation between autoantibody levels and clinical disease. This argument becomes less convincing as the relationship between autoantibodies and disease is analysed in conditions such as the anti-phospholipid syndrome (APLS) and necrotizing vasculitis [13,14]. It is now clear that standard serological tests give a very crude measure of the pathogenic potential of autoantibodies. Close correlations can only be expected when we understand the importance of such factors as autoantibody isotype, subclass, fine specificity, germline gene usage (dictating framework regions), and interactions with cofactors, such as serum β2 glycoprotein in APLS [13,14]. RF assays have justifiably been criticized as having little clinical value. However, this relates to issues about probabilities in medical decision making. The correlation between RF and disease is at least as good as that seen in other syndromes in which the pathogenic role of antibody is difficult to challenge.

Interest in T cells in RA started when it was found that most of the lymphocytes in RA synovium are T cells, even if outnumbered by plasma cells [15,16]. However, this pattern of cell populations is common to most chronic inflammation. What is unusual about rheumatoid synovium to the histopathologist is the presence of follicles containing B lymphocytes, sometimes with germinal centres [17]. T cells in rheumatoid synovium show little evidence of responding to antigen [18], and no consistent T-cell responses to synovial, or other, antigens have been identified despite prolonged search. Joint damage correlates with macrophage numbers, rather than T-cell numbers [19], and the activated intimal macrophages characteristic of early disease [20] are rarely in close contact with T cells. Everything points away from direct T-cell involvement in macrophage activation and cytokine release.

RA is associated with major histocompatibility complex (MHC) class II allotype [21]. This association implicates T cells in the process. However, antigen presentation to T cells occurs in all adaptive immune responses [22]. The suggestion that T cells extracted from rheumatoid joints show a 'Th1' phenotype *in vitro* adds little [23]. B-cell survival and differentiation and autoantibody synthesis are clearly occurring in rheumatoid synovium and whatever T cells are present must be providing the help required, presumably through a mechanism that involves antigen presentation via MHC class II.

The stochastic (random) element in RA

Any pathogenic model must explain the epidemiology of RA. Although it has been suggested that the onset of RA may be triggered by an environmental agent such as infection, the evidence is firmly against this. Disease onset is at random through adult life. In contrast to Reiter's syndrome or rheumatic fever, there are neither epidemics nor a clear temporal relationship to external events [24,25]. Most animal models of inflammatory arthritis are induced by external agents such as antigen or adjuvant and may tell us more about seronegative arthropathies than RA.

This lack of relationship between RA and external events, and the low concordance rate in monozygotic twins [24] suggests that a major element of causality is neither genetic, nor environmental, but stochastic. The stochastic element of causality is familiar in neoplasia, in the form of an accumulation of random mutations [26]. Despite claims that fibroblasts may appear 'transformed' in rheumatoid synovium [5] there is no consistent evidence of neoplastic change in any cell lineage in RA. However, the coexistence of hypergammaglobulinaemia, autoantibodies and B-cell maltomas in Sjögren's syndrome [27] highlights the fact that the life history of the B lymphocyte provides an opportunity for the dividing line between neoplasia and the immune response to become blurred. Cumulative somatic mutation occurs throughout life in B-cell immunoglobulin (Ig) genes [28]. In contrast, random T cell receptor gene rearrangement occurs chiefly in early life and is not cumulative. Ig gene mutation normally occurs in a temporal relationship to exposure to foreign antigen. However, as discussed by Pulendran and Nossal [29,30], responses to more or less trivial foreign antigens occur all the time and the random nature of Ig gene mutation means that, at any time, a B-cell clone may arise with an antibody specificity to a completely unrelated antigen. If this unrelated antigen is an autoantigen, and for some reason the clone is not deleted, an autoimmune process will develop, with no apparent temporal relationship to external events.

RFs from rheumatoid joints show repeated somatic mutations [31]. Moreover, it seems that RA may represent the outcome of the gradual accumulation of multiple B-cell clones of RF specificity, only some of which are capable of inducing clinical disease. High levels of autoantibodies and total IgG in RA may precede disease onset by several years [6]. The fluctuating course of RA is consistent with continued shifts in the spectrum of RF molecular species with variable re-establishment of control mechanisms, unlike the situation in true neoplasia or transformation.

This idea that humoral autoimmunity is a random spin-off of Ig gene mutation has several attractions. It may be the only model that is reasonably consistent with the epidemiology. It also raises difficult questions, as reviewed by MacLennan [32]. Why should B cells, recognizing soluble autoantigens such as IgG, survive, when soluble antigen should give a signal to B cells to undergo cell death [30]? Why should T-cell help be available? These questions lead directly to the issue of how B cells survive and how B cells of RF specificity may use aberrant survival strategies.

Control of B-cell survival

Ig gene mutation normally confers survival advantage to a B-cell clone if the resulting surface Ig binds to molecules identified as 'foreign' either by their ability to recruit T-cell help [22], or by their association with the complement fragment C3d [33]. Within the lymphoid follicle antigen alone conveys a negative survival signal to B cells, but, when bound to C3d, a positive signal [30,33,34]. Autoreactive B cells arising at random during an immune response to foreign antigen should normally die, because of the negative signal from native antigen and T-cell anergy. There are, however, two obvious loopholes in the system. If Ig gene mutation leads to the production of an antibody either to complement components or to IgG itself, the rules may change and control mechanisms may fail.

   Davies, Walport and others [35,36] have proposed that antibodies to C1q play a key role in systemic lupus. Anti-C1q antibodies can initiate complement activation and depletion, leading to impaired clearance of immune complexes. A disturbance of complement activation is also likely to impair B-cell clonal selection by altering the availability of C3d. This may contribute to the inappropriate survival of autoantibody producing clones of a wide variety of specificities.

   Moreover, it is becoming clear that both IgG RF and IgG anti-C1q antibodies may have unusual means of recruiting T cell or C3d-dependent signals for their parent B cells.

Survival of RF-specific B-cell clones

B-cell clones with RF specificity can potentially make use of two abnormal survival strategies.

Mechanism 1

This mechanism has been demonstrated by Roosnek and Lanzavecchia [37]. B cells of RF specificity can bind, through their surface Ig (i.e. RF), any IgG-based immune complex, internalize the antigen and present it to T cells

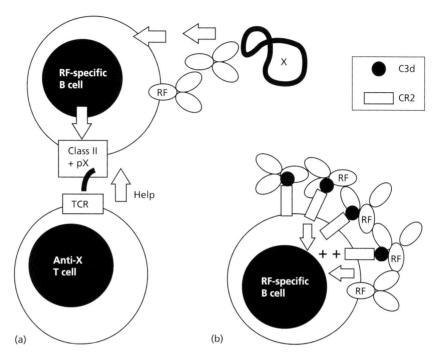

Fig. 1.3 (a) Mechanism 1 in which a B cell utilizes surface RF to obtain help from a T cell responsive to irrelevant antigen X. (b) Mechanism 2 in which a B cell receives a potent positive survival signal from IgG RFs bound to C3d.

(Fig. 1.3a). If the antigen is foreign, as it should normally be, the RF-specific B cell will receive T-cell help.

This mechanism is independent of the Ig isotype to which the B cell is committed. It is likely to be the mechanism driving IgM RF production following a normal response to foreign antigen. Its effects should, however, be short lived, being dependent on the presence of foreign antigen. Except where antigen is available for long periods, as in subacute bacterial endocarditis, the RF produced should remain largely of IgM isotype. On its own, this mechanism appears not to lead to a persistent autoimmune state.

Mechanism 2

This mechanism depends on the fact that IgG RFs can, in themselves, form immune complexes capable of binding to the surface Ig present on their parent B-cell clones (Fig. 1.3b). These complexes may acquire covalently bound C3d and confer survival advantage to the parent B cells [31]. Potentially, these complexes can form necklaces of indefinite length, encrusted with C3d, similar to artificial complexes described by Fearon and colleagues

[33], which could increase the survival signal given to the B cell by several orders of magnitude. A key point is that this mechanism will only operate in the context of IgG RF production.

This second mechanism is theoretically available to all autoantibody-producing B cells. However, for most autoantigens negative control mechanisms should be foolproof. T-cell help, as envisaged in mechanism 1, should not be available. Surface Ig on isolated autoantibody-producing clones should have to compete for the antigenic epitope already bound by soluble antibody. The clone should preferentially receive a negative signal from native antigen rather than a positive signal from complexed antigen. This does not necessarily apply to binding via RF (Fig. 1.3b). B-cell clones producing IgG RF in a confined space, such as a joint, would also, by generating high local levels of antibody which is also antigen, create optimal conditions for complex formation.

Even for IgG RF, mechanism 2 may only operate effectively for clones producing RF with very specific steric characteristics. IgG RFs may occur in bacterial endocarditis, but are neither perpetual nor pathogenic. This suggests that at least a proportion of the RF generated in RA are different from those occurring as an extension of 'physiological' RF production. This is precisely what has been found by Børretzen and colleagues [31]. Whereas 'physiological' RFs from normal individuals responding to tetanus immunization arise from a common germline sequence, RFs synthesized in RA joints arise from unrelated Ig genes. So far, this has only been demonstrated for IgM RF, but it is reasonable to assume that IgG RFs in RA will also differ in their germline origin.

The association with MHC class II allotype and the role of T-cell help

It is likely that to become self-perpetuating IgG RF-producing B-cell clones must take advantage of both T-cell help and the positive signal from C3d. The indiscriminate T-cell help provided by mechanism 1 [37] should fail if the only immune complexes around are self–self RF complexes. There would be no foreign antigen to present to T cells. Moreover, although mechanism 1 provides a role for T cells in the process, it is not clear why it should be class II allotype dependent. A solution to this problem, which would allow mechanisms 1 and 2 to act synergistically, would be available if RA subjects had T-cell responses either to IgG Fab-derived peptides in general, or to specific IgG RF Fab sequences. In preliminary studies, Elson and colleagues found anti-Fab T-cell responses in RA subjects (C. Elson, pers. comm., 1997). Responses to RF-specific Fab peptides are not documented. However, if the IgG Fc-binding peptides in at least a proportion of the IgG RF in RA are similar or identical to those in bacterial IgG Fc-binding proteins such as staphylococcal protein A, then such responses would be expected to be present.

The association of RA with class II DRβ allotype may relate to either RF-specific or general anti-Fab responses. Fab peptides shared with staphylococcal protein might bind preferentially to risk-associated class II allotypes [38]. An alternative explanation is that DRβ allotype influences antigen processing [39] and may thereby influence the likelihood of IgG Fab peptides being presented to T cells, in particular when the IgG is endocytosed in the guise of antigen.

This analysis suggests that the genesis of self-perpetuating IgG RF-producing B-cell clones is likely to be dependent on the background T-cell repertoire, and, in particular, responses to bacterial proteins. It is intriguing to note that close contact with domestic animals during childhood, perhaps with broader exposure to commensal bacteria, appears to be associated with an increased risk of developing RA in later life [40].

Ironically, if RF-specific B-cell clones in RA can take advantage of both mechanisms 1 and 2 because of the presence of anti-Fab T-cell responses, then conditions will also be ideal for the generation of a persistent and high level 'physiological' IgM RF response. Self-perpetuating IgG RFs would assist the survival of physiological RF-secreting B-cell clones just as readily as they would support their parent B-cell clones. Thus, the IgM RF in RA sera measured by routine assays may be largely an irrelevant smoke screen, just as the T-cell advocates would have us believe. This adds to the difficulty in studying RF pathogenicity. Although the crystal structure of an RA-derived RF Fab bound to IgG4 Fc has recently been reported [41], and the binding involves the staphylococcal protein A binding site, but via an unrelated peptide sequence, there is, at present, no way of knowing whether this represents a potentially pathogenic interaction.

To summarize so far: current understanding of B-lymphocyte biology provides a credible basis for implicating anti-C1q and anti-IgG Fc antibodies in systemic lupus and RA, respectively. IgG RF production may become self-perpetuating through a mechanism distinct from that which generates 'physiological' RF. However, this mechanism may require T-cell responses to Fab peptides. The critical test of these arguments lies in an extension of the experiments initiated by Elson.

IgG RF complexes and inflammation

Self-perpetuating IgG RF production may occur without clinical outcome, if the resulting immune complexes fail to induce cellular activation or are cleared. If, however, IgG RF complexes do induce disease, then a mechanism has to be found which explains the pattern of features listed in Table 1.1.

Under normal conditions circulating complexes are cleared by complement receptor 1 on red cells [35]. This clearance may fail if the system is overloaded, as in serum sickness, if low complement levels reduce the efficiency of clearance, as proposed in systemic lupus [36], or if the complexes are too small to fix complement, but can still generate inflammation through other means. This third option may apply in RA.

Immune complexes can generate inflammation, without involving complement, by binding Ig Fc receptors (FcγR) in normal non-lymphoid tissues chiefly present on macrophages [42]. FcγR can bind free IgG, but only induce signalling when cross-linked by at least two IgG molecules as part of a complex.

The dominant form of immune complex described in RA serum is an IgG RF dimer [1]. It is poor at fixing complement [11], which is probably why it persists long enough in the circulation to be detected. Moreover, unlike most immune complexes, being only twice the size of IgG, IgG RF dimers should have significant access to the extravascular tissue space. Thus, these complexes can be predicted to cause, not vascular injury, but cell activation in tissues in which FcγR are expressed. This marries with the current view that the production of cytokines such as tumour necrosis factor alpha (TNF-α) and interleukin-1 by activated tissue macrophages is central to the genesis of inflammation in RA [43].

Macrophages can carry three classes of FcγR [42]. FcγRI has a high affinity for free IgG. However, it is not expressed at high level in normal tissues. Moreover, it may be saturated with free IgG under most physiological conditions. Binding of soluble immune complexes is chiefly ascribed to FcγRII and FcγRIII.

FcγRII is expressed by all macrophages, but is of lowest affinity. Moreover, monoclonal antibodies to FcγRII, which should in theory cross-link pairs of receptors, do not induce cell signalling [44]. Whether for reasons of affinity or a requirement for multiple cross-linking, it appears that, at least on polymorphs, cell signalling in response to dimeric complexes requires the additional presence of FcγRIII [45].

A proportion of macrophages carry the FcγRIIIa isoform of FcγRIII, which signals through the common Fc receptor γ chain [42,46]. Ligation of FcγRIIIa, with agents that include a monoclonal antibody which acts as a dimeric ligand, is known to induce the release of both reactive oxygen species [47] and cytokines such as TNF-α [48]. At least on natural killer (NK) cells immune complexes from rheumatoid serum will induce TNF-α production via FcγRIIIa [12]. The prediction from the conventional dogma is therefore that IgG RF dimers will chiefly exert their effects in the extravascular compartment via binding to the surface of macrophages which express, not only FcgRII, but also FcγRIIIa, with the production of TNF-α and other mediators.

FcγRIII expression in normal tissues

Studies of macrophages in synovium have often attempted to identify differences between macrophages in RA and control tissues. However, since the administration of antigen into the knee of a sensitized rabbit will produce the same histological changes in macrophage and fibroblast populations seen in RA, it seems likely that any change in phenotype of these cell types in RA will simply reflect the existence of an immune response [49]. In the context of the preceding discussion, a new question needs to be asked: do normal synovial macrophages differ from macrophages in other normal tissues in their Fc receptor status, and hence, susceptibility to the effects of small immune complexes?

Synovium contains two macrophage populations: intimal and subintimal [50]. Intimal macrophages were known as type A synoviocytes when their relationship to other macrophages was uncertain [51]. One of the most consistent features of rheumatoid synovitis is an increase in size and number of intimal macrophages, largely responsible for what was previously termed 'lining hyperplasia' [52].

Although monocytes which have 'matured' into macrophages *in vitro* express FcγRIIIa [46], recent studies have indicated that expression of FcγRIIIa by macrophages in normal tissues *in vivo* is restricted to specific sites, one of which is the synovial intima [53]. Most strikingly, in fetal limbs, synovial intima is the only site of significant FcγRIIIa expression. The consensus from published reports on adult tissues is that Kupffer cells, alveolar macrophages, cells in lymphoid organs and bone marrow and placental macrophages express most FcγRIIIa [54–56]. Recent studies indicate that to these can be added pericardial and salivary gland macrophages [53] (Table 1.2). In dermis, expression is minimal, with the exception of sites of mechanical stress, where rheumatoid nodules form. At these sites the majority of macrophages were found to express FcγRIIIa [53]. A wide range of other normal tissues show minimal FcγRIIIa expression.

FcγRIIIa expression by macrophages is induced by transforming growth factor beta (TGF-β) [57,58] and interleukin 10 (IL-10) *in vitro* [59]. Many cell types produce TGF-β in response to mechanical stress [60] and induction of FcγRIIIa by TGF-β would provide a convenient explanation for the recognized link between physical stress, both in synovium and skin, and inflammation in RA. The detailed pattern of synovial and dermal lesions suggests that tissue is particularly susceptible when stretched over bone within a restricted space: in metacarpophalangeal joints, metatarsophalangeal joints (where synovium is compressed between bone and ground) and skin over the olecranon. Expression of FcγRIIIa in liver, lung and salivary gland may reflect local availability of active TGF-β, but may also reflect other factors including availability of IL-10.

Table 1.2 Correspondence between sites of FcγRIIIa expression and lesions in rheumatoid arthritis.

Sites of FcγRIIIa expression on macrophages in normal tissue	Pathological lesions in rheumatoid arthritis
Synovium—intimal macrophages only	Erosive synovitis—centered on the intima
Liver—intrasinusoidal Kupffer cells	Acute-phase response (and amyloid) Abnormalities of liver enzymes Nodular regenerative hyperplasia in Felty's syndrome
Lung—alveolar macrophages	Alveolitis—severe in a few CT evidence in many Common in Felty's
Pericardial macrophages, probably other serosae	Pericarditis in 10%, pleuritis common
Bone marrow	Suppression of erythropoeiesis Osteopenia, subchondral erosion
Lymph node	Lymphadenopathy
Dermis exposed to stress	Subcutaneous nodules—20% of cases, specific to sites of stress Nailfold microinfarcts
Salivary gland macrophages	Sjögren's syndrome
Placental (Hofbauer) macrophages	?Subfertility

Other cells expressing FcγRIII	Isoform	Correlate in rheumatoid arthritis
Granulocytes	FcγRIIIb	Reduced cell half life due to immune complex binding in Felty's?
Large granular lymphocytes (LGL) (CD57+ T cells or CD56+ NK cells)	FcγRIIIa	Proliferation of LGL driven by ligation of FcγRIII by complexes in circulation or marrow? Further effects on myelopoeisis in Felty's?

CT, computed tomography.

Correlation between lesions in RA and sites of FcγRIIIa expression

The pattern of FcγRIIIa expression is therefore a very reasonable map of pathological changes in RA (see Table 1.2): synovitis, subcutaneous lesions at sites of stress, a prominent acute phase response, suppressed haemato-poiesis, lymphadenopathy, pericarditis, alveolitis and, probably, impaired fertility [61]. Although the acute phase response and anaemia of RA are often thought to be secondary to joint disease, they would also be consistent with a direct interaction between immune complexes and FcγRIIIa on Kupffer cells and cells in bone marrow. TNF-α released from Kupffer cells would be expected to stimulate hepatocyte production of acute phase proteins, either directly or via induction of IL-6 [62]. TNF-α produced locally in bone marrow would have a more potent suppressant effect on erythropoiesis than circulating cytokine.

The common manifestations of RA are consistent with ligation of macrophage FcγRIIIa, but some features of Felty's syndrome suggest ligation of FcγRIIIa on other cells, such as large granular lymphocytes (LGL) [63]. Felty's syndrome is associated with very high levels of RF and circulating complexes, and a corresponding high prevalence of systemic features. LGL activation in bone marrow may contribute to neutropenia, together with coating of granulocytes with complexes bound to FcγRIIIb, leading to shortened half-life. FcγRIIIa ligation on LGL can induce proliferation [64], and a significant proportion of Felty's patients have oligoclonal LGL expansions which may resemble leukaemia [63].

Why should synovitis overshadow all other features?

The preceding discussion suggests that both synovial and extra-articular features in RA are driven by the same process; binding of IgG RF complexes to FcγRIII. This is in keeping with the impression of many who have studied the microarchitecture of rheumatoid synovitis and nodules in detail, notably Palmer and colleagues [65]. With two caveats, rheumatoid nodules and synovitis are the same thing: a sheet of activated macrophages dividing a collection of necrotic debris from vascularized chronic inflammatory tissue. The macrophages of nodule palisades and synovial intima have an identical phenotype which includes prominent expression of FcγRIIIa. However, in the synovium there are more B lymphocytes and the fibroblasts express markers specific to synovium [50]. Recent studies suggest that these two features are related and may indicate why synovitis tends to overshadow other features of the disease.

Synovial intimal fibroblasts are unusual amongst fibroblasts in their very high level of expression of vascular cell adhesion molecule 1 (VCAM-1) and complement decay-accelerating factor (DAF) in normal tissue [50,66,67]. *In vitro*, synovial fibroblasts, as a whole, differ from fibroblasts from other tissues in their readiness to respond to cytokines such as TNF-α with the expression of not only VCAM-1 and DAF, but also the C3d receptor (CR2) [68–70].

VCAM-1, DAF and CR2 are all present in lymphoid follicle centres on follicular dendritic cells and have all been implicated in B-cell survival and/or differentiation [66,71–74]. VCAM-1 binds to very late antigen 4 (VLA-4), which is carried by several mononuclear leucocyte populations, including B lymphocytes. DAF protects cells from complement-mediated damage, and also NK cell killing [75]. CR2 is involved in retention of C3d-bearing immune complexes capable of providing a survival signal to B cells [72]. *In vitro*, synovial fibroblasts have been shown to be superior to fibroblasts from other tissues in supporting B-cell differentiation into plasma cells [76]. Thus, the predicted outcome of TNF-α production by intimal macrophages in response to immune complex ligation of FcγRIIIa is the expression of molecules on subintimal fibroblasts, perhaps most critically VCAM-1, which will favour local B-cell survival and differentiation. The involvement of subintimal fibroblasts is probably essential, since immunohistochemical evidence suggests that intimal fibroblasts *in vivo* will not support B-cell survival [70]. This may be explained by the fact that the same intimal cells that express VCAM-1 and DAF in normal tissue also synthesize large amounts of hyaluronan, which is a potent inhibitor of cell–cell adhesion [50].

These properties of synovial fibroblasts would explain the tendency of synovium to become colonized by B cells, a significant proportion of which, in RA, generate RF [77]. High local levels of IgG RF should assist survival of the parent B-cell clones. They are also associated with the formation of larger multimeric complexes which are likely to be responsible, not only for further Fc receptor binding but also, together with IgM RF-based complexes, activation of complement, with both pro-inflammatory and B-cell stimulatory consequences [1,78]. In some patients, particularly those seronegative for RF, the entire disease process may persist within the confines of synovium.

VCAM-1 may also be implicated in the activation of T cells [79–81]. Fibroblasts are capable of supporting T-cell survival, but this effect is not specific to synovial fibroblasts and is probably mediated through soluble factors [82]. VCAM-1 may also support T-cell survival indirectly by bringing T cells into contact with other VLA-4-positive cells. These could include macrophages, other T-cell subsets or B cells. The fact that the distribution of VCAM-1 in tissues tends to match sites of B-cell accumulation suggests that such an influence on T-cell survival may be chiefly through enhanced interaction with B cells, perhaps involving antigen presentation [83,84]. Thus, the weight of evidence suggests that synovial fibroblasts are above average at supporting B-cell survival, but might also contribute to inappropriate T-cell survival, particularly if that survival required antigen presentation by B cells.

The broader context of synovitis

Figure 1.1 gives a diagrammatic overview of how RF may be involved in

RA pathogenesis. Although at first sight complex, each step is consistent with both conventional immunological dogma and available data and goes a long way to explaining the features in Table 1.1.

Neither the activation of FcγRIIIa+ macrophages by small complexes, nor the survival of B cells in synovium under the influence of cytokine-stimulated fibroblasts need necessarily involve RF. However, the persistent and destructive nature of RA may reflect the fact that RF-producing B-cell clones are ideally suited to exploiting both pathways.

Other small complexes probably reach synovial macrophages in a wide range of syndromes which include synovitis—most obviously systemic lupus erythematosus. Some cases of RA seronegative for RF may represent the survival of B-cell clones producing other complex-forming autoantibodies.

Inappropriate B-cell survival in synovium may follow any persistent irritation of the tissue. In syndromes in which pericarditis, alveolitis, nodules and sicca syndrome do not occur, B-cell survival in synovium may have nothing to do with autoantibodies. Lymphoid follicles are occasionally seen even in tissue from cases apparently of simple osteoarthritis. This may represent no more than normal lymphoid tissue becoming established at a site of trauma-induced cytokine release.

In the seronegative spondarthropathies synovitis may be secondary to events at the enthesis [85]. These events, in turn, are likely to be dependent on recognition of MHC class I, presumably often in the form of B27 [86], either by T cell receptors on CD8+ T cells or a range of newly recognized receptors on both NK and CD8+ cytotoxic cells [87]. Accumulation of both B and T cells in synovium may lead to amplification events, in which B cells may play a lesser or greater role.

The test of the involvement of RF in the pathogenesis of RA is not therefore a demonstration of a one to one match between serum RF levels and synovitis. It lies in predictions about the detailed functional properties of very small immune complexes and interactions between synovial cells and lymphocytes, and in therapeutic studies designed to abrogate the synthesis of autoantibodies forming small complexes.

Persisting difficulties with RF pathogenicity

Although RF may appear ideally suited to the generation of a disorder with the clinical features of RA, there remain genuine doubts about the reasons for RF-specific B-cell survival and factors determining the ability of IgG RF complexes to induce signalling through FcγRIIIa.

The ability of IgG RF complexes to reach FcγRIIIa+ macrophages in tissues such as synovium may be critically dependent on their small size, both to allow access to the tissue and to evade complement binding. On the other hand, for IgG RF complexes to support the survival of their parent B cells they must fix complement and carry C3d. The original interpretation of work from Kunkel's colleagues was that at high local concentration IgG RF dimers would polymerize [1]. However, this would require IgG Fc to act as a divalent antigen (see Fig. 2.2: structure 2), a matter about which there is considerable doubt. An alternative is that at high concentration a different complex species forms which is branching rather than reciprocal in binding format (see Fig. 2.2: structure 3). There is also the question as to whether an IgG RF Fc that is engaged by another IgG RF Fab as part of a dimer could also engage FcγRIIIa.

Another problem is why IgG RFs in subjects with bacterial endocarditis never cause polyarthritis. Børretzen's work [31] would suggest that they may have a different structure from IgG RF in rheumatoid subjects if they result from class switching of IgM RF involved in a physiological RF response. This difference in structure would have to determine whether or not dimers could form which could engage FcγRIIIa but not complement.

These detailed steric problems need to be resolved. They may be dependent on a range of factors including IgG subclass, fine specificity, framework region structure and glycosylation [88,89]. The work of Natvig's group, at the nucleic acid level, needs to be extended. There is also considerable scope for the application of techniques such as X-ray crystallography and atomic force microscopy.

There is also a paradox relating to the polyclonality of RFs in RA. If the genesis of an autoantibody capable of perpetuating its own production is a rare chance event, why are RFs in RA not monoclonal or from closely related clones, all using a common IgG gene combination? The problem is not that this is difficult to explain. Invocation of various combinations and permutations of mechanisms 1 and 2 will readily provide an explanation. The weakness is that at present it is so easy to explain almost any pattern of Ig gene usage by RFs in RA that there is no critical test of this link in the theoretical model.

Lastly, nodular RA has been described in a subject with hyper-IgM syndrome [90], in which class switching to IgG is blocked by a defect in the interaction between CD40 and its ligand. This would seem inconsistent with an IgG-based immune-complex-driven process. However, it is not clear that this patient did not have complex-forming IgG or even IgG RF, since low but significant levels of IgG were present (1 g/L). Moreover, there are reasons for thinking that autoantibodies might be overrepresented in the IgG populations generated in the presence of defective B–T-cell cooperation.

Therapeutic tests of RF pathogenicity

The implication of self-perpetuating IgG RFs as mediators in RA leads to the concept that permanent remission can only be achieved by the removal of B-cell clones generating pathogenic IgG RFs. If these clones arise, as suggested, via a protracted process of affinity maturation to an irrelevant antigen, followed by a chance switch to RF activity, then, if destroyed, the risk of them reappearing may be small. In contrast, B-cell clones specific for foreign antigen should regenerate by normal affinity-based selection under T-cell control. This suggests that the logical thing to do is to destroy all B cells and allow B cells recognizing foreign antigen, but not IgG RF-producing clones, to re-emerge. If B-cell clones generating RF need to be present in a critical mass to support their own survival, then there is the added advantage that it may not be necessary to kill every single B cell to induce complete involution of the autoimmune process.

This approach might fail if expanded anti-Fab T-cell clones facilitated re-emergence of IgG RF-producing B cells. However, recent reports indicate that indiscriminate destruction of memory B cells can be effective and could be entirely safe. Long-term remission has been described in RA patients treated with high doses of cyclophosphamide prior to bone marrow transplantation [91]. Although this regimen is designed to ablate all immune cells, its key action may be subtotal clearance of B cells and plasma cells. B cells can now be depleted with anti-CD20 antibodies with few or no unwanted effects [92]. It seems not unrealistic to propose that results achieved with cyclophosphamide might therefore be achievable using a protocol acceptable for the treatment of all RA patients.

Conclusion

The issue is far from settled, but it appears that Henry Kunkel might have been right after all. He and his colleagues may not have identified the effector mechanisms in RA purely because the heterogeneity of IgG Fc receptors, the detailed mechanisms of T-cell help and the role of C3d in B lymphocyte survival were not known at the time.

Rheumatoid factor deserves another look.

References

1 Mannik M, Nardella FA. IgG rheumatoid factors and self association of these antibodies. *Clin Rheum Dis* 1985; 11: 551–72.

2 Lachmann PJ, Peters K, Rosen FS, Walport MJ, eds. *Clinical Aspects of Immunology*, 5th edn. Oxford: Blackwell, Scientific Publications, 1993.

3 Janossy G, Duke O, Poulter LW, Panayi G, Bofill M, Goldstein G. Rheumatoid arthritis: a disease of T lymphocyte–macrophage immunoregulation. *Lancet* 1981; ii: 839–42.

4 Burmester GR, Stuhlmuller B, Keyszer G, Kinne RW. Mononuclear phagocytes and rheumatoid synovitis. Mastermind or workhorse in arthritis? *Arthritis Rheum* 1997; 40: 5–18.

5 Muller-Ladner U, Kriegsmann J, Gay RE, Gay S. Oncogenes in rheumatoid arthritis. *Rheum Dis Clin North Am* 1995; 21: 675–90.

6 Aho K, Palusuo T, Kurki P. Marker antibodies of rheumatoid arthritis: diagnostic and pathogenetic implications. *Semin Arthritis Rheum* 1994; 23: 379–87.

7 Da Silva JA, Hall GM. The effects of gender and sex hormones on outcome in rheumatoid arthritis. *Baillière's Clin Rheumatol* 1992; 6: 196–219.

8 Williams DG. Autoimmunity in rheumatoid arthritis. In: Klippel JH, Dieppe PA, eds. *Rheumatology*. London: Mosby–Year Book Europe, 1994: 3.9.1–3.9.14.

9 Winchester RJ, Agnello V, Kunkel HG. Gamma globulin complexes in synovial fluids of patients with rheumatoid arthritis. *Clin Exp Immuol* 1970; 6: 689–706.

10 Male D, Roitt IM, Hay FC. Analysis of immune complexes in synovial effusions of patients with rheumatoid arthritis. *Clin Exp Immunol* 1980; 39: 297–306.

11 Brown PB, Nardella FA, Mannik M. Human complement activation by self-associated IgG rheumatoid factors. *Arthritis Rheum* 1982; 25: 1101–7.

12 Hendrich C, Kuipers JG, Kolanus W, Hammer M, Schmidt RE. Activation of CD 16+ effector cells by rheumatoid factor complex. *Arthritis Rheum* 1991; 34: 423–31.

13 Cabral AR, Cabiedes J, Alarcon-Segovia D, Sanchez-Guerrero J. Phospholipid specificity and requirement of beta 2-glycoprotein-I for reactivity of antibodies from patients with primary antiphospholipid syndrome. *J Autoimmun* 1992; 5: 787–801.

14 Schultz DR, Tozman EC. Antineutrophil cytoplasmic antibodies: major autoantigens, pathophysiology, and disease associations. *Semin Arthritis Rheum* 1995; 25: 143–59.

15 van Boxel JA, Paget SA. Predominantly T-cell infiltrate in rheumatoid synovial membranes N *Engl J Med* 1975; 293: 517–20.

16 Meijer CJLM, van de Putte LBA, Eulderink F *et al.* Characteristics of mononuclear cell populations in chronically inflamed synovial membranes. *J Pathol* 1976; 21: 1–11.

17 Gardner DL, ed. Rheumatoid arthritis: cell and tissue pathology. In: *Pathological Basis of Connective Tissue Diseases*. London: Edward Arnold, 1992: 444–526.

18 Breedveld FC, Verweij CL. T-cells in rheumatoid arthritis. *Br J Rheumatol* 1997; 36: 617–8.

19 Mulherin D, Fitzgerald O, Bresnihan B. Synovial tissue macrophage populations and articular damage in rheumatoid arthritis. *Arthritis Rheum* 1996; 39: 115–24.

20 Fassbender HG. Rheumatoid arthritis. *Pathology of Rheumatic Diseases*. Springer-Verlag, 1975: 109–19.

21 Stastny P. Association of the B cell alloantigen DRw4 with rheumatoid arthritis. *N Engl J Med* 1978; 298: 869–72.

22 Mitchison NA. Cell–cell interactions. In: Lachmann PJ, Peters K, Rosen FS, Walport MJ, eds. *Clinical Aspects of Immunology*, 5th edn. Oxford: Blackwell Scientific Publications, 1993: 637–50.

23 Dolhain RJEM, van der Heiden AN, ter Haar NT, Breedveld FC, Miltenburg AAM. Shift toward T lymphocytes with a T helper 1 cytokine-secretion profile in the joints of patients with rheumatoid arthritis. *Arthritis Rheum* 1996; 12: 1961–9.

24 Ollier WE, MacGregor A. Genetic epidemiology of rheumatoid disease. *Br Med Bull* 1995; 51: 267–85.

25 Conway SC, Creed FH, Symmons DP. Life events and the onset of rheumatoid arthritis. *J Psychosom Res* 1994; 38: 837–47.

26 Morgan SE, Kastan MB. p53, ATM. cell cycle, cell death, and cancer. *Adv Cancer Res* 1997; 71: 1–25.

27 Bahler DW, Miklos JA, Swerdlow SH. Ongoing Ig gene hypermutation

in salivary gland mucosa-associated lymphoid tissue-type lymphomas. *Blood* 1997; 89: 3335–44.

28 Rabbitts TH. Human immunoglobulin genes and associated chromosomal abnormalities. In: Lachmann PJ, Peters K, Rosen FS, Walport MJ, eds. *Clinical Aspects of Immunology*, 5th edn. Oxford: Blackwell Scientific Publications, 1993: 131–48.

29 Pulendran B, van Driel R, Nossal GJV. Immunological tolerance in germinal centres. *Immunol Today* 1997; 18: 27–32.

30 Pulendran B, Kannourakis G, Nouri S, Smith KGC, Nossal GJV. Soluble antigen can cause enhanced apoptosis of germinal-centre B cells. *Nature* 1995; 375: 331–4.

31 Børretzen M, Randen I, Natvig JB, Thompson KM. Structural restriction in the heavy chain CDR3 of human rheumatoid factors. *J Immunol* 1995; 155: 3630–7.

32 MacLennan-IC. B-cells. Avoiding autoreactivity. *Nature* 1995; 375: 281.

33 Dempsey PW, Allison ME, Akkaraju S, Goodnow CC, Fearon DT. C3d of complement as a molecular adjuvant: bridging innate and acquired immunity. *Science* 1996; 271: 348–50.

34 Walport MJ, Lachmann PJ. Complement. In: Lachmann PJ, Peters K, Rosen FS, Walport MJ, eds. *Clinical Aspects of Immunology*, 5th edn. Oxford: Blackwell Scientific Publications, 1993: 347–76.

35 Davies KA, Hird V, Stewart S *et al.* A study of *in vivo* immune complex formation and clearance in man. *J Immunol* 1990; 144: 4613–20.

36 Davies KA. Complement, immune complexes and systemic lupus erythematosus. *Br J Rheumatol* 1996; 35: 5–23.

37 Roosnek E, Lanzavecchia A. Efficient and selective presentation of antigen antibody complexes by rheumatoid factor B cells. *J Exp Med* 1991; 173: 487–9.

38 Silverman GJ, Carson DA. Rheumatoid arthritis. In: Lachmann PJ, Peters K, Rosen FS, Walport MJ, eds. *Clinical Aspects of Immunology*, 5th edn. Oxford: Blackwell, Scientific Publications, 1993: 1133–60.

39 Nicolle MW, Hawke S, Willcox N, Vincent A. Differences in processing of an autoantigen by DR4:Dw4.2 and DR4:Dw14.2 antigen-presenting cells. *Eur J Immunol* 1995; 25: 2119–22.

40 Bond C, Cleland LG. Rheumatoid arthritis: are pets implicated in its etiology? *Semin ArthritisRheum* 1996; 25: 308–17.

41 Corper AL, Sohi MK, Bonagura VR *et al.* Structure of human IgM rheumatoid factor Fab bound to its autoantigen IgG Fc reveals a novel topology of antibody–antigen interaction. *Nat Struct Biol* 1997; 4: 374–81.

42 van de Winkel JG, Capel PJA. Human IgG Fc receptor heterogeneity: molecular aspects and clinical implications. *Immunol Today* 1993; 14: 215–21.

43 Maini RN, Elliott M, Brennan FM, Williams RO, Feldmann M. TNF blockade in rheumatoid arthritis: implications for therapy and pathogenesis. *APMIS* 1997; 105: 257–63.

44 Debets JM, van de Winkel JG, Ceuppens JL, Dieteren IE, Buurman WA. Cross-linking of both Fc gamma RI and Fc gamma RII induces secretion of tumor necrosis factor by human monocytes, requiring high affinity Fc–Fc gamma R interactions. *J Immunol* 1990; 144: 1304–10.

45 Huizinga TW, van Kemenade F, Koenderman L *et al.* The 40-kDa Fc gamma receptor (FcRII) on human neutrophils is essential for the IgG-induced respiratory burst and IgG-induced phagocytosis. *J Immunol* 1989; 142: 2365–9.

46 Terstappen LW, Buescher S, Nguyen M, Reading C. Differentiation and maturation of growth factor expanded human hematopoietic progenitors assessed by multidimensional flow cytometry. *Leukemia* 1992; 6: 1001–10.

47 Trezzini C, Jungi TW, Spycher MO, Maly FE, Rao P. Human monocytes CD36 and CD16 are signaling molecules. Evidence from studies using antibody-induced chemiluminescence as a tool to probe signal transduction. *Immunology* 1990; 71: 29–37.

48 Abrahams VM, Cambridge G, Edwards JCW. FcgRIIIa mediates TNFa secretion

by human monocytes/macrophages. *Br J Rheumatol* 1988; 37 (Abstracts Suppl. 1): 90.

49 Dumonde DC, Glynn LE. The production of arthritis in rabbits by an immunological reaction to fibrin. *Br J Exp Pathol* 1962; 43: 373–83.

50 Edwards JCW. The synovium. In: Klippel JH, Dieppe PA, eds. *Rheumatology*. St Louis: Mosby–Year Book, 1997: 5.6.1–5.6.11.

51 Barland P, Novikoff AB, Hamerman D. Electron microscopy of the human synovial membrane. *J Cell Biol* 1962; 14: 207–16.

52 Henderson B, Revell P, Edwards JCW. Synovial lining cell hyperplasia in rheumatoid arthritis: dogma and fact. *Ann Rheum Dis* 1988; 47: 348–9.

53 Bhatia A, Blades S, Cambridge G, Edwards JCW. Differential distribution of FcγRIIIa in normal human tissues and co-localization with DAF and fibrillin-1: implications for immunological microenvironments. *Immunology* 1998; 94: 56–63.

54 van Ravenswaay Claasen HH, Kluin PM, Fleuren GJ. Tumor infiltrating cells in human cancer. On the possible role of CD16+ macrophages in antitumor cytotoxicity. *Lab Invest* 1992; 67: 166–74.

55 Tuijnman WB, Van Wichen DF, Schuurman HJ. Tissue distribution of human IgG Fc receptors CD16, CD32 & CD64: an immunohistochemical study. *APMIS* 1993; 101: 319–29.

56 Bordessoule D, Jones M, Gatter KC, Mason DY. Immunohistological patterns of myeloid antigens. *Br J Haematol* 1993; 83: 370–83.

57 Wahl SM, Allen JB, Welch GR, Wong HL. Transforming growth factor-beta in synovial fluids modulates FcgRIII (CD16) expression on mononuclear phagocytes. *J Immunol* 1992; 148: 485–90.

58 Wong HL, Welch GR, Brandes ME, Wahl SM. IL-4 antagonizes induction of Fc gamma RIII (CD16) expression by transforming growth factor-beta on human monocytes. *J Immunol* 1991; 147: 1843–8.

59 Calzada-Wack JC, Frankenberger M, Ziegler-Heitbrock HW. Interleukin-10 drives human monocytes to CD16 positive macrophages. *J Inflamm* 1996; 46(2): 78–85.

60 Zhuang H, Wang W, Tahernia AD, Levitz CL, Luchetti WT, Brighton CT. Mechanical strain-induced proliferation of osteoblastic cells parallels increased TGF-beta 1 mRNA. *Biochem Biophys Res Commun* 1996; 229: 449–53.

61 Maini RN, Zvaifler N. Rheumatoid arthritis. In: Klippel JH, Dieppe PA, eds. *Rheumatology*. London: Mosby–Year Book Europe, 1994: 3.1.1–3.15.6.

62 Husby G. The acute phase response and the pathogenesis of reactive myloid A amyloidosis. In: Lachmann PJ, Peters K, Rosen FS, Walport MJ, eds. *Clinical Aspects of Immunology*, 5th edn. Oxford: Blackwell Scientific Publications, 1993: 411–31.

63 Loughran TP, Starkebaum G, Kidd P, Neiman P. Clonal proliferation of large granular lymphocytes in rheumatoid arthritis. *Arthritis Rheum* 1988; 31: 31–6.

64 Hoshino S, Oshimi K, Teramura M, Mizoguchi H. Activation via the CD3 and CD16 pathway mediates interleukin-2-dependent autocrine proliferation of granular lymphocytes in patients with granular lymphocyte proliferative disorders. *Blood* 1991; 78: 3232–40.

65 Palmer DG, Hogg N, Highton J, Hessian PA, Denholm I. Macrophage migration and maturation within rheumatoid nodules. *Arthritis Rheum* 1987; 30: 729–36.

66 Rice GE, Munro JM, Corless C, Bevilacqua MP. Vascular and non-vascular expression of INCAM-110; a target for mononuclear leucocyte adhesion in normal and inflamed human tissues. *Am J Pathol* 1991; 38: 385–93.

67 Medof ME, Walter EI, Rutgers JL, Knowles DM, Nussenzweig V. Identification of the complement decay accelerating factor on epithelium and glandular cells and in body fluids. *J Exp Med* 1987; 165: 848–64.

68 Morales Ducret J, Wayner E, Elices MJ *et al.* α4/β1 integrin (VLA-4) ligands in arthritis: Vascular cell adhesion molecule expression in synovium and on fibroblast-like

synoviocytes. *J Immunol* 1992; 149: 1424–31.

69 Marlor CW, Webb DL, Bombara MP, Greve JM, Blue ML. Expression of vascular cell adhesion molecule-1 in fibroblast-like synoviocytes after stimulation with tumor necrosis factor. *Am J Pathol* 1992; 140: 1055–60.

70 Edwards JCW, Leigh RD, Cambridge G. Expression of molecules involved in B lymphocyte survival and differentiation by synovial fibroblasts. *Clin Exp Immunol* 1997; 108: 407–14.

71 Lampert IA, Schofield JB, Amlot P, Van Noorden S. Protection of germinal centres from complement attack. *J Pathol* 1993; 170: 115–20.

72 Lindhout E, de Groot C. Follicular dendritic cells and apoptosis: life and death in the germinal centre. *Histochem J* 1995; 27: 167–834.

73 Freedman AS, Munro JM, Rice GE *et al.* Adhesion of human B cells to germinal centres *in vitro* involves VLA-4 and INCAM-110. *Science* 1990; 249: 1030–2.

74 Lindhout E, Mevissen ML, Kwekkeboom JM, de Groot C. Direct evidence that human follicular dendritic cells rescue germinal centre B cells from death by apoptosis. *Clin Exp Immunol* 1993; 91: 330–4.

75 Finberg RW, White W, Nicholson-Weller A. Decay-accelerating factor expression on either effector or target cells inhibits cytotoxicity by human natural killer cells. *J Immunol* 1992; 149: 2055–60.

76 Dechanet J, Merville P, Durand I, Banchereau J, Miossec P. The ability of synoviocytes to support terminal differentiation of activated B cells may explain plasma cell accumulation in rheumatoid synovium. *J Clin Invest* 1995; 95: 456–63.

77 Youinou PY, Morrow JW, Lettin AWF, Lydyard PM, Roitt IM. Specificity of plasma cells in the rheumatoid synovium I. *Scand J Immunol* 1984; 20: 307–15.

78 Guc D, Gulati P, Lemercier C, Lappin D, Birnie GD, Whaley K. Expression of the components and regulatory proteins of the alternative complement pathway and the membrane attack complex in normal and diseased synovium. *Rheum Int* 1993; 13: 139–46.

79 Bombara MP, Webb DL, Conrad P *et al.* Cell contact between T cells and synovial fibroblasts causes induction of adhesion molecules and cytokines. *J Leuk Biol* 1993; 54: 399–406.

80 Burkly C, Jakubowski A, Newman BM *et al.* Signalling by vascular cell adhesion molecule-1 through VLA-4 promotes CD3 dependent T cell proliferation. *Eur J Immunol* 1991; 21: 2871–5.

81 Damle NK, Aruffo A. Vascular cell adhesion molecule 1 induces T cell antigen receptor dependent activation of CD4 positive lymphocytes. *Proc Natl Acad Sci USA* 1991; 88: 6403–7.

82 Gombert W, Borthwick NJ, Wallace DL *et al.* Fibroblasts prevent apoptosis of IL-2-deprived T cells without inducing proliferation: a selective effect on Bcl-XL expression. *Immunology* 1996; 89: 397–404.

83 Wilkinson LS, Edwards JCW, Poston R, Haskard DO. Cell populations expressing VCAM-1 in normal and diseased synovium. *Lab Invest* 1993; 68: 82–8.

84 Edwards JCW, Wilkinson LS, Speight P, Isenberg DA. Vascular cell adhesion molecule 1 and a4 and b1 integrins in lymphocyte aggregates in Sjögren's syndrome and rheumatoid arthritis. *Ann Rheum Dis* 1993; 52: 806–11.

85 McGonagle D, Pease C, Geen MJ *et al.* Knee synovitis in reactive arthritis is strongly associated with the presence of knee enthesopathy. *Br J Rheumatol* 1997; 36 (Suppl. 1): 171.

86 Brewerton DA, Hart FD, Nicholls A *et al.* Ankylosing spondylitis and HL-A 27. *Lancet* 1973; i: 904–7.

87 Long EO, Burshtyn DN, Clark WP *et al.* Killer inhibitory receptors: diversity, specificity and function. NK cells, MHC class I antigens and missing self. *Immunol Rev* 1991; 155: 135–44.

88 Parekh RB, Roitt IM, Isenberg DA *et al.* Galactosylation of IgG associated oligosaccharides: reduction in patients with adult and juvenile onset rheumatoid arthritis and relation to disease activity. *Lancet* 1988; i: 966–9.

89 Jefferis R. Rheumatoid factors, B cells and immunoglobulin genes. *Br Med Bull* 1995; 51: 312–31.

90 Sibilia J, Durandy A, Schaeverbeke T, Fermand JP. Hyper-IgM syndrome associated with rheumatoid arthritis: report of RA in a patient with primary impaired CD40 pathway. *Br J Rheumatol* 1996; 35: 282–4.

91 Wicks I, Cooley H, Szer J. Autologous hemopoietic stem cell transplantation: a possible cure for rheumatoid arthritis? *Arthritis Rheum* 1997; 40: 1005–11.

92 Maloney DG, Liles TM, Czerwinski DK *et al.* Phase I clinical trial using escalating single-dose infusion of chimeric anti-CD20 monoclonal antibody (IDEC-C2B8) in patients with recurrent B-cell lymphoma. *Blood* 1994; 84: 2457–66.

2: The role of apoptosis in rheumatoid arthritis

M. Salmon and A.N. Akbar

Why should people with rheumatoid arthritis care about apoptosis?

Apoptosis is fashionable and like all fashionable things it has evoked a fair degree of controversy. This has ranged from the biochemical specifics of whether caspase 3 is upstream or downstream of protein kinase C delta (PKC-δ), through to questions like 'why should patients with rheumatoid arthritis care about apoptosis?' Actually both of these extremes are healthy and constructive areas of debate, except where the protagonists hold significantly divergent views to our own. In this discussion we will try to focus on the role of apoptosis in perpetuating chronic rheumatoid synovitis, and also suggest that chronic inflammation is a distinct physiological-cum-pathological process that is an unfortunate side-effect of immunological memory for T lymphocytes.

The advantage of a fashionable scientific area is rapid progress. A considerable amount of work will be done simultaneously by people coming to the area from different backgrounds, with different perspectives. Unfortunately this is also the downside of such fashions, because it leads to a great deal of confusion. Similar data may be interpreted very differently because of the particular sets of prejudices that workers bring to their research, or apparently conflicting data may be produced because not enough is known about the field to design unequivocal experiments or reconcile discrepancies. For these reasons, we believe it is best to view controversies in a rapidly developing field such as this with tolerant good humour; a clearer position will inevitably emerge within a few years. In other words, the sensible and rational explanation for persistent rheumatoid synovitis, that we will describe here, will ultimately become the universally accepted model.

Apoptosis is a physiological mechanism for eliminating unwanted cells [1,2]. In the course of embryonic development this is vital. Indeed, significant mutations in apoptosis-related genes almost invariably have severe pathological consequences that are apparent very early in life and are

frequently embryonically lethal. Consequently primary genetic abnormalities in apoptosis-related genes are unlikely to play a role in most chronic
rheumatological conditions, which tend to occur in adulthood or adolescence.
Research into systemic lupus erythematosus (SLE) has illustrated this clearly.
Several years ago, the nature of the *lpr* gene defect in MRL mouse was
identified as non-functional Fas, a receptor that can transduce a signal for
apoptosis; similar defects in its counter-receptor were identified in the gld
strain [3,4]. These mouse strains develop a wide range of autoantibodies,
and have consequently been used by many as a model for SLE. These observations precipitated a torrent of papers looking for Fas defects in SLE. This
only subsided when it became quite clear that an *lpr*-like defect in human
Fas produces a lymphoproliferative disease in very young children that is
remarkably similar to that seen in MRL-*lpr* mice; but nothing like SLE [5,6].
More recent research in SLE has focused on the opposite side of the
apoptosis spectrum, i.e. too much apoptosis, or rather inefficient clearance
of apoptotic cells by phagocytes [7–9]. This is thought to result from acquired
complement deficiencies leading to poor recognition of apoptotic cells
through the important C1q receptor pathway and subsequent release of free
antigen [10]. Even a marginal reduction in clearance of apoptotic cells is
likely to be significant, without any need for increasing the numbers of
cells that die, because in the blood, and the immune system in general,
apoptosis is a continuous process in normal day-to-day function. For example the half-life of neutrophils in blood is about 8 h, which means that
the total neutrophil pool is synthesized (and destroyed) about twice a day.

These and related areas of research suggest that if disorders of
apoptosis play a part in chronic diseases of adulthood, such as rheumatoid
arthritis (RA), they are likely to be subtle, acquired abnormalities, or
peculiarities of the lesional microenvironment.

Immunological abnormalities in RA

One of the most intriguing features of RA is that it does not resolve. During
their lifetime most people will suffer from transient events of synovitis or
even arthritis, usually associated with infections, but almost invariably these
will resolve spontaneously after a short time. In RA, the inflammation becomes chronic and persistent. Numerous abnormalities of the rheumatoid
immune system were described in trying to address this issue during the
1980s [11]. These could obviously not all be primary genetic peculiarities
of the disease for two reasons: first, such a large and complex genetic requirement would make RA an extremely rare condition, yet approximately 1%
of the population worldwide suffers from this crippling disease. Secondly,
many of the 'abnormalities' were equally apparent in patients with other

chronic inflammatory conditions [12]. This latter observation suggested that the apparent down-regulation of immune responses in chronic inflammation may be a perfectly normal response to excessive stimulation in specific microenvironments.

A role for T cells in RA?

The question of whether T lymphocytes play a significant role in the pathology of RA has proved controversial [11,13,14]. Two prominent arguments in favour of a role for T cells in this disease are:

1   the observation that there are quite a lot of them in the inflamed joints of most patients with RA [11];

2   that the only clearly mapped genetic association with this condition is a class II HLA motif within the third hypervariable region of the DR-β chain. This short stretch of amino acids forms part of the α helix bordering the antigen-binding cleft [15–17]. As the only known function of class II HLA molecules is to present antigens to CD4+ helper T cells, this strongly supports a role for T cells at some point in the disease process. This amino acid sequence is shared, or highly conserved, among HLA alleles that show a positive association with RA, but not those that show no association. Intriguingly, although the association is principally with several subtypes of HLA-DR4, a number of completely unrelated molecules that share this sequence also show a strong association with RA. We and others have shown that the association between the conserved HLA motif and RA only holds for patients with severe and persistent disease and also that patients who express two different HLA molecules that both bear the motif do very badly [18–22]. We have previously suggested that this implies a role for class II HLA (and indirectly for T cells) in the switch to persistent and erosive disease [17–19]. However, it is equally plausible that the American College of Rheumatology (ACR) criteria for RA do not define a single disease entity [23]. Patients with severe HLA-DR-associated RA may actually have a quite separate disease to those who present with mild symptoms. No satisfactory mechanism has been advanced to explain this extremely complex association between the conserved class II HLA motifs and RA [17]. On balance it seems that the HLA association does imply a role for T cells in the initiation of RA, but does not really address the issue of chronicity.

T-cell populations in rheumatoid joints show a largely polyclonal antigen receptor usage and precursors specific for most T-cell recall antigens can be found in this compartment [24–28]; indeed, when patients with RA were immunized with influenza vaccine, T cells recognizing this antigen were recovered from affected joints within weeks [28]. However, even in experimental lesions induced by a known antigen, the number of cells found within the lesion that actually recognize the causative antigen is very low: between 1 : 500 and 1 : 5000 [29,30]. T-cell responses are therefore highly specific in their induction, but rapidly lose this specificity by recruitment of unrelated cells to the lesion. In long-standing chronic inflammation, the original causative antigen is likely to remain elusive, and perhaps irrelevant to the persistent process. Having said this, removing T cells was shown many years ago to have a beneficial effect on rheumatoid synovitis [31,32], which does suggest an active role for these cells in the continuing disease process. Antigenically irrelevant cells recruited to the synovium in a non-specific manner but in an activated state may well produce potent levels of inflammatory cytokines for short periods of time, sufficient to drive a macrophage/fibroblast-based inflammatory process [11].

T cells removed from rheumatoid synovial tissue or fluid are difficult to stimulate and produce cytokines in very low levels, particularly interleukin 2 (IL-2) and interferon gamma (IFN-γ) [11,12,14,33]. These cytokines might have been expected to be prominent in a chronic inflammatory response driven by T cells. Indeed, in the mid 1980s it was argued that this seemingly deficient function of synovial T cells was responsible for the persistence of rheumatoid synovial inflammation, because such a 'defective' response would be unable to resolve spontaneously [11]. In fact, as we will discuss later, this apparent deficiency in T-cell responsiveness almost certainly reflects the state of differentiation of synovial T cells.

The progressive differentiation of primed T cells is associated with increasing susceptibility to apoptosis

Synovial T lymphocytes in RA are almost exclusively antigen-experienced primed cells, expressing the lowest molecular weight isoform of the leucocyte common antigen: CD45RO [34,35]. This results from a well-documented preference for migration of primed cells to tissue lesions [34,36]. Until recently no markers were available to distinguish newly primed cells from long-established clones. This severely hampered attempts to determine the functional role of T cells in synovial joints. We have described a spectrum of primed CD4+ T cells characterized by an inverse relationship between the expression of two CD45 epitopes: CD45RB and CD45RO [37]. Primed CD4+ T cells progress through many cycles of division from a CD45RB^{bright}O^{dull} to a CD45RB^{dull}O^{bright} state. This progressive differentiation defined by the shift from CD45RB^{bright} to CD45RB^{dull} is paralleled by the gradual loss of bcl-2 (an intracellular protein that inhibits apoptosis) and gain of Fas (CD95) expression. Fas is a surface receptor for specific signals that induce apoptosis; consequently these two features are associated with an increased propensity for apoptosis. At the same time, these highly differentiated CD45RB^{dull} cells selectively lose the capacity to synthesize IL-2, a cytokine which is particularly effective in preventing T-cell apoptosis and also, to a lesser extent, IFN-γ. This leads to the apoptosis of primed CD45RB^{dull} cells, when they are stimulated in the absence of exogenous IL-2 [37]. This process is likely to be an important mechanism contributing to the maintenance of T-cell homeostasis *in vivo*, preventing excessive increase in the size of the immune system.

Rheumatoid synovial T cells are very highly differentiated

T lymphocytes from the synovial fluid of patients with RA represent an extreme limit of differentiation. These cells express higher levels of CD45RO and lower levels of CD45RB than any cells found in the blood of the same patients [25]. RA blood T cells are very similar to healthy controls in this respect although here also there is a slightly increased proportion of highly differentiated cells in rheumatoid patients. It is currently unclear whether cells are recruited to the synovium in a recently primed CD45RB^{bright} state, in a highly differentiated CD45RB^{dull} state, or indeed whether any such selectivity occurs at all. However, in recent experiments we have shown that CD45RB^{dull} cells preferentially cross endothelial barriers *in vitro*, suggesting that CD45RB^{dull} cells may be specifically recruited to inflammatory lesions [38]. The highly differentiated CD45RB^{dull} character of rheumatoid synovial T cells explains many of the apparent functional discrepancies reported for this population, such as poor proliferative responses to stimulation and limited cytokine production [11], because peripheral blood CD45RB^{dull} T cells behave in a very similar way [37].

As rheumatoid synovial T cells are very highly differentiated, we would expect them to be very susceptible to apoptosis and unstable, a process that should contribute towards resolution of inflammatory lesions. Yet T cells in the rheumatoid synovium show no evidence of apoptosis, using any currently available techniques [39]. We eliminated the possibility that synovial T cells in RA are intrinsically resistant to apoptosis, because these cells die spontaneously and quite rapidly when cultured *in vitro* without any stimulus. Another possibility was that the cells did indeed apoptose, but were phagocytosed rapidly, before we could detect them. Macrophages recognize apoptotic T cells using the αVβ3 integrin-CD36 structure [40,41]. An alternative recognition structure expressed by all apoptotic cells is surface exposure of phosphatidyl-serine [42]. This molecule appears not to be used by macrophages during phagocytosis of apoptotic T cells [40], but detection of phosphatidyl-serine exposure using the serum protein Annexin V is a useful tool that allows us to identify apoptotic cells at least as early as phagocytes can [39,42]. We found no evidence of phosphatidyl-serine exposure on synovial T cells in RA. However, in most rheumatoid synovial samples, apoptotic neutrophils were readily detected, suggesting that the methods used were very sensitive [39]. An intriguing serendipitous observation confirmed that phagocytosis of apoptotic T cells was not a likely explanation for our failure to detect apoptosis of T cells in RA synovium: patients with acute uric acid crystal-induced arthritis actually show very high levels of T-cell apoptosis *in vivo*. We found up to three-quarters of the T cells in these patients' synovia to be apoptotic [39]. This might explain the neutrophil dominance of these acute inflammatory lesions. So why should chronic rheumatoid inflammation be different? Could this apparent failure to remove lymphoid cells be involved in the process of chronic inflammation itself?

The regulation of T-cell apoptosis by γ-chain cytokines and stromal cells

Apoptosis of T cells can be induced actively by ligation of molecules such as Fas/Apo-1 (CD95) [43,44] or passively, by inadequate levels of stimulatory cytokines [45,46]. Previous reports have shown genes such as *Bcl-2* can prevent apoptosis, either through altering cell-cycle rates or by antioxidant-associated mechanisms [47–50]. Products of a related gene, *Bcl-x*, can be differentially spliced to generate large (Bcl-x_L) and small (Bcl-x_S) mRNA transcripts which code for proteins that either prevent or induce apoptosis, respectively [51]. In humans, no Bcl-x_S protein has been detected; Bcl-x_L is the only protein observed [52]. Bcl-2 and Bcl-x_L appear to repress a common pathway leading to apoptosis [53]. We found that although Bcl-2 expression was low in synovial T cells, Bcl-x_L remained at levels comparable to those seen in peripheral blood lymphocytes from the same patients [39]. This suggested that one reason for the lack of apoptosis in synovial T cells may be maintenance of high Bcl-x_L expression. This observation also indicated that factors present in the synovial microenvironment could differentially regulate Bcl-x_L expression relative to Bcl-2. In accordance with this observation, T cells from gout patients who showed significant *in situ* apoptosis expressed low levels of both Bcl-2 and Bcl-x_L.

We have previously described two mechanisms by which apoptosis of cytokine-deprived T cells can be retarded. When IL-2 is withdrawn from T cells the expression of both Bcl-2 and Bcl-x_L which are inhibitors of apoptosis falls sharply, while expression of apoptosis promoters such as Bax (an inhibitory ligand for Bcl-2) or Fas does not change significantly [52]. If T cells are subsequently cultured with any member of a class of cytokines that use the shared γ-chain signalling component of the IL-2 receptor (including IL-2, IL-4, IL-7, IL-13 and IL-15), apoptosis is prevented and

Bcl-2 and Bcl-x$_L$ expression are up-regulated, indicating that these cyto-kines coordinate the expression of these genes [52]. The second mechanism for rescue involves co-culture of the T cells with fibroblast monolayers; this system induced survival without proliferation. An important observation was that Bcl-2 expression was reduced during fibroblast-mediated rescue, but Bcl-x$_L$ expression was maintained, indicating that this mechanism of survival uncouples the expression of these genes [46,54].

Although early reports suggested significant quantities of IL-15 to be present in rheumatoid synovium [55], more recent data from the same group suggests that the original values were an overestimate by several orders of magnitude [56]. The limited T-cell proliferation observed *in situ* and the low Bcl-2 expression observed suggest that IL-2R γ-chain cytokines are unlikely to be the principal mechanism preventing apoptosis of T cells in the rheumatoid joint [39]. However, the low Bcl-2 but high Bcl-x$_L$ expression of the synovial T cells *in vivo* suggests that the stromal cell-mediated route of rescue is likely to operate *in vivo*. Culture experiments *in vitro* supported this possibility and showed that co-culture with fibroblast-conditioned medium maintained the *in vivo* phenotype of synovial T cells (Bcl-2^{low}, Bcl-x$_L^{high}$). In contrast, addition of IL-15 led to high Bcl-2 and Bcl-x$_L$ expression. Proliferating pannus tissue in rheumatoid joints contains a high density of fibroblasts [57], but synovial thickening in patients with acute crystal-induced-arthritis is usually much less marked or even absent, with considerably less evidence of fibroblast proliferation. Synovial T cells from patients with gout could be rescued by either IL-15 or fibroblast-conditioned medium, but the phenotype produced was in each case that predicted, i.e. IL-15 induced Bcl-2^{high}Bcl-x$_L^{high}$ and stromal rescue induced a Bcl-2^{low}Bcl-x$_L^{high}$ phenotype. However, gout T cells *in vivo* express a Bcl-2^{low}Bcl-x$_L^{low}$ phenotype and die by apoptosis. These results suggest strongly that apoptosis of T cells in the rheumatoid synovium is actively inhibited by stromal cells present in the proliferating pannus tissue.

Stromal mediators of survival

So what is it that the inflammatory microenvironment, or stromal cells, provide to keep T cells alive? Hyaluronic acid is present in extremely high levels in synovial fluid; intriguingly this molecule has been reported to block Fas-mediated activation-induced apoptosis in mouse T-cell hybridomas [58]. Unfortunately for those of us who like elegant solutions, hyaluronic acid does not inhibit spontaneous synovial T-cell apoptosis *in vitro* [39]. This does not necessarily exclude an active role for hyaluronate in modu-lating activation-induced apoptosis *in situ*, as any Fas-derived signals gen-erated are likely to be transient and not persist in culture [53]. Many integrin molecules bind to specific ligands through a motif consisting of Arg-Gly-Asp [59,60]. *In vitro* the peptide Arg-Gly-Asp-Ser (RGDS) has been used to inhibit such interactions for many years; Arg-Gly-Glu-Ser (RGES) is used as a control. We showed that the ability of fibroblast-conditioned medium to rescue synovial T cells from apoptosis was markedly 'inhibited' by the RGDS but not the RGES peptide, suggesting that an integrin interaction was likely to be involved [39]. This is actually completely wrong. We have now shown that the effect of RGD peptides in biological experiments is almost exclusively independent of integrins. The peptides enter cells directly, bind to caspase 3 and induce a conformational change that leads to the autocatalytic cleavage of this molecule [63]. Caspase 3 plays a pivotal role in the effector stage of apoptosis, analogous in many respects to C3 in the complement cascade. Not surprisingly RGD peptides directly induce apoptosis in target cells. While this observation considerably alters our perception of adhesion molecule biology, it also suggests a very powerful therapeutic tool. RGD peptides have been used in preliminary therapeutic trials, intended to target adhesion and migration of cells in tumour meta-stasis, angiogenesis and several related conditions. Intriguingly, the effects of these peptides was dramatic, even at doses too low to significantly affect integrin function, and the effects persisted after the peptides had been cleared. It seems very likely that what was detected in these experiments was induc-tion of apoptosis.

So what is it in stromal cells that keeps T cells alive? IFN-β [64]. We have now shown that both IFN-α and -β are capable of maintaining T-cell survival. Inhibitory-antibody and cell-signalling experiments suggest that only IFN-β is produced by fibroblasts in sufficient quantity to affect survival. IFN-α is a prominent product of macrophages, which of course make up about half of pannus tissue. We have shown that these cytokines are abundant in rheumatoid, but not in acute inflammatory synovium, and also that the cells at these sites appear to have been rescued by their actions. The identification of type I interferons as the principal agent for survival enabled us to study its effects on other cells in the synovial microenviron-ment. We found that its effects are not restricted to T cells. Neutrophil survival and also fibroblast survival is extended markedly by its action. The stromal-mediated rescue of T cells appears to be a fundamental process in the generation and maintenance of T-cell memory, providing the only currently known mechanism for inducing a resting G0/G1 state in activated T cells, without apoptosis. Precisely the same mechanism under certain circumstances induces persistence of chronic inflammatory cells.

The mechanism by which type I interferons prolong survival seems to be complex. Many cytokine receptors are closely related and are associ-ated with one or more members of the JAK family of tyrosine kinases [65].

JAKs couple cytokine receptors to a variety of signalling proteins including Ras, PI-3-kinase, phospholipase C-γ (PLC-γ) and the STAT family of transcription factors. JAK-1 kinase interacts specifically with the IL-2R β chain while JAK-3 interacts with the γ chain, activating the STAT-5 transcription factor [66]. We have shown that the signalling pathway employed by IFN-β in up-regulating Bcl-x$_L$ in T cells is through dimerization of STAT-1 and activation of the interferon stimulated response element (ISRE)–STAT complex. The latter is completely specific for type I interferons. We identified a putative STAT binding sequence in the Bcl-x gene regulatory sequence, and have now shown that this interacts with the IFN-induced IRES complex, leading to transcription activation (Pilling, Girdlestone & Salmon, unpublished). The specific induction of STAT-1 and IRES complexes by fibroblast-conditioned medium was mimicked by synovial fluid [64] suggesting that this is a key mechanism in the rescue of synovial cells from apoptosis. Intriguingly, no STAT-5-inducing signals were identified, which would have been the expected mechanism for γ-chain cytokines such as IL-15.

There is, however, a problem with the STAT-1/Bcl-x pathway as the principal mediator of rescue from apoptosis. It is too slow. Activation of STATs and translocation to the nucleus takes about 15 min [64]. Transcription, processing and translation of the gene product will then take several hours before functional Bcl-x$_L$ protein can successfully inhibit apoptosis. Yet IFN-β prevents Fas-mediated apoptosis when added at the initiation of the induction process [64]. Fas-mediated apoptosis proceeds too quickly to be blocked by the Bcl-x$_L$ induction route. Furthermore IFN-β also retards neutrophil apoptosis, with a significant delay to apoptosis seen within 3 h and prior to any detectable changes in Bcl-x expression. The STAT-1/IRES pathway therefore appears fundamentally to be a mechanism for reducing susceptibility to apoptosis, not for blocking its effector function.

Our current understanding of intracellular signalling events involved in the regulation of apoptosis suggests that there are several distinct or 'private' pathways that converge to effect a common apoptotic programme [67]. A majority of these pathways can be regulated downstream by members of the Bcl-2 family of proteins. An alternative and much more rapid route for inhibition of apoptosis by IFN-β may lie in the modulation of one or more of these pathways. Fas-induced apoptosis involves ceramide signalling, initiated by the activation of a neutral sphingomyelinase which causes the hydrolysis of membrane sphingomyelin to generate ceramide. Ceramide modulates the activity of several targets including PKC, ceramide-activated protein kinase and ceramide-activated protein phosphatase. To identify how interferons block the progression of apoptosis we needed to investigate alternative upstream regulatory processes, that do not require *de novo* protein synthesis.

PKC regulates a large number of intracellular signalling events, including cell proliferation and apoptosis, with its pleiotropic actions mediated by the distinct actions of the 11 isoenzymes of PKC [68]. Three such isoforms, PKC-α, PKC-βII and PKC-δ, appear to actively regulate apoptosis. The first two inhibit apoptosis, while active PKC-δ induces apoptosis [69]. We deprived T cells of survival factors and after varying intervals fractionated the cells into their cytoplasmic, membrane and cytoskeletal constituents. Translocation of PKC to membrane or cytoskeletal compartments is an indicator of enzyme activation. Western blot analysis showed that PKC-δ accumulated in the cytoskeletal fraction in the early stages of apoptosis [70]. Addition of IFN-β inhibited this translocation. Immunofluorescence staining of cytospin preparations indicated that in the early stages of apoptosis PKC-δ accumulated at the nuclear envelope. This is consistent with previous data suggesting that the primary target for PKC-δ is lamin B [71], a cytoskeletal component of the nuclear envelope. Addition of IFN-β to T cells already deprived of survival factors showed a rapid retranslocation of PKC-δ to the cytoplasm, suggesting that this is a reversible step in the signalling pathway to apoptosis. PKC-δ can also be activated by proteolytic degradation by caspase 3, which releases the catalytic (40-kDa) fragment from the control of the regulatory domain. IFN-β also actively inhibited the downstream activation of PKC-δ by caspase 3. Interestingly, preliminary data also revealed that IFN-β induced translocation of PKC-α and this may contribute to T-cell survival [70]. Furthermore, inhibition of neutrophil apoptosis by IFN β was also associated with a delay in the appearance of caspase-activated PKC-δ. These results suggest at least a bimodal signalling route for the regulation of apoptosis by type I interferons and also that PKC isoenzymes offer a potential therapeutic target in the control of RA and other forms of chronic inflammation.

Infiltrating T cells persist in chronic inflammation through active suppression of apoptosis by stromal cells

The available data suggest that T cells in the rheumatoid synovium are a perfectly normal population of very highly differentiated cells. Our results suggest that the inflammatory T-cell infiltrate persists principally because apoptosis is actively suppressed by the synovial microenvironment [39]. It is very unlikely that T-cell apoptosis is completely blocked. We suggest that during active flares of rheumatoid disease activity, probably associated with random infections, cells are actively recruited to the joint in a largely non-specific manner. During more stable periods of disease, the suppression of T-cell apoptosis will maintain the infiltrating population for extended periods of time. The stromal (IFN-β) mediated rescue of activated T cells from apoptosis is essentially a physiological mechanism for the generation and maintenance of T-cell memory, that under certain circumstances is subverted to the perpetuation of chronic inflammation.

It is unclear at the moment whether synovial pannus formation is a semi-neoplastic process of self-driven proliferation of fibroblasts, or is itself a product of the chronic inflammatory process [61]. However, it seems wise to be cautious in proposing a fundamental defect in synovial fibroblasts as the likely cause of the rheumatoid lesion at this stage. Chronic inflammation in many respects is a very similar process wherever it is found. In our studies we have compared RA patients with uric acid-induced crystal arthritis, but chronic and acute inflammation may be more appropriate labels, because the characteristic of persistence sustained by interaction of immune cells with the stromal microenvironment is likely to be a feature of all chronic inflammation. A recent study has shown that inflammatory T-cell infiltrates are not cleared by apoptosis in patients with a range of chronic inflammatory myopathies [62]. The authors suggested that T cells in muscle fail to receive positive signals for apoptosis. We would suggest that these cells like those in the rheumatoid synovium may actually receive positive signals to stay alive. The role of the inflammatory fibroblast in perpetuating the immunological aspects of chronic inflammation deserves considerable attention, and offers important new approaches for treating these intractable diseases.

Apoptosis of non-lymphoid cells in RA?

Several groups have studied apoptosis in the rheumatoid synovium, both as a biological process, as a way to understand the disease, but also as a simple therapeutic tool. Like ourselves, Firestein and colleagues have reported unexpectedly low levels of apoptosis in the synovium [72], particularly noting the absence of T-cell death. Others concentrated instead on mechanisms to induce apoptosis in synovial cells therapeutically; including cytotoxic drugs and gene-therapy approaches [73,74]. Intriguingly others have shown that drugs commonly used in RA may operate through induction of apoptosis, including steroids and sulphasalazine. Firestein's group has developed the hypothesis that synovial fibroblasts are inhibited from dying by apoptosis by mutations in control genes, such as p53 [75]. Such mutations are a prerequisite, but are insufficient for the development of malignancy. Intriguingly, many of the mutations they identified were identical to those found previously in malignant cells. They propose that oxygen free radicals produced as part of the inflammatory process lead to mutations in p53 in fibroblasts, rendering them less susceptible to apoptosis. Actually this integrates very effectively with the model for chronic inflammation derived from our own studies described earlier; because the proliferating fibroblasts would then maintain survival of inflammatory cells within the lesion. Oxidant-induced somatic mutations of p53 in fibroblasts would then provide the point at which a specific acute inflammatory process switches to a chronic phase and loses its specificity. At this point it simply becomes chronic inflammation, within a site determined by the primary reaction. Synovitis will therefore persist in the joints, inflammatory bowel disease in the gut, myositis in the muscles. So by this point in the proceedings, it seems, chronic inflammation is chronic inflammation.

Acknowledgements

We would like to thank our colleagues who have contributed to the various studies discussed here. This work was funded by the Arthritis and Rheumatism Council UK (SO190, SO130, SO185, HO156) and the Medical Research Council (G9218555MA, G931916MA).

References

1 Kerr JFR, Wyllie AH, Currie AH. Apoptosis: a basic biological phenomenon with wide-ranging implications in tissue kinetics. *Br J Cancer* 1972; 26: 239–57.

2 Williams GT, Smith CA. Molecular regulation of apoptosis—genetic-controls on cell-death. *Cell* 1993; 74: 777–9.

3 Chu JI, Drappa J, Parnassa A, Elkon KB. The defect in Fas mRNA expression in Mrl lpr mice is associated with insertion of the retrotransposon, etn. *J Exp Med* 1993; 178: 723–30.

4 Elkon KBJ. Apoptosis in SLE—too little or too much? *Rheumatology* 1997; 24: 6–7.

5 Rieux-Laucat F, le Deist F, Hivroz C *et al.* Mutations in Fas associated with human lymphoproliferative syndrome and autoimmunity. *Science* 1995; 268: 1347–9.

6 Wu JG, Wilson J, He J *et al.* Fas ligand mutation in a patient with systemic lupus erythematosus and lymphoproliferative disease. *J Clin Invest* 1996; 98: 1107–13.

7 Salmon M, Pilling D, Akbar AN. The role of apoptosis in autoimmunity. *R Soc Med CML* 1995; 14: 63–9.

8 Herrmann M, Voll RE, Zoller OM *et al.* Impaired phagocytosis of apoptotic cell material by monocyte-derived macrophages from patients with systemic lupus erythematosus. *Arthritis Rheum* 1998; 41: 1241–50.

9 Casciola-Rosen L, Rosen A, Petri M, Schlissel M. Surface blebs on apoptotic cells are sites of enhanced procoagulant activity: Implications for coagulation events and antigenic spread in systemic lupus erythematosus. *Proc Natl Acad Sci USA* 1996; 93: 1624–9.

10 Botto M, DellAgnola C, Bygrave AE *et al.* Homozygous C1q deficiency causes glomerulonephritis associated with multiple apoptotic bodies. *Nature Genet* 1998; 19: 56–9.

11 Salmon M, Gaston JSH. The role of T lymphocytes in rheumatoid arthritis. *Br Med Bull* 1995; 51: 332–45.

12 Kitas GD, Salmon M, Farr M, Young SP, Bacon PA. T cell functional defects in RA. intrinsic or extrinsic. *J Autoimmun* 1988; 1: 339–51.

13 Panayi GS, Lanchbury JS, Kingsley GH. The importance of the T-cell in initiating and maintaining the chronic synovitis of rheumatoid-arthritis. *Arthritis Rheum* 1992; 35: 729–35.

14 Firestein GS, Zvaifler NJ. How important are T cells in chronic rheumatoid
synovitis? *Arthritis Rheum* 1990; 33:
768–73.

15 Wordsworth BP, Lanchbury JSS, Sakkas
LI *et al*. HLA-DR4 subtype frequencies
in rheumatoid-arthritis indicate that
DRB1 is the major susceptibility locus
within the HLA class-II region. *Proc
Natl Acad Sci USA* 1989; 86:
10049–53.

16 Winchester RJ, Gregerson PK. The
molecular-basis of susceptibility to
rheumatoid-arthritis—the conformational equivalence hypothesis. *Springer
Semin Immunopathol* 1988; 10:
119–39.

17 Salmon M. The immunogenetic
component of susceptibility to
rheumatoid arthritis. *Curr Opin
Rheumatol* 1992; 4: 342–7.

18 De Jongh BM, Van Romunde LKJ,
De Valkenburg HA, Lange GG, Van
Rood JJ. Epidemiological-study of HLA
and GM in rheumatoid-arthritis and
related symptoms in an open Dutch
population. *Ann Rheum Dis* 1984;
43: 613–19.

19 Salmon M, Emery P, Wordsworth BP
et al. HLA Dw4 is associated with
persistence rather than the induction of
rheumatoid arthritis. *Br J Rheumatol*
1993; 32: 628–30.

20 Gough A, Faint J, Salmon M *et al*.
Genetic typing of patients with inflammatory arthritis at presentation is predictive
of outcome. *Arthritis Rheum* 1994; 34:
1166–70.

21 Van Zeben D, Hazes LMW,
Zwinderman AH *et al*. Association
of HLA-DR4 with a more progressive
disease course in patients with
rheumatoid-arthritis—results of a
follow-up-study. *Arthritis Rheum* 1991;
34: 822–30.

22 Wordsworth P, Pile K, Buckley JD *et al*.
HLA heterozygosity contributes to
susceptibility to rheumatoid-arthritis.
Am J Hum Genet 1992; 51: 585–91.

23 Arnett FC, Edworthy SM, Bloch DA
et al. The American Rheumatism
Association 1987 revised criteria for the
classification of rheumatoid-arthritis.
Arthritis Rheum 1988; 31: 315–24.

24 Uematsu Y, Wege H, Straus A *et al*.
The T-cell-receptor repertoire in the
synovial fluid of a patient with
rheumatoid arthritis is polyclonal. *Proc
Natl Acad Sci USA* 1991; 88: 8534–8.

25 Pluschke G, Ricken G, Taube H *et al*.
Biased T-cell receptor V alpha region
repertoire in the synovial fluid of
rheumatoid arthritis patients. *Eur J
Immunol* 1991; 21: 2749–54.

26 Fischer HP, Sharrock CEM, Colston
MJ, Panayi GS. Limiting dilution
analysis of proliferative T-cell responses
to mycobacterial 65-KDa heat-shock
protein fails to show significant
frequency differences between synovial
fluid and peripheral blood of patients
with rheumatoid arthritis. *Eur J
Immunol* 1991; 21: 2937–41.

27 Marguerie C, Lunardi C, So A.
PCR-based analysis of the Tcr
repertoire in human autoimmune
diseases. *Immunol Today* 1992;
13: 336–8.

28 Pelton BK, Harvey AR, Denman AM.
The rheumatoid synovial membrane
participates in systemic anti-viral
immune responses. *Clin Exp Immunol*
1985; 62: 657–61.

29 Sun JB, Link H, Olsson T, Xiao BG
et al. T-cell and B-cell responses to
myelin-oligodendrocyte glycoprotein
in multiple-sclerosis. *J Immunol* 1991;
146: 1490–5.

30 Offner H, Buenafe AC, Vainiene M
et al. Where, when, and how to detect
biased expression of disease—relevant
V-beta-genes in rats with experimental
autoimmune encephalomyelitis.
J Immunol 1993; 151: 506–17.

31 Paulus HE, Machleder HI, Levine S,
Yu DTY, McDonald NS. Lymphocyte
involvement in rheumatoid arthritis.
Arthritis Rheum 1977; 20: 1249–62.

32 Karsh J, Klippel JH, Plotz PH *et al*.
Lymphophoresis in rheumatoid
arthritis. *Arthritis Rheum* 1981;
24: 867–73.

33 Aaron S, Paetku V. Synovial cell
secretion of Il-2 *in vitro*, a limiting
dilution analysis. *Clin Exp Rheumatol*
1991; 9: 113–18.

34 Pitzalis C, Kingsley GH, Covelli M
et al. Selective migration of the
human helper-inducer memory T-cell
subset—confirmation by *in vivo* cellular
kinetic-studies. *Eur J Immunol* 1991;
21: 369–76.

35 Matthews N, Emery P, Pilling D, Akbar A, Salmon M. CD45RB exon expression by T lymphocytes from patients with rheumatoid arthritis. *Arthritis Rheum* 1993; 36: 603–7.

36 Mackay CR, Marston WL, Dudler L. Naive and memory T-cells show distinct pathways of lymphocyte recirculation. *J Exp Med* 1990; 171: 801–17.

37 Salmon M, Pilling D, Borthwick NJ *et al*. The progressive differentiation of primed T cells is associated with an increasing susceptibility to apoptosis. *Eur J Immunol* 1994; 24: 892–9.

38 Borthwick NJ, Akbar AN, MacCormac LP *et al*. Selective migration of highly differentiated primed T cells, defined by low expression of CD45RB, across human umbilical vein endothelial cells: Effects of viral infection on transmigration. *Immunology* 1997; 90: 272–80.

39 Salmon M, Scheel-Toellner D, Huissoon AP *et al*. Inhibition of T cell apoptosis in the rheumatoid synovium. *J Clin Invest* 1997; 99: 439–46.

40 Akbar AN, Savill J, Gombert W *et al*. The specific recognition by macrophages of CD8⁺CD45RO⁺ T cells undergoing apoptosis: a mechanism for T cell clearance during resolution of viral infections. *J Exp Med* 1994; 180: 1943–7.

41 Savill J, Fadok V, Henson P, Haslett C. Phagocyte recognition of cells undergoing apoptosis. *Immunol Today* 1993; 14: 131–6.

42 Martin SJ, Reutelingsperger CPM, Mcgahon AJ *et al*. Early redistribution of plasma-membrane phosphatidylserine is a general feature of apoptosis regardless of the initiating stimulus—inhibition by overexpression of bcl-2 and abl. *J Exp Med* 1995; 182: 1545–56.

43 Dhein J, Walczak H, Baumler C, Debatin KM, Krammer PH. Autocrine T cell suicide mediated by Apo-1/(Fas/CD95). *Nature* 1995; 373: 438–41.

44 Brunner T, Mogil RJ, Laface D *et al*. Cell-autonomous fas (CD95) Fas–ligand interaction mediates activation-induced apoptosis in T-cell hybridomas. *Nature* 1995; 373: 441–4.

45 Cohen JJ, Duke RC, Fadok VA, Sellins KS. Apoptosis and programmed cell-death in immunity. *Ann Rev Immunol* 1992; 10: 267–93.

46 Akbar AN, Borthwick N, Salmon M *et al*. The significance of low bcl-2 expression by CD45RO-T-cells in normal individuals and patients with acute viral-infections—the role of apoptosis in T-cell memory. *J Exp Med* 1993; 178: 427–38.

47 Mazel S, Burtrum D, Petrie HTJ. Regulation of cell division cycle progression by bcl-2 expression: a potential mechanism for inhibition of programmed cell death. *J Exp Med* 1996; 183: 2219–26.

48 O'Reilly LA, Huang DCS, Strasser A. The cell death inhibitor Bcl-2 and its homologues influence control of cell cycle entry. *EMBO J* 1996; 15: 6979–90.

49 Korsmeyer SJ, Shutter JR, Veis DJ, Merry DE, Oltvai ZN. Bcl-2/bax—a rheostat that regulates an antioxidant pathway and cell-death. *Semin Cancer Biol* 1993; 4: 327–32.

50 Hyde H, Salmon M, Janossy G, Akbar AN. Upregulation of intracellular glutathione by fibroblast-derived factors: prevention of activated T cell apoptosis in the presence of low Bcl-2. *Blood* 1997; 89: 2453–60.

51 Boise LH, Gonzalezgarcia M, Postema CE *et al*. Bcl-x, a bcl-2-related gene that functions as a dominant regulator of apoptotic cell-death. *Cell* 1993; 74: 597–608.

52 Akbar AN, Borthwick N, Wickremasinghe RG *et al*. Interleukin-2 receptor common γ-chain cytokines regulate activated T cell apoptosis in response to growth factor withdrawal: selective induction of anti-apoptotic (bcl-2, bcl-x$_L$) but not pro-apoptotic (bax, bcl-x$_S$) gene expression. *Eur J Immunol* 1996; 26: 294–9.

53 Hale AJ, Smith CA, Sutherland LC *et al*. Apoptosis—molecular regulation of cell death. *Eur J Biochem* 1996; 236: 1–26.

54 Gombert W, Wallace DL, Borthwick NJ *et al*. Fibroblasts prevent apoptosis of IL-2 deprived T cells without inducing proliferation: a selective effect on Bcl-x$_L$

expression. *Immunology* 1996; 86: 397–404.

55 McInnes IB, Al-Mughales J, Field M *et al.* The role of interleukin-15 in T cell migration and activation in rheumatoid arthritis. *Nature Med* 1996; 2: 175–82.

56 McInnes IB, Leung BP, Sturrock RD, Field M, Liew FY. Interleukin 15 mediates T cell dependent regulation of tumor necrosis factor alpha production in rheumatoid arthritis. *Nature Med* 1997; 3: 189–95.

57 Fassbender HG. *Pathology of Rheumatic Diseases.* New York, Springer-Verlag, 1975.

58 Ayroldi E, Cannarile L, Migliorati G *et al.* CD44 (pgp-1) inhibits CD3 and dexamethasone-induced apoptosis. *Blood* 1995; 86: 2672–8.

59 Yokota K, Murata N, Saiko O *et al.* High avidity state of leukocyte function-associated antigen-1 on rheumatoid synovial-fluid T-lymphocytes. *J Immunol* 1995; 155: 4118–24.

60 Stewart M, Thiel M, Hogg N. Leukocyte integrins. *Curr Opin Cell Biol* 1995; 7: 690–6.

61 Firestein GS. Invasive fibroblast-like synoviocytes in rheumatoid-arthritis —passive responders or transformed aggressors. *Arthritis Rheum* 1996; 39: 1781–90.

62 Schneider C, Gold R, Dalakas MC *et al.* MHC Class-I mediated cytotoxicity does not induce apoptosis in muscle fibres nor in inflammatory T cells—studies in patients with polymyositis, dermatomyositis and inclusion body myositis. *J Neuropathol Exp Neurol* 1996; 55: 1205–9.

63 Buckley CD, Pilling D, Henriquez NV *et al.* RGD peptides induce apoptosis by direct caspase-3 activation: a ubiquitous motif for cell death. *Nature* 1998 (In press).

64 Pilling D, Akbar AN, Girdlestone J *et al.* Interferon-β is the principle mediator of stromal cell rescue of T cells from apoptosis. *Eur J Immunol* 1998 (In press).

65 Salmon M, Pilling D, Mappin C, Akbar AN. Human T cell differentiation and cytokine regulation. In: Gordon & Whetton, eds. *Haemopoeitic Cell Growth Factors.* Plenum. *Blood Cell Biochemistry* 1996; 7: 203–15.

66 Taher TE, Smit L, Griffioen AW *et al.* Signaling through CD44 is mediated by tyrosine kinases—association with p56(lck) in T lymphocytes. *J Biol Chem* 1996; 171: 2863–7.

67 Hale AJ, Smith CA, Sutherland LC *et al.* Apoptosis—molecular regulation of cell death. *Eur J Biochem* 1996; 236: 1–26.

68 Dekker LV, Parker PJ. Protein-kinase-C—a question of specificity. *Trends Biochem Sci* 1994; 19: 73–7.

69 Ghayur T, Hugunin M, Talanin RV *et al.* Proteolytic activation of protein kinase C delta by an ICE/CED 3-like protease induces characteristics of apoptosis. *J Exp Med* 1996; 184: 2399–404.

70 Scheel-Toellner D, Pilling D, Hardie D *et al.* Inhibition of T-cell apoptosis by interferon-β reverses nuclear translocation of protein kinase C-delta. 1998 (Submitted).

71 Lord JM, Garrone B, Griffiths G, Watters D. Protein-kinase-C—a family of isoenzymes with distinct roles in pathogenesis. *J Cell Biochem* 1995; S19B: 275.

72 Firestein GS, Yeo M, Zvaifler NJ. Apoptosis in rheumatoid-arthritis synovium. *J Clin Invest* 1995; 96: 1631–8.

73 Migita K, Eguchi K, Ichinose Y *et al.* Effects of rapamycin on apoptosis of rheumatoid synovial cells. *Clin Exp Immunol* 1997; 108: 199–203.

74 Okamoto K, Asahara H, Kobayashi T *et al.* Induction of apoptosis in the rheumatoid synovium by Fas ligand gene transfer. *Gene Therapy* 1998; 5: 331–8.

75 Firestein GS, Echeverri F, Yeo M, Zvaifler NJ, Green DR. Somatic mutations in the p53 tumor suppressor gene in rheumatoid arthritis synovium. *Proc Natl Acad Sci USA* 1997; 94: 10895–900.

3: Are cytokines directly involved in pathogenesis?

A. Cope and A.G. Wilson

Cytokines comprise a large number of proteins that regulate a diverse range of physiological processes such as cellular activation, differentiation, division and death. They are analogous to hormones but characteristically they mediate their effects locally, both intra- and intercellularly. Activity is generally mediated by interaction with specific high-affinity receptors.

Each cytokine tends to be produced by a limited number of cell types. For example, tumour necrosis factor alpha (TNF-α) is classically macrophage derived. However, significant amounts are also produced by T and B cells, whereas the two TNF receptors are expressed on virtually all nucleated cells. Much current research activity involves the unravelling of the intracellular signals generated by the different cytokine receptors.

Attempts to classify cytokines have proved difficult. Some groups such as the TNF superfamily share common regions of homology, whereas others have been grouped according to the predominant cellular sources. Thus, monokines, such as interleukin 1 (IL-1) and TNF-α, are derived predominantly, but not exclusively, from monocytes/macrophages, while lymphokines, such as IL-2, interferon gamma (IFN-γ) and lymphotoxin beta, are produced by lymphocytes. A large number of cytokines have been detected in the rheumatoid joint, for example, and have been grouped into those with predominantly pro- or anti-inflammatory actions: the former includes TNF-α, IL-1, IL-6, IL-8, IL-12 and the latter includes transforming growth factor beta (TGF-β), IL-4, IL-10 and IL-13. It has been suggested that an imbalance in the relative production of these two groups, perhaps due to genetic polymorphism within cytokine genes, may lead to the chronic inflammatory process typical of rheumatoid arthritis (RA).

The initiating event in RA is unknown but probably results from activation of a T cell by arthritogenic antigen(s). The strong association with particular major histocompatibility complex (MHC) class II antigens, particularly with HLA-DR alleles encoding a common, or shared epitope, is strongly supportive of this hypothesis. This activation is followed by the pathological features of joint inflammation including cellular recruitment, activation and proliferation, as well as angiogenesis and progressive bone and cartilage destruction leading to joint failure. As we discuss below, cytokines have been shown to mediate many of these effects.

Are the pathological features of RA compatible with cytokine-driven disease?

The patient with severe, active, chronic RA will present to their physician with acutely hot, swollen and tender joints, subcutaneous nodules, widespread lymphadenopathy, and perhaps even fever, together with a history to match the signs. Invariably, the disease has immobilized the patient through joint pain and profound stiffness. While these clinical features indicate that the disease has both local and systemic components, are they compatible with a pathological process driven by the overproduction of cytokines?

The pathological process of severe, active RA is most obvious in the lining membrane of inflamed synovial joints [1]. Unlike the synovial lining of healthy joints, which is only a few cells in thickness and contains scanty cells of haemopoetic origin, the chronically inflamed synovial joint is packed with infiltrates of haemopoetic cells, including T and B lymphocytes, macrophages, dendritic cells and plasma cells. Also prominent are fibroblast-like cells and increased numbers of blood vessels, around which cluster aggregates of infiltrating mononuclear cells. Polymorphonuclear neutrophils, in contrast, are the predominant cell type of synovial fluid. In both acute and chronic disease, the overriding characteristic of the inflammatory infiltrate is a cell with an activated phenotype, as defined by the expression of activation antigens such as HLA-DR, very late antigen 1 (VLA-1), CD69 and IL-2Rα on the cell surface of T cells [2–5]. Other cell types express effector molecules such as B7, Fc receptors and metalloproteinases [6–8]. Closer inspection reveals evidence of cell-cycle progression, senescence and varying degrees of apoptosis, indicating that resident cells may undergo the full transition from activation, growth and differentiation, to cell death [9].

Irreversible joint damage occurs at the junction of the synovial lining layer with cartilage and bone known as pannus, an area particularly enriched with cells of macrophage lineage. These cells are thought to migrate over the cartilage and erode into subchondral bone, leading ultimately to the formation of bony erosions visible on radiographs [10]. As well as areas of destruction, there are transitional zones showing evidence of resorption and repair. The chronic inflamed joint therefore is a site of multiple pathological processes including cell activation and growth, chemotaxis and cell trafficking, clustering and organization of cells into lymphoid follicles, as well as new blood vessel formation. To achieve this level of complexity within the confined space of the synovial joint, there must exist multiple networks of growth and activation factors, chemotactic and angiogenic factors of comparable complexity, capable of perpetuating the chronic inflammatory response. The infiltrating cells are thought to be both the source and target of these cytokine networks for many of these processes. Thus, through autocrine and paracrine loops these factors have been described as both the orchestrators and effectors of the immuno-inflammatory response.

In simple terms, these findings would predict that the synovial joint should express a vast array of different inflammatory mediators. Furthermore, one might anticipate that some factors could spill over into the systemic circulation. What is the evidence for this? The last decade and a half of research in this field has revealed an impressive range of cytokines expressed in the joints of patients with RA (Table 3.1). The earliest studies documented the expression of cytokines such as IL-1 and TNF in synovial fluid from inflamed joints [11–13]. For other cytokines, such as IL-6, serum levels can be detected easily and are often associated and correlate closely with the acute-phase response [14,15]. In circumstances where cytokine protein expression has been difficult to detect, Northern blotting analysis of synovial fluid cell or synovial tissue derived mRNA has revealed transcripts for a large number of different cytokines including pro-inflammatory cytokines of monocyte/macrophage origin [16], cytokines produced exclusively by T lymphocytes [17], and more recently a panoply of chemokines (see Table 3.1). In the case of T-cell-derived cytokines, IL-2, IL-4 and IFN-γ mRNA expression has not always correlated with protein production which is often undetectable [17,18]. As a result, more attention has focused on the spontaneous production of cytokine protein by cells of monocyte/ macrophage lineage [19]. Studies of cultures of dissociated, unstimulated synovial tissue mononuclear cells have been the most informative and, in retrospect, perhaps most representative of the ongoing disease process [16,17].

Compelling evidence to support a biological role for cytokines in the inflammatory process within synovial joints has been the histopathological localization of inflammatory cytokines at the cartilage–pannus junction, the leading edge of the inflammatory destructive process [20–22]. Dual colour immunofluorescence or staining of serial sections has allowed the expression of specific families of cytokines such as the monokines IL-1 and TNF to be correlated with distinct cell subsets such as the CD14+ subset [20,23]. More recently, the cognate cell-surface receptors for these soluble ligands have been found to be co-expressed with ligand not only in the tissues of the inflamed target organ [24–26], but at levels significantly higher than those expressed on cells of the same lineage found in the peripheral blood from the same patient [27]. These studies were important, because they confirmed that synovial mononuclear cells were indeed potential targets of cytokine action *in vivo*.

Table 3.1 Cytokine expression in the synovial joint.

| | Expression dominant cell | | |
Cytokine group	mRNA	protein	source
Pro-inflammatory			
IL-1α,β	+	+	M
TNF	+	+	M
IL-6	+	+	M,F,T
GM-CSF	+	+	M
M-CSF	+	+	M
LIF	+	+	M
Oncostatin M	?	?	
LT	+	±	T
IL-2	+	±	T
IL-3	–	–	
IL-7	?	?	
IL-9	?	?	
IL-12	+	+	M
IL-15	+	+	M
IFN-α,β	+	+	F
IFN-γ	+	±	T
VEGF	+	+	M
Immunoregulatory			
IL-4	±	–	T
IL-10	+	+	M,T
IL-11	+	+	M,F
IL-13	+	+	T
TGF-β	+	+	F,M
IL-1Ra	+	+	M
Chemokines			
IL-8	+	+	M,F
Gro-α	+	+	?
MIP-1α,β	+	+	M,F
MCP-1	+	+	M
ENA-78	+	+	M
RANTES	+	+	M
Mitogens			
BDGF	+	+	M
FGF	+	+	M,F
PDGF	+	+	M

M, macrophages; T, T lymphocytes; F, fibroblasts. Chondrocytes also contribute to the expression of factors such as TGF-β and MCP-1.
IL, interleukin; TNF, tumour necrosis factor; GM-CSF, granulocyte–macrophage colony-stimulating factor; M-CSF, macrophage colony-stimulating factor; LIF, leukaemia inhibitor factor; LT, lymphotoxin; IFN, interferon; VEGF, vascular endothelial growth factor; TGF, transforming growth factor; MIP, macrophage inflammatory protein; MCP, monocyte chemoattractant protein; ENA, epithelial neutrophil activating peptide; RANTES, regulated upon activation normal T cell expressed and secreted; BDGF, bone derived growth factor; FGF, fibroblast growth factor; PDGF, platelet derived growth factor.

A new dimension to the study of pro-inflammatory cytokines in chronic inflammatory diseases such as RA has been the finding of significantly increased expression of naturally occurring cytokine inhibitors. These include inhibitors which neutralize the cognate ligand either by binding directly, such as soluble TNF receptors, or by blocking cell-surface receptors such as the IL-1 receptor antagonist protein (reviewed in [28]). These too are up-regulated in the joint [29–31]. There are also a number of cytokines with known potent anti-inflammatory properties, including IL-4, IL-10, IL-13 and TGF-β. Of these, IL-10 and TGF-β are abundant in the joint [32,33]. These findings have raised some intriguing questions about the aetiology and progression of the chronic inflammatory process. Clearly there is evidence for an attempt at homeostasis. Specifically, they raise the possibility that the chronic phase of the disease may persist not just because of over-production of pro-inflammatory cytokines, but perhaps because of inadequate anti-inflammatory or inhibitory responses. The balance of these factors is therefore thought to exert a profound influence on disease progression.

In summary, therefore, the detection of cytokines and their cognate receptor ligands at sites of joint damage have provided strong evidence to suggest that the disease is cytokine driven. What evidence is there to suggest that cytokines may be directly involved?

Does disease remission correlate with down-modulation of cytokine expression?

A further step in an attempt to establish whether cytokine expression is related to disease pathogenesis has been to document cytokine expression at different stages of disease activity. Given the long list of cytokines whose expression has been shown to be increased in RA (see Table 3.1), this approach has had the advantage of examining whether there exist expression patterns of some inflammatory mediators which more closely reflect the disease process. The prediction therefore would be that those cytokines most consistently down-regulated during disease remission may be more intimately involved in disease pathogenesis. Following on from this, it becomes possible to attribute mechanisms of action of some disease-modifying agents directly or indirectly, at least in part, to the down-regulation of cytokine expression.

Several experimental approaches have been employed. Perhaps the most common has been to compare serum levels of cytokines in groups of patient previously shown in retrospective studies to have active or inactive disease. This approach has not always met with success. Studies have reported highly varied results, partly because of the disadvantages associated with single samples and the heterogeneous nature of the disease, as well as the limitations associated with detecting by immuno- or bioassay meaningful changes or differences in levels of cytokine in serum (often at the lower limit of detection) at sites distant from the inflamed target organ [34]. Not surprisingly, the more consistent results have been achieved with the detection of cytokines such as IL-6, which are expressed at significant levels even in healthy individuals [35]. Implicit in these results has been the suggestion that expression and abundance correlate directly with pathogenicity. This has turned out to be a misguided concept. Indeed, the detection of circulating as well as local joint expression of cytokines depends on a balance between production and consumption. RA is a chronic inflammatory disease in which consumption is likely to be significant. In this context, conventional assays are likely to underestimate cytokine expression. This may be especially true for T-cell-derived cytokines.

Where cytokines themselves are undetectable in serum, levels of soluble cytokine receptors have also been studied. The experience with soluble IL-1, IL-2, and TNF receptors indicates that while levels are detectable in all individuals, including the healthy control population, and increases correlate well with disease activity [29,36,37], the results at best may only reflect indirectly levels of the cognate ligand. Perhaps more likely they provide some indication of the activation status of mononuclear cells such as T cells (for sIL-2R) and macrophages (sTNF-R), respectively. There is a similar experience with sIL-6R and sIFN-γR [38].

An alternative approach has been the longitudinal prospective evaluation of serial serum samples obtained in controlled trials. The inclusion of well-documented control subjects under these circumstances is a distinct advantage. Studies have been reported in the literature showing, over periods of up to 6 months, that some disease-modifying agents down-regulate the levels of cytokine detected in serum when compared with baseline levels (reviewed in [39]). More recently, the effects of combination therapy have been of interest, especially where combined treatments show evidence of synergistic effects on down-regulating cytokine expression [40]. In addition to studying serum levels, spontaneous cytokine production by peripheral blood mononuclear cells *in vitro* or following stimulation with mitogens have been studied. Spontaneous cytokine production is usually indicative of cell activation assuming that the culture conditions are lipopolysaccharide (LPS)/mitogen free. Whether fractionated suspensions of cells in culture truly reflect cytokine expression *ex vivo*, when compared with whole blood, is yet to be determined [41]. Clearly these and related issues are of importance when evaluating cytokine expression in patients, and more importantly the effects of therapeutic intervention *in vivo*, in prospective trials.

One of the limitations of longitudinal evaluation of cytokine expression in patients is the availability of sequential joint tissue samples. Even

in the case of synovial fluid, serial sampling is not always possible. However, repeated needle biopsy of synovial tissue, or repeated biopsy under
direct vision using fine bore arthroscopy of the knee can provide sufficient
material for sequential histological analysis. An alternative approach has
been to study the effects of drugs on cytokine expression by synovial tissue
in vitro [42].

These limitations have inevitably led to the use of animal disease
models of arthritis to study cytokine expression in the context of disease and
therapeutic intervention, in a more controlled fashion. Such models have
the advantage of evaluating cytokine levels both before, at the onset and
throughout the progression of disease [43]. The initiating arthritogen is well
defined and in most cases there are clear and relevant disease endpoints.
Inbred strains of mice also provide a more homogeneous population for
study. Expression of cytokines in rat adjuvant arthritis and collagen-induced
arthritis have been documented in detail (reviewed in [44]). Animal models
have provided important information about the kinetics of cytokine expression, and in particular have provided evidence for a hierarchy of cytokine
expression, as well as evidence *in vivo* for cytokine networks.

In summary, there is clear evidence that cytokine expression is down-
regulated during disease remission and that several disease-modifying agents
can suppress cytokines expressed by cells of many lineages. Furthermore,
it would appear that, during disease remission, the balance of cytokines and
their cytokine inhibitors would favour the production of cytokine inhibitors, indicating that homeostasis has been restored at least to some extent
(reviewed in [45]). Even though the data demonstrate that where the
disease is less active, cytokine expression is down-modulated, this still does
not prove that overexpression of cytokines is pathological. Accordingly, more
detailed functional studies have been necessary to provide more direct evidence for the link.

Defining the key mediators

Over the last 5 years, much emphasis has shifted towards addressing not
whether cytokines are up-regulated at sites of inflammation, but which
cytokines are the critical pro-inflammatory mediators expressed in joints.
For example, as the functions of many cytokines have become clear, and
the processes central to the inflammatory process have become better
defined, it has been possible to evaluate the effects of a large number of
recombinant cytokines. Culture systems *in vitro* can be used to define
which cytokines are driving synovial proliferation and cell activation, as well
as chemotaxis and cell trafficking (reviewed in [45,46]). By neutralizing
pro-inflammatory cytokines such as IL-1 and TNF *in vitro*, it has been

possible to show that blockade of these cytokines down-regulates the spontaneous production of other pro-inflammatory cytokines such as IL-1 and TNF themselves, or IL-6, IL-8 and granulocyte–macrophage colony-stimulating factor (GM-CSF) in synovial tissue cultures [19,47,48]. While IL-1 blockade can also down-regulate IL-6 and IL-8 production, the effects observed with anti-TNF appear to be more pronounced, since IL-1Ra does not appear to suppress TNF or IL-1 production [48]. The combination of TNF and IL-1 blockade may turn out to have more potent effects than either neutralizing regimen alone.

The original observations that IL-1 and TNF enhance cartilage destruction and bone resorption in explants of joint tissue *in vitro* have provided some of the most compelling evidence to suggest a direct role for these pro-inflammatory mediators in the destructive process [49–51]. At that time, the mechanisms were not understood. Analysis of synovial fluid as well as cultures of dissociated synovial membrane cells *in vitro* has since identified monocyte-derived cytokines such as IL-1 and TNF as being dominant producers of cartilage matrix-destroying proteinases, known as metalloproteinases (MMPs) [52,53]. Of particular interest from a therapeutic standpoint is the finding that cytokines such as IL-10, IL-4, and possibly IL-13 down-regulate the production of these enzymes [54], while in some cases up-regulating their natural inhibitors, the tissue inhibitors of metalloproteinases (TIMPS) [54].

To test further the hypothesis that these and related cytokines are intimately involved in joint destruction, monoclonal antibody therapy has been tested in animal models, particularly collagen-induced arthritis, an animal model which resembles RA and in which there is clear evidence for both immune and inflammatory responses being involved in the destruction of joints [55]. In this model whole joints can be obtained and evaluated by histochemistry. This approach therefore allows a detailed evaluation of the effects of each therapy on the destructive process. The results have been informative. Neutralization of anti-TNF and also IL-1 reduce the severity of disease, particularly the severity of inflammatory process, but more importantly the number of erosions in inflamed joints [56–59]. Indeed, comparative studies of TNF, IL-1α or IL-1β blockade *in vivo* indicate that these cytokines have subtle but distinct roles at different stages of the disease [60]. Significantly these effects can also be observed when therapy is commenced after the onset of disease, analogous and more representative of the situation in patients in the clinic [56,60].

A converse approach has been taken in the same experimental system. Thus far, regulatory cytokines such as IL-4, IL-10 and TGF-β have all been tested for their capacity to replace the supposedly deficient levels of these anti-inflammatory cytokines, with varying degrees of success. These experiments have been inspired largely by the anti-inflammatory effects that these cytokines exhibit in *in vitro* culture systems [45]. Both IL-4 and IL-10 appear to be chondroprotective [60]. The role of IFN-γ and TGF-β, on the other hand has been more controversial, appearing to be involved in different phases of the disease process [61–64]. Of perhaps more interest is the role of IL-12. Significantly, it has been shown that in collagen arthritis IL-12 injections can replace the use of mycobacteria in complete Freund's adjuvant [65]. The findings suggest that IL-12 may be responsible in part for driving the T-cell response towards a Th1 pro-inflammatory phenotype. This takes on particular significance given the data which suggest that T-cell responses appear to differentiate toward a pro-inflammatory Th1 rather than a Th2-like response in RA joints [66–68]. Combinations of anti-IL-12 and other cytokine inhibitors are currently being evaluated in animal models [69]. It is of interest that low levels of IL-12 have been detected in synovial joint cell cultures from RA patients at levels well within the biological range for this cytokine [45] (Brennan *et al.*, unpublished data). Whether it is involved early or late in RA needs further investigation.

A similar approach has been taken with IL-15, a cytokine reported to be important in driving TNF production and cultures [70]. Recent evidence suggests that neutralizing IL-15 with soluble IL-15Rα injections in the collagen arthritis model also has powerful therapeutic affects (M. Field, personal communication, 1998). In this context the study of factors which drive the production of cytokines such as TNF suggest evidence of T-cell dependency. For example, depleting T cells from synovial joint cultures dramatically reduces the amount of TNF produced (Brennan *et al.*, unpublished data). Although IL-15 is an attractive candidate [71], it would appear that this cytokine is not the only factor involved. Indeed studies from the group of Dayer and colleagues strongly suggest that cell-surface molecules are involved in driving this process [72]. This notion has been confirmed in studies where T cells and macrophages have been co-cultured in dual chambers, and in experiments demonstrating that cell-membrane preparations from T lymphocytes can themselves enhance TNF production *in vitro* [73–75]. Several candidates have been suggested including CD69 and CD11. However, blocking the interactions of these cell-surface receptors with their cognate ligands only partially suppresses pro-inflammatory cyto-kine production. What is known is that the proteins responsible, collectively termed SAFTS, are expressed at high levels on synovial T cells compared with levels expressed on peripheral blood. Expression also appears to be dependent on T stimulation with antigen, monoclonal anti-CD3 antibody (OKT3) or PMA-phorbol ester/PHA-phytohaemagglutinin [76]. Defining the molecular nature of SAFTS should provide some attractive targets for therapy in the near future.

Collectively, these data indicate that several candidate inflammatory and anti-inflammatory mediators contribute significantly (by their over- or underexpression) to disease severity. Accordingly, these data have prompted studies to examine whether polymorphisms encoded within these candidate genes might be over-represented in populations of patients with RA.

The genetic approach—studies in mice and humans

While the genome-wide search for susceptibility genes using microsatellite markers is eagerly awaited, much work has focused on the candidate gene approach, defining polymorphic genes of possible functional relevance which may contribute to the susceptibility or severity of RA.

Tumour necrosis factor alpha

TNF-α is a particularly attractive candidate gene in RA because of its biological activities and the location of the TNF-α gene in the MHC, approximately 1 megabase telomeric of the HLA-DRB1 locus. Production of TNF-α has been correlated with particular DR alleles: the carriage of DR2 being associated with low production, while DR3 and DR4 are associated with high production, with the latter phenotype being dominant in heterozygous individuals [77]. The association of DR4 with high production is intriguing since certain subtypes of this allele are associated with severe, seropositive, destructive RA.

A number of polymorphisms within the TNF locus have been identified in RA: five microsatellites and two biallelic promoter polymorphisms have been intensively studied [78]. The microsatellites are particularly useful in genetic studies because of the large number of alleles and high heterozygosity. However, there is no evidence that they have a direct effect on gene expression. Conversely the biallelic markers are less useful in genetic studies, but because of their location in the promoter are more likely to have direct effects on gene expression.

Two major studies involving the microsatellites have given different results. A linkage study of 50 multiplex RA families suggested a contribution from the TNF locus that was independent of class II alleles [79]. However, this was not supported by an association study [80].

The two promoter polymorphisms, at -308 and -238, have also been studied in RA. No association of alleles of -308 have been demonstrated in a number of studies [81,82]. However, one report did show an association of carriage of the -238A allele with decreased radiologically detectable progression, which was independent of HLA-DR4 [82]. This result will need to be confirmed.

Overall therefore, the TNF locus does not seem to contribute significantly, if at all, to the genetic background of RA.

Interleukin 6

Recently, three polymorphisms have been described in the promoter region of the IL-6 gene. Association between an allele, -174G, and systemic juvenile chronic arthritis has been reported [83]. Transfection of the human epithelial cell line, HeLa, with plasmids encoding a reporter gene under the control of the two promoter alleles, has demonstrated a threefold higher reporter expression from the -174G allele, suggesting that this polymorphism has direct effects on gene expression. Studies of this polymorphism in RA are awaited.

Interleukin 10

Three biallelic polymorphisms have been described within the IL-10 promoter region. The -1082A allele has been correlated with low IL-10 production. An initial report has suggested that this allele is associated with the presence of IgA rheumatoid factors, which are associated with more severe forms of RA [80].

Chromosome 5q31.1

The genes for IL-3, -4, -5, -9, -13, GM-CSF and several cytokine receptors all lie on 5q. A genetic study using intercrosses between B10.D2 and BALB/c mice, displaying Th1 and Th2 phenotypes respectively, has identified a locus on chromosome 11 that controls these phenotypic differences, the syntenic region in the humans being 5q31.1 [84].

A recent study of this region in humans has identified a biallelic polymorphism in the IL-4 receptor (alpha) chain involving an amino acid switch at position 576 involving a substitution from glutamine to arginine [85]. Carriage of R576 is associated with higher expression of CD23 (the low-affinity IgE receptor) on B cells, due to an alteration in signal transduction due to the polymorphism.

Imbalance between Th1 and Th2 cytokine production has been proposed to be important in the development, or maintenance, of a number of auto-immune disorders, including RA. It will therefore be interesting to see if this region contains polymorphisms that contribute to the development of RA.

What has transgenic and knockout technology taught us?

Transgenic technology has made a major contribution to our understanding of the role of selected cytokines in the arthritic process. Much work has focused on TNF and IL-1, for the reasons outlined above. Transgenic mice engineered to overexpress a human TNF gene under the influence of its own promoter, but including an altered 3′ untranslated region (UTR) develop a severe chronic inflammatory polyarthritis with 100% penetrance [86]. The pathological features are similar in many respects to those of RA. They include proliferative synovial inflammatory infiltrates and, during the chronic phase of the disease, deposition of fibrous tissue, the formation of pannus and subsequently cartilage destruction and bone erosion. Interestingly, severity depends on the strain of mice in which the transgene is expressed. For example in the original F1 cross between C57BL/6 and CBA strains, mice develop arthritis between 4 and 6 weeks of age. On the arthritis-prone DBA1/J background, mice develop a severe arthritis at 3 weeks of age [87]. In this strain, the disease is more rapidly progressive and systemic features are prominent, suggesting that there may be differences in the regulatory elements in different strains which influence either the level of transgene expression, its persistence or its biological effects.

A similar phenotype is seen in mice overexpressing a mutant TNF transgene which is only expressed as a cell-membrane cytokine, as well as mice which have a mutant endogenous gene in which the AU-rich sequence in the 3′ UTR has been deleted (Kollias, unpublished data). The finding that these transgenic mice on RAG-deficient background develop severe disease supports the idea that TNF provides an important inflammatory component with proliferation of activated synoviocytes and the production of factors that ultimately destroy cartilage, which is independent of T- and B-cell responses (D. Kioussis and G. Kollias, personal communication, 1998). The reasons why TNF targets the joints and not other tissues such as pancreatic islets or the thyroid gland remain a mystery that may relate to specific and selective effects that TNF has on fibroblast-like cells in synovial joints.

The role of the IL-1 system has been studied using both transgenic and gene deletion technology. An IL-1α transgenic mouse develops synovial cell hypertrophy and cartilage and bony destruction [88]. Furthermore an IL-1 receptor antagonist transgenic mouse was resistant to the induction of collagen-induced arthritis [89]. However, surprisingly, in view of these results, an IL-1α-deficient mouse did not show any evidence of attenuation of antigen-induced arthritis compared with wild-type control animals. By contrast, transgenic mice overexpressing IL-6 [90] and IL-8 do not develop spontaneous arthritis.

Gene knockouts

Knockout technology has also provided some important clues as to how cytokines may be involved in the induction or regulation of the inflammatory process *in vivo* (reviewed in [91]). Perhaps the best examples are mice deficient in IL-10 or TGF-β. These knockout mice develop widespread systemic inflammatory disease [92–94]. In TGF-β-deficient mice there is an arthritic component but other organs are also involved, most notably the gut. Interestingly, IL-2 knockout mice also develop chronic inflammatory disease [95], a phenotype suggesting that IL-2 is in some way involved in T-cell homeostasis, perhaps through regulation of the apoptotic pathway, consequent upon T-cell-receptor ligation [96]. The phenotype of mice knockout for TNF or its receptors in inducible animal models of arthritis is under investigation. The prediction would be that mice deficient in TNF or the p55 TNF receptor would not be susceptible to the development of collagen-induced arthritis.

These findings indicate that the cellular and molecular basis for the arthritic process is complex and multifactorial. Animal models confirm that both overexpression of pro-inflammatory cytokines and a deficiency in the expression of immunoregulatory factors such as IL-10 and TGF-β may be important in pathogenesis of chronic inflammatory disease, including arthritis.

What have clinical trials taught us?

The data summarized above suggest that a spectrum of cytokines produced locally in inflamed synovial joints, and the imbalance between the production of cytokine ligands and their cognate inhibitors, could provide a molecular basis for the observed pathology. Clinical trials of cytokine blockade in patients with RA have provided unique opportunities to validate the direct role of several of the key players in the disease.

Therapeutic strategies have taken the form of humanized/chimeric monoclonal antibodies [97,98], soluble TNF-R fusion proteins [99] or receptor antagonists [100], where the targets are the cytokine itself or its receptor, depending on the therapeutic agent. Aside from isolated reports, the published studies to date are confined principally to the neutralization of TNF; fewer data are available for IL-1, IL-6 and IL-10. More experience with anti-IL-6 is needed to evaluate its effect, especially as the monoclonal antibody induces an increase in IL-6 levels [101], which may in turn have anti-inflammatory effects. The features of some of these trials are summarized in Table 3.2. Notable among these multicentre, randomized, double-blind, placebo-controlled trials is the enrolment of patients with severe, chronic disease, who have failed multiple attempts at suppression of the disease with disease-modifying agents. Thus, interpretation of the results has to be taken in this context, together with an appreciation that the variable route, dosing and frequency of each agent, as well as variation in the affinity

Table 3.2 Clinical trials of cytokine blockade in rheumatoid arthritis.

Agent	Trial design	No. patients recruited	Regimen	% achieving benefit (> 20% Paulus)	Acute-phase response
cA2 anti-TNF IgG1 mAb	Multicentre, randomized, double blind, placebo controlled	73	Single i.v. dose: 1 or 10 mg/kg	79% @ 4 weeks with 10 mg/kg dose	Reduced
CDP571 anti-TNF IgG4 mAb	Randomized, double blind, placebo controlled	36	Single i.v. dose: 0.1, 1 or 10 mg/kg	nd	Reduced
p75 TNF-R Fc fusion protein IgG1	Multicentre, randomized, double blind, placebo controlled	180	Loading dose 2/week s.c. 0.25, 2 or 16 mg/m^2	75% @ 3 months with 16 mg/kg dose	Reduced
rhuIL-1Ra	Multicentre, randomized, double blind, placebo controlled	175	20, 70, or 200 mg 1, 3, or 7/week for 3 weeks, then 1/week for 4 weeks	nd	Reduced
Anti-IL-6 IgG1 mAb	Open label	5	10 mg/day i.v. for 10 days	nd	Reduced

TNF, tumour necrosis factor; mAb, monoclonal antibody.

and half-life of the therapeutics make direct comparisons of efficacy difficult.

Taken as a whole, the results from these trials are striking in several respects. First, all treatments are well tolerated. Secondly, a single infusion of antibody can profoundly influence subjective and objective disease parameters for many weeks, even when vigorous criteria are applied [98,102]. Thirdly, the high frequency of responders to intervention indicates that cytokines such as TNF and IL-1 must be important components of the inflammatory response in *most* patients. One can only conclude therefore, that these and related cytokines are central to the pathogenesis of the inflammatory component of arthritis.

There are many other findings of interest. A comparison of TNF blockade vs. IL-1Ra in relation to the frequency of dosing, reflects to a large extent a requirement for > 90% IL-1R to be engaged for effective IL-1 blockade. In this context, cost becomes an issue. The relative efficacy of different IgG antibody isotypes, regardless of whether they are monoclonal antibodies or as soluble receptor Fc fusion proteins, raises the issue of Fc binding and complement fixation. For example, it has been suggested that since membrane TNF may be an important component of TNF bioactivity *in vivo*, Fc binding (± complement fixation) may contribute to the observed therapeutic effects. Likewise, cytotoxicity of membrane-TNF-expressing cells might be more efficient with IgG1 compared with IgG4 monoclonal antibody therapy.

Finally, given the therapeutic benefits afforded by these new treatment strategies, we now need to learn more about how these agents work. Cytokines such as TNF and IL-1 are pleiotropic, and so it becomes all the more important that mechanisms of action are incorporated into the therapeutic monitoring process. For example, how much of the effects of TNF blockade are due to the down-regulation of cell trafficking [103], and how much can be attributed to suppressing the production of other cytokines, and MMPs? Or are all these processes modulated? Is the impressive reduction in the acute phase response of direct therapeutic relevance, or merely a feature secondary to disease modification? Perhaps the critical question is: to what extent are these agents chrondroprotective? The prediction would be that where IL-1 is down-regulated—either directly or through TNF blockade—cartilage protection might be expected. *In vitro* animal data would favour this idea [60], as would the finding that MMP-1 and -3 are down-regulated in patients receiving anti-TNF therapy [104]. Long-term prospective studies are necessary to address this. Either way, we may have to await licensing of these agents before this crucial information becomes available. Where mechanisms of action clearly differ, it should be possible to combine these and alternative therapies, and strive to achieve synergism at the clinical level.

References

1 Edwards JCW. Structure of synovial lining. In: *The Synovial Lining in Health and Disease*. London: Chapman & Hall, 1987: 17–40.

2 Burmester GR, Yu DT, Irani AM, Kunkel HG, Winchester RJ. Ia+ T cells in synovial fluid and tissues of patients with rheumatoid arthritis. *Arthritis Rheum* 1981; 24: 1370–6.

3 Duke O, Panayi GS, Janossy G, Poulter LW. An immunohistological analysis of lymphocyte subpopulations and their microenvironment in the synovial membranes of patients with rheumatoid arthritis using monoclonal antibodies. *Clin Exp Immunol* 1982; 49: 22–30.

4 Klareskog L, Forsum U, Wigren A, Wigzell H. Relationship between HLA-DR-expressing cells and T lymphocytes of different subsets in rheumatoid synovial tissue. *Scand J Immunol* 1981; 15: 501–7.

5 Cush JJ, Lipsky PE. Phenotypic analysis of synovial tissue and peripheral blood lymphocytes isolated from patients with rheumatoid arthritis. *Arthritis Rheum* 1988; 31: 1230–8.

6 Broker BM, Edwards JC, Fanger MW, Lydyard PM. The prevalence and distribution of macrophages bearing Fc gamma R I, Fc gamma R II, and Fc gamma R III in synovium. *Scand J Rheumatol* 1990; 19: 123–35.

7 McCachren SS. Expression of metalloproteinases and metalloproteinase inhibitor in human arthritic synovium. *Arthritis Rheum* 1991; 34: 1085–93.

8 Ranheim EA, Kipps TJ. Elevated expression of CD80 (B7/BB1) and other accessory molecules on synovial fluid mononuclear cell subsets in rheumatoid arthritis [see comments]. *Arthritis Rheum* 1994; 37: 1637–46.

9 Salmon M, Scheel-Toellner D, Huissoon A.P. *et al.* Inhibition of T cell apoptosis in the rheumatoid synovium. *J Clin Invest* 1997; 99: 439–46.

10 Allard SA, Muirden KD, Camplejohn KL, Maini RN. Chondrocyte-derived cells and matrix at the rheumatoid cartilage–pannus junction identified with monoclonal antibodies. *Rheumatol Int* 1987; 7: 153–9.

11 Fontana A, Hengartner H, Weber E *et al.* Interleukin 1 activity in the synovial fluid of patients with rheumatoid arthritis. *Rheumatol Int* 1982; 2: 49–53.

12 Di Giovine FS, Nuki G, Duff GW. Tumour necrosis factor in synovial exudates. *Ann Rheum Dis* 1988; 47: 768–72.

13 Saxne T, Palladino MA Jr, Heinegard D, Talal N, Wollheim FA. Detection of tumor necrosis factor alpha but not tumor necrosis factor beta in rheumatoid arthritis synovial fluid and serum. *Arthritis Rheum* 1988; 31: 1041–5.

14 Hirano T, Matsuda T, Turner M *et al.* Excessive production of interleukin 6/B cell stimulatory factor-2 in rheumatoid arthritis. *Eur J Immunol* 1988; 18: 1797–801.

15 Houssiau FA, Devogelaer JP, Van Damme J, de Deuxchaisnes CN, Van Snick J. Interleukin-6 in synovial fluid and serum of patients with rheumatoid arthritis and other inflammatory arthritides. *Arthritis Rheum* 1988; 31: 784–8.

16 Buchan G, Barrett K, Turner M *et al.* Interleukin-1 and tumour necrosis factor mRNA expression in rheumatoid arthritis: prolonged production of IL-1 alpha. *Clin Exp Immunol* 1988; 73: 449–55.

17 Buchan G, Barrett K, Fujita T *et al.* Detection of activated T cell products in the rheumatoid joint using cDNA probes to Interleukin-2 (IL-2) IL-2 receptor and IFN-gamma. *Clin Exp Immunol* 1988; 71: 295–301.

18 Firestein GS, Xu WD, Townsend K *et al.* Cytokines in chronic inflammatory arthritis. I. Failure to detect T cell lymphokines (interleukin 2 and interleukin 3) and presence of macrophage colony-stimulating factor (CSF-1) and a novel mast cell growth factor in rheumatoid synovitis. *J Exp Med* 1988; 168: 1573–86.

19 Brennan FM, Chantry D, Jackson AM, Maini RN, Feldmann M. Cytokine production in culture by cells isolated

from the synovial membrane. *J Autoimmun* 1989; 2: 177–86.

20 Chu CQ, Field M, Feldmann M, Maini RN. Localization of tumor necrosis factor alpha in synovial tissues and at the cartilage–pannus junction in patients with rheumatoid arthritis. *Arthritis Rheum* 1991; 34: 1125–32.

21 Field M, Chu C, Feldmann M, Maini RN. Interleukin-6 localisation in the synovial membrane in rheumatoid arthritis. *Rheumatol Int* 1991; 11: 45–50.

22 Deleuran B, Lemche P, Kristensen M et al. Localisation of interleukin 8 in the synovial membrane, cartilage–pannus junction and chondrocytes in rheumatoid arthritis. *Scand J Rheumatol* 1994; 23: 2–7.

23 Wood NC, Dickens E, Symons JA. Duff GW. *In situ* hybridization of interleukin-1 in CD14-positive cells in rheumatoid arthritis. *Clin Immunol Immunopathol* 1992; 62: 295–300.

24 Deleuran BW, Chu CQ, Field M et al. Localization of tumor necrosis factor receptors in the synovial tissue, cartilage–pannus junction in patients with rheumatoid arthritis. Implications for local actions of tumor necrosis factor alpha. *Arthritis Rheum* 1992; 35: 1170–8.

25 Deleuran BW, Chu CQ, Field M et al. Localization of interleukin-1 alpha, type 1 interleukin-1 receptor and interleukin-1 receptor antagonist in the synovial membrane and cartilage/pannus junction in rheumatoid arthritis. *Br J Rheumatol* 1992; 31: 801–9.

26 Field M, Clinton L. Expression of GM-CSF receptor in rheumatoid arthritis [letter; comment]. *Lancet* 1993; 342: 1244.

27 Brennan FM, Gibbons DL, Mitchell T et al. Enhanced expression of tumor necrosis factor receptor mRNA and protein in mononuclear cells isolated from rheumatoid arthritis synovial joints. *Eur J Immunol* 1992; 22: 1907–12.

28 Arend WP, Dayer JM. Cytokines and cytokine inhibitors or antagonists in rheumatoid arthritis. *Arthritis Rheum* 1990; 33: 305–15.

29 Cope AP, Aderka D, Doherty M et al. Increased levels of soluble tumor necrosis factor receptors in the sera and synovial fluid of patients with rheumatic diseases. *Arthritis Rheum* 1992; 35: 1160–9.

30 Roux-Lombard P, Modoux C, Vischer T, Grassi J, Dayer JM. Inhibitors of interleukin 1 activity in synovial fluids and in cultured synovial fluid mononuclear cells. *J Rheumatol* 1992; 19: 517–23.

31 Firestein GS, Berger AE, Tracey DE et al. IL-1 receptor antagonist protein production and gene expression in rheumatoid arthritis and osteoarthritis synovium. *J Immunol* 1992; 149: 1054–62.

32 Fava R, Olsen N, Keski-Oja J, Moses H, Pincus T. Active and latent forms of transforming growth factor beta activity in synovial effusions. *J Exp Med* 1989; 169: 291–6.

33 Katsikis PD, Chu CQ, Brennan FM, Maini RN, Feldmann M. Immuno-regulatory role of interleukin 10 in rheumatoid arthritis. *J Exp Med* 1994; 179: 1517–27.

34 Cope AP, Brennan FM. Cytokine measurements in biological fluids. *Br J Rheumatol* 1992; 31: 721–2.

35 Uson J, Balsa A, Pascual-Salcedo D et al. Soluble interleukin 6 (IL-6) receptor and IL-6 levels in serum and synovial fluid of patients with different arthropathies. *J Rheumatol* 1997; 24: 2069–75.

36 Keystone EC, Snow KM, Bombardier C et al. Elevated soluble interleukin-2 receptor levels in the sera and synovial fluids of patients with rheumatoid arthritis. *Arthritis Rheum* 1988; 31: 844–9.

37 Symons JA, Eastgate JA, Duff GW. Purification and characterization of a novel soluble receptor for interleukin 1. *J Exp Med* 1991; 174: 1251–4.

38 Desgeorges A, Gabay C, Silacci P, et al. Concentrations and origins of soluble interleukin 6 receptor-alpha in serum and synovial fluid. *J Rheumatol* 1997; 24: 1510–16.

39 Barrera P, Boerbooms AM, van de Putte LB, van der Meer JW. Effects of antirheumatic agents on cytokines.

Semin Arthritis Rheum 1996;
25: 234–53.

40 Barrera P, Haagsma CJ, Boerbooms
    AM *et al.* Effect of methotrexate alone
    or in combination with sulphasalazine
    on the production and circulating
    concentrations of cytokines and their
    antagonists. Longitudinal evaluation in
    patients with rheumatoid arthritis. *Br J
    Rheumatol* 1995; 34: 747–55.

41 Swaak AJ, van den Brink HG, Aarden
    LA. Cytokine production in whole
    blood cell cultures of patients with
    rheumatoid arthritis. *Ann Rheum Dis*
    1997; 56: 693–5.

42 Ounissi-Benkalha H, Pelletier JP,
    Tardif G *et al. In vitro* effects of 2
    antirheumatic drugs on the synthesis
    and expression of proinflammatory
    cytokines in synovial membranes from
    patients with rheumatoid arthritis. *J
    Rheumatol* 1996; 23: 16–23.

43 Connolly KM, Stecher VJ, Danis E,
    Pruden DJ, LaBrie T. Alteration of
    interleukin-1 activity and the acute
    phase response in adjuvant arthritic
    rats treated with disease modifying
    antirheumatic drugs. *Agents Actions*
    1988; 25: 94–105.

44 Brennan FM. Role of cytokines in
    experimental arthritis. *Clin Exp
    Immunol* 1994; 97: 1–3.

45 Feldmann M, Brennan FM, Maini RN.
    Role of cytokines in rheumatoid
    arthritis. *Ann Rev Immunol* 1996;
    14: 397–440.

46 Ivashkiv LB. Cytokine expression
    and cell activation in inflammatory
    arthritis. *Adv Immunol* 1997;
    63: 337–76.

47 Haworth C, Brennan FM, Chantry D
    et al. Expression of granulocyte-
    macrophage colony-stimulating factor
    in rheumatoid arthritis: regulation by
    tumor necrosis factor-alpha. *Eur J
    Immunol* 1991; 21: 2575–9.

48 Butler DM, Maini RN, Feldmann M,
    Brennan FM. Modulation of
    proinflammatory cytokine release in
    rheumatoid synovial membrane cell
    cultures. Comparison of monoclonal
    anti TNF-alpha antibody with the
    interleukin-1 receptor antagonist. *Eur
    Cytokine Netw* 1995; 6: 225–30.

49 Saklatvala J, Sarsfield SJ, Townsend Y.
    Pig interleukin 1. Purification of two

immunologically different leukocyte
proteins that cause cartilage
resorption, lymphocyte activation,
and fever. *J Exp Med* 1985;
162: 1208–22.

50 Gowen M, Wood DD, Ihrie EJ,
    McGuire MK, Russell RG. An
    interleukin 1 like factor stimulates
    bone resorption *in vitro*. *Nature* 1983;
    306: 378–80.

51 Saklatvala J. Tumour necrosis factor
    alpha stimulates resorption and
    inhibits synthesis of proteoglycan in
    cartilage. *Nature* 1986; 322: 547–9.

52 Dayer JM, Beutler B, Cerami A.
    Cachectin/tumor necrosis factor
    stimulates collagenase and
    prostaglandin E2 production by
    human synovial cells and dermal
    fibroblasts. *J Exp Med* 1985;
    162: 2163–8.

53 Dayer JM, de Rochemonteix B, Burrus
    B, Demczuk S, Dinarello CA. Human
    recombinant interleukin 1 stimulates
    collagenase and prostaglandin E2
    production by human synovial cells.
    J Clin Invest 1986; 77: 645–8.

54 Lacraz S, Nicod LP, Chicheportiche
    R, Welgus HG, Dayer JM. IL-10
    inhibits metalloproteinase and
    stimulates TIMP-1 production in
    human mononuclear phagocytes.
    J Clin Invest 1995; 96, 2304–10.

55 Holmdahl R, Andersson M,
    Goldschmidt TJ *et al.* Type II collagen
    autoimmunity in animals and
    provocations leading to arthritis.
    Immunol Rev 1990; 118: 193–232.

56 Williams RO, Feldmann M, Maini
    RN. Anti-tumor necrosis factor
    ameliorates joint disease in murine
    collagen-induced arthritis. *Proc Natl
    Acad Sci USA* 1992; 89: 9784–8.

57 Piguet PF, Grau GE, Vesin C *et al.*
    Evolution of collagen arthritis in
    mice is arrested by treatment with
    anti-tumour necrosis factor (TNF)
    antibody or a recombinant soluble
    TNF receptor. *Immunology* 1992;
    77: 510–14.

58 Wooley PH, Dutcher J, Widmer MB,
    Gillis S. Influence of a recombinant
    human soluble tumor necrosis factor
    receptor FC fusion protein on type II
    collagen-induced arthritis in mice.
    J Immunol 1993; 151: 6602–7.

59 Wooley PH, Whalen JD, Chapman DL
et al. The effect of an interleukin-1
receptor antagonist protein on type
II collagen-induced arthritis and
antigen-induced arthritis in mice.
Arthritis Rheum 1993; 36: 1305–14.

60 Joosten LA, Lubberts E, Durez P
et al. Role of interleukin-4 and
interleukin-10 in murine collagen
induced arthritis. Protective effect
of interleukin-4 and interleukin-10
treatment on cartilage destruction.
Arthritis Rheum 1997; 40: 249–60.

61 Allen JB, Manthey CL, Hand AR et al.
Rapid onset synovial inflammation and
hyperplasia induced by transforming
growth factor beta. J Exp Med 1990;
171: 231–47.

62 Brandes ME, Allen JB, Ogawa Y,
Wahl SM. Transforming growth factor
beta 1 suppresses acute and chronic
arthritis in experimental animals. J
Clin Invest 1991; 87: 1108–13.

63 Williams RO, Williams DG,
Feldmann M, Maini RN. Increased
limb involvement in murine collagen-
induced arthritis following treatment
with anti-interferon-gamma. Clin Exp
Immunol 1993; 92: 323–7.

64 Boissier MC, Chiocchia G, Bessis N et
al. Biphasic effect of interferon-gamma
in murine collagen-induced arthritis.
Eur J Immunol 1995; 25: 1184–90.

65 Germann T, Szeliga J, Hess H et al.
Administration of interleukin 12 in
combination with type II collagen
induces severe arthritis in DBA/1
mice. Proc Natl Acad Sci USA 1995;
92: 4823–7.

66 Miltenburg AM, van Laar JM, de
Kuiper R, Daha MR, Breedveld FC. T
cells cloned from human rheumatoid
synovial membrane functionally
represent the Th1 subset. Scand J
Immunol 1992; 35: 603–10.

67 Simon AK, Seipelt E, Sieper J.
Divergent T-cell cytokine patterns in
inflammatory arthritis. Proc Natl Acad
Sci USA 1994; 91: 8562–6.

68 Cohen SB, Katsikis PD, Chu CQ et al.
High level of interleukin-10 production
by the activated T cell population
within the rheumatoid synovial
membrane. Arthritis Rheum 1995;
38: 946–52.

69 Malfait AM, Butler DM, Presky et al.

Blockade of IL-12 during the induction
of collagen-induced arthritis (CIA)
markedly attenuates the severity of the
arthritis. Clin Exp Immunol 1998;
111: 377–83.

70 McInnes IB, al-Mughales J, Field M
et al. The role of interleukin-15 in
T-cell migration and activation in
rheumatoid arthritis. Nat Med 1996;
2: 175–82.

71 McInnes IB, Leung BP, Sturrock RD,
Field M, Liew FY. Interleukin-15
mediates T cell-dependent regulation
of tumor necrosis factor-alpha
production in rheumatoid arthritis.
Nat Med 1997; 3: 189–95.

72 Lacraz S, Isler P, Vey E, Welgus HG,
Dayer JM. Direct contact between T
lymphocytes and monocytes is a major
pathway for induction of metalloproteinase expression. J Biol Chem
1994; 269: 22027–33.

73 Vey E, Burger D, Dayer JM.
Expression and cleavage of tumor
necrosis factor-alpha and tumor
necrosis factor receptors by human
monocytic cell lines upon direct
contact with stimulated T cells. Eur J
Immunol 1996; 26: 2404–9.

74 Lou J, Dayer JM, Grau GE, Burger D.
Direct cell/cell contact with stimulated
T lymphocytes induces the expression
of cell adhesion molecules and
cytokines by human brain micro-
vascular endothelial cells. Eur J
Immunol 1996; 26: 3107–13.

75 Vey E, Dayer JM, Burger D. Direct
contact with stimulated T cells
induces the expression of IL-1beta,
IL-1 receptor antagonist in
human monocytes. Involvement of
serine/threonine phosphatases in
differential regulation. Cytokine 1997;
9: 480–7.

76 Miltenburg AM, Lacraz S, Welgus
HG, Dayer JM. Immobilized anti-CD3
antibody activates T cell clones to
induce the production of interstitial
collagenase, but not tissue inhibitor
of metalloproteinases, in monocytic
THP-1 cells and dermal fibroblasts.
J Immunol 1995; 154: 2655–67.

77 Jacob CO, Fronek Z, Lewis GD et al.
Heritable major histocompatibility
complex class II-associated differences
in production of tumour necrosis

factor α: Relevance to genetic predisposition to systemic lupus erythematosus. *Proc Natl Acad Sci USA* 1990; 87: 1233–7.

78 Wilson AG, di Giovine FS, Duff GW. Genetics of tumour necrosis factor-α in autoimmune, infectious, and neoplastic illnesses. *J Inflamm* 1995; 45: 1–12.

79 Mulcahy B, Waldron-Lynch F, McDermott MF *et al.* Genetic variability in the tumor necrosis factor-lymphotoxin region influences susceptibility to rheumatoid arthritis. *Am J Hum Genet* 1996; 59: 676–83.

80 Hajeer AH, Worthington J, Silman AJ, Ollier WER. Association of tumor necrosis factor microsatellite polymorphisms with HLA-DRB1*04-bearing haplotypes in rheumatoid arthritis patients. *Arthritis Rheum* 1996; 39: 1109–14.

81 Wilson AG, de Vries N, van de Putte LBA, Duff GW. A tumour necrosis factor alpha polymorphism is not associated with rheumatoid arthritis. *Ann Rheum Dis* 1995; 54: 601–3.

82 Brinkman BMN, Huizinga TWJ, Kurban SS *et al.* Tumour necrosis factor a gene polymorphisms in rheumatoid arthritis: association with susceptibility to, or severity of, disease? *Br J Rheumatol* 1997; 36: 516–21.

83 Fishman D, Woo P. A polymorphism of the interleukin-6 (IL-6) gene conferring high IL-6 production is associated with systemic-onset JCA. *Arthritis Rheum* 1997; 40: 249 (Abstract).

84 Gorham JD, Guler ML, Steen RG *et al.* Genetic-mapping of a murine locus controlling development of T-helper-1 T-helper-2 type responses. *Proc Natl Acad Sci USA* 1996; 93: 12467–72.

85 Hershey GKK, Friedrich MF, Esswein LA, Thomas ML, Chatila TA. The association of atopy with a gain-of-function mutation in the alpha subunit of the interleukin-4 receptor. *N Engl J Med* 1997; 337: 1720–5.

86 Keffer J, Probert L, Cazlaris H *et al.* Transgenic mice expressing human tumour necrosis factor: a predictive genetic model of arthritis. *EMBO J* 1991; 10: 4025–31.

87 Butler DM, Malfait AM, Mason LJ *et al.* DBA/1 mice expressing the human TNF-alpha transgene develop a severe, erosive arthritis: characterization of the cytokine cascade and cellular composition. *J Immunol* 1997; 159: 2867–76.

88 Takaishi H, Yamada H, Hotta H *et al.* Induction of inflammatory arthropathy resembling rheumatoid arthritis in mice transgenic for IL-1 alpha overexpression. *Arthritis Rheum* 1997; 40: 1455 (Abstract).

89 Ma Y, Hirsch R, Hirsh D, Hirsch E. Protection from collagen induced arthritis in transgenic mice over-producing IL-1 receptor antagonist. *Arthritis Rheum* 1997; 40: 897 (Abstract).

90 De Benedetti F, Moretta A, Martini A. IL-6 causes stunted growth in transgenic mice through a decrease in insulin-like growth-factor-1 (IGF-1)—A model for stunted growth in children with chronic inflammation. *Arthritis Rheum* 1996; 39: 1661.

91 Cope AP. What can we learn from gene 'knockout mice'? In: *Role of Cytokines in Autoimmunity*. Austin, Texas: RG Lands Co., 1996: 201–26.

92 Shull MM, Ormsby I, Kier AB *et al.* Targeted disruption of the mouse transforming growth factor-β gene results in multifocal inflammatory disease. *Nature* 1992; 359: 693–99.

93 Kulkarni AB, Huh CG, Becker D *et al.* Transforming growth factor beta 1 null mutation in mice causes excessive inflammatory response and early death. *Proc Natl Acad Sci USA* 1993; 90: 770–4.

94 Kuhn R, Lohler J, Rennick D *et al.* Interleukin-10 deficit mice develop chronic enterocolitis. *Cell* 1993; 75: 263–74.

95 Sadlack B, Merz H, Schorle H *et al.* Ulcerative colitis-like disease in mice with a disrupted interleukin-2 gene [see comments]. *Cell* 1993; 75: 253–61.

96 Lenardo MJ. Interleukin-2 programs mouse alpha beta T lymphocytes for apoptosis. *Nature* 1991; 353: 858–61.

97 Elliott MJ, Maini RN, Feldmann M
et al. Treatment of rheumatoid
arthritis with chimeric monoclonal
antibodies to tumor necrosis factor
alpha. *Arthritis Rheum* 1993; 36:
1681–90.

98 Rankin EC, Choy EH, Kassimos D
et al. The therapeutic effects of an
engineered human anti-tumour
necrosis factor alpha antibody
(CDP571) in rheumatoid arthritis.
Br J Rheumatol 1995; 34: 334–42.

99 Moreland LW, Baumgartner SW,
Schiff MH et al. Treatment of
rheumatoid arthritis with a
recombinant human tumor necrosis
factor receptor (p75) -Fc fusion
protein. *N Engl J Med* 1997;
337: 141–7.

100 Campion GV, Lebsack ME,
Lookabaugh J, Gordon G, Catalano
M. Dose-range and dose-frequency
study of recombinant human
interleukin-1 receptor antagonist in
patients with rheumatoid arthritis. The
IL-1ra Arthritis Study Group. *Arthritis
Rheum* 1996; 39: 1092–101.

101 Wendling D, Racadot E, Wijdenes J.
Treatment of severe rheumatoid
arthritis by anti-interleukin 6
monoclonal antibody. *J Rheumatol*
1993; 20: 259–62.

102 Elliott MJ, Maini RN, Feldmann M
et al. Randomised double-blind
comparison of chimeric monoclonal
antibody to tumour necrosis factor
alpha (cA2) versus placebo in
rheumatoid arthritis. *Lancet* 1994;
344: 1105–10.

103 Paleolog EM, Hunt M, Elliott MJ
et al. Deactivation of vascular
endothelium by monoclonal anti-tumor
necrosis factor alpha antibody in
rheumatoid arthritis. *Arthritis Rheum*
1996; 39: 1082–91.

104 Brennan FM, Browne KA, Green PA
et al. Reduction of serum matrix
metalloproteinase 1 matrix
metalloproteinase 3 in rheumatoid
arthritis patients following
anti-tumour necrosis factor-alpha
(cA2) therapy. *Br J Rheumatol* 1997;
36: 643–65.

4: Has research on lymphocytes hindered progress in rheumatoid arthritis?

T. Pap, J. Franz, R.E. Gay and S. Gay

Introduction

Rheumatoid arthritis (RA) is a chronic, systemically spreading disorder that, as the most prominent feature, results in the progressive destruction of affected joints. The aetiology of RA remains elusive and has puzzled researchers for several decades. Although it is well recognized that RA is characterized by the mutually interacting phenomena of synovial hyperplasia, chronic inflammation and pathological immune response, and the last decade has brought considerable progress in elucidating the molecular and cellular basis of rheumatoid joint destruction, key questions about the aetiopathogenesis of RA have not been elucidated. What is the initiating step and what the perpetuating force in RA? What are the differences between early and late stages of disease? And which of the characteristic features of RA are primary and which secondary?

The observations of massive lymphocyte accumulation in rheumatoid synovium as well as abnormal production of rheumatoid factors (RFs), and the association of certain major histocompatibility complex (MHC) class II molecules with susceptibility to and severity of RA, have prompted several authors to put autoimmunity at the centre of RA. Thus, it has been postulated that recognition of an arthritogenic antigen by synovial T cells, which are restricted to the associated HLA-DR alleles, then subsequent induction of an autoimmune reaction represent the initiating steps in the pathogenesis of RA. In view of some additional evidence that B lymphocytes are also specifically activated and expanded clonally in RA synovium, lymphocytes in general have been assigned a key role in the pathophysiology of disease.

Therefore, in the past years considerable efforts have been made in identifying potential (auto)antigens as well as in investigating alterations in the immune response of RA patients including activation of T and B cells, changes in T-cell receptor (TCR) repertoire, chronic oligoclonal expansion of T cells, and defective mechanisms of lymphocyte apoptosis. Although these studies have increased substantially our knowledge about human immune response mechanisms, they have not given satisfactory answers to aforementioned questions.

To explore the role of T cells in initiating the progressive destruction of joints in an animal model, our laboratory has been studying MRL-lpr/lpr arthritis. However, pathohistological studies on a light and electron microscopical level have revealed that initial joint damage in this model is mediated by proliferating synovial cells [1,2]. Cartilage and bone destruction occurs at sites of synovial attachment to these tissues, after cartilage and/or bone are degraded, inflammatory cells migrate into the synovium and accelerate the process. The finding that synovial lining cells mediate the initial destructive process in the absence of inflammatory cells and that autoimmunity to collagen type II occurs as a consequence of cartilage damage rather than preceding it [3], has prompted us to search for the molecular and cellular mechanisms of joint destruction in RA [4]. Based on the observation of Fassbender [5], we explored the role of proto-oncogenes in synovial cells [4]. Therefore, it needs to be stressed at this point that a search of the role of lymphocytes in the MRL-lpr/lpr mouse [1] has stimulated our laboratory to investigate pathways of synovial cell activation and resulted subsequently in the hypothesis that two pathways, a T-cell-dependent as well as a T-cell-independent pathway, are operating in the pathogenesis of RA [6,7].

Advances in molecular biology techniques as well as the development of novel animal models and the opportunity of investigating early stages of human RA, have given growing evidence that T-cell-independent mechanisms contribute significantly to the pathogenesis of this disease. Thus, as we will show, research on lymphocytes has not hindered but rather promoted the discovery of molecular and cellular mechanisms in RA which are different, and more than complementary to concepts that have long been thought to dominate exclusively an immunopathogenesis of RA.

Characteristics of rheumatoid synovium

In contrast to normal synovial membrane, which is a thin, rather unremarkable appearing membrane covering loose connective tissue, RA synovium appears dramatically changed. Most prominently, it becomes considerably thickened with multiple cell layers.

Lining cell hyperplasia

It has been understood that thickening of RA synovium is mostly due to lining layer hyperplasia. In the course of disease, the lining increases up to 10 cell layers and is characterized by the presence of proliferating synovial cells as well as of large numbers of infiltrating cells [2,8]. Immunohisto-logical studies revealed about 70% of lining cells to be derived from the monocyte/macrophage (MØ) lineage. These cells are called macrophage-like or type A synoviocytes and characteristically express various macrophage markers such as CD11b, CD14, CD33, and CD68 [9,10]. A smaller propor-tion of lining cells (about 25%) appears to originate from resident synovial cells. Due to their specific, fibroblast-like appearance and their lack of specific surface markers these cells are called synovial fibroblasts or type B synoviocytes [7,8,11]. They can be identified by antibodies recognizing prolyl 4-hydroxylase, an enzyme that is involved in collagen synthesis [12]. Both type A and type B synoviocytes have been found activated in RA [4,7,10]. The lining layer plays a central role in the pathogenesis of RA as in the course of disease it attaches to the cartilage and mediates progressive destruction of the joint [13]. While the debate continues as to whether hyper-plasia of the lining is caused by cell proliferation or by alterations in cell death mechanisms, growing evidence suggests that defective apoptosis plays an important role in this process [14].

With respect to synovial cell proliferation, Aicher and colleagues have clearly shown that synovial cells from patients with RA are activated but do not proliferate faster than those from osteoarthritis patients [15]. More-over, as determined by thymidine incorporation, only 1–5% of synovial cells have been found to proliferate [16]. Mitosis is also rarely found in RA synovial tissue and immunohistochemistry for specific proliferation markers such as Ki-67 reveals only a very low number of positive cells [17]. Interestingly, those few Ki-67-positive cells are located predominantly within lymphocytic infiltrates, whereas negligible numbers of Ki-67-positive cells are detectable in the lining layer [18,19]. In contrast, numerous reports have described changes of apoptotic pathways in RA synovium, in par-ticular within the lining layer. When examined by ultrastructural methods, fewer than 1% of lining cells exhibit morphological features of apoptosis [20,21]. In related studies, anti-apoptotic molecules such as bcl-2 have been found expressed in synovial lining cells [22]. Recently described somatic mutations of p53 tumour-suppressor gene in RA synovial cells may also contribute significantly to reduced apoptosis in these cells [23]. Moreover, a novel anti-apoptotic molecule, sentrin [24], has been demonstrated in RA synovium most recently [25]. Sentrin, which was termed after its guardian function against cell death signalling, interacts with the signal-competent forms of Fas/APO-1 and tumour necrosis factor (TNF) receptor 1 death domains, and overexpression of sentrin in transfected BJAJ cells protects against apoptosis [24]. As Franz and colleagues could show, sentrin is abund-ant in RA synovial lining cells, whereas normal synovium cells express only very little sentrin mRNA [25].

This picture has been clouded by reports on the expression of Fas, a pro-apoptotic molecule, in synovial lining cells [20,21]. However, most recent findings, indicating a dual function of the Fas molecule, may shed a new light on the role of Fas in the balanced action of pro- and anti-apoptotic molecules. Apart from its pro-apoptotic function, Fas appears to be involved in pathways leading to proliferation [26,27]. Therefore, intracellular signalling pathways, following Fas activation, appear to be modified by additional stimuli, which determine whether the affected cell undergoes apoptosis or proliferates [28]. These findings may also explain the fact that cultured synovial fibroblasts are resistant to Fas-induced apoptosis, despite the surface expression of Fas molecules [29].

Changes in the sublining layer

In the course of RA, the sublining also undergoes considerable changes. It becomes massively infiltrated by mononuclear cells such as T cells, B cells and macrophages. In contrast to the macrophages, lymphocyte infiltration is mainly perivascular with a clear dominance of T cells. Interestingly, lymphocytes often organize into aggregates, which resemble those seen in lymph nodes or in extralymphatic sites such as Peyer's patches [11]. However, within the T-cell population the majority of cells are CD4+ and express CD29/CD45R0 antigens, which characterizes them as memory T cells [30]. This clearly distinguishes RA synovium from lymphatic tissues. While lymph nodes contain larger numbers of suppressor/cytotoxic lymphocytes, in RA synovium CD8+ cells represent only a minority and are located at the periphery of the aggregates. This might contribute to local B-cell hyperreactivity and increased synthesis of immunoglobulins such as RF [11].

In addition, changes in synovial architecture are accompanied by an increase in vascularization which appears critical to synovial hyperplasia. The overall increase in the number of blood vessels results from both high endothelial venule formation, which may facilitate the trafficking of mononuclear cells into the synovium and new vessel formation, also called neoangiogenesis. As neoangiogenesis is believed to be mainly stimulated by the cells of the activated synovium, interest has been focused on the regulation of new blood-vessel formation within RA synovium. Based on the findings that synovial fibroblasts of the lining express significant amounts of vascular cell adhesion molecule 1 (VCAM-1) [31] and that VCAM-1 has been shown to induce angiogenesis [32], it might be postulated that the activated synovial fibroblast contributes significantly to the induction of angiogenesis in the synovium.

However, changes in the sublining layer in general are highly variable among different patients, which appear to be related to different stages of disease as well as to interindividual differences. In addition, histological evaluation of sublining [11] reveals considerable overlap with other chronic arthritides especially clearly antigen-driven conditions such as reactive arthritis [33].

T cells in RA

As the presence of lymphocytes, in particular that of T cells, is a prominent feature of synovial changes in RA, many researchers have set out to characterize T-cell infiltrates [34] and to identify potential candidate auto-antigens in RA.

Numerous cartilage-derived proteins have been proposed for functioning as autoantigens in RA. Among these, collagen type II, which is mainly produced by chondrocytes, has been suggested a candidate autoantigen. Londei and colleagues demonstrated that 12% of T-cell clones were reactive with collagen type II [35]. In addition, collagen type II degradation products have been shown to be present in RA joints [36]. However, such T-cell clones do not occur in all RA patients and collagen-specific T and B cells from RA patients as well as those with other specificities are not invariable. Thus, it might be hypothesized, that such lymphocytes may arise secondary to joint destruction rather than being primarily involved into the pathogenesis of RA.

Apart from the general question of what T cells might be responding to in RA, interest has been focused on isolating and characterizing disease-relevant T-cell clones. Understanding of the molecular basis of T-cell specificity and the genetic organization of TCRs has further promoted research on T-cell-dependent mechanisms. Thus, it has been hypothesized that T cells in different patients may respond to the same antigen(s) which are present(ed) in the joint and that therefore T cells in different patients would use at least similar TCRs to recognize these relevant antigens [37,38]. Focusing on the overexpression of certain Vβ elements, numerous studies have made quite unsuccessful attempts to identify shared clones within single as well as among different patients.

At present, there is no clear evidence that a specific antigen is initiating and driving RA. In contrast, T-cell infiltrates in RA synovium are highly heterogeneous and T-cell-mediated immune responses within the joint might reflect an attempt of tissue repair being naturally directed against an array of different antigen determinants [37].

The hypothesis of primary local T-cell activation due to (super)antigen exposure has been further challenged by the observation that at best only a minority of T cells appear activated within RA synovium and that only negligible amounts of T-cell-derived cytokines could be detected within the

RA synovium [39]. The latter observation has been the basis for questioning the role of T cells in the pathogenesis of RA [40], and anergy has been proposed to be a dominant feature of synovial T cells [41].

T cells in RA synovium do not only appear anergic but appear also highly resistant to apoptosis. By investigating synovial fluids from 28 RA patients Salmon and colleagues were unable to demonstrate apoptosis in synovial T cells, whereas substantial cell death could be found in non-T-cell populations in all of the samples [42]. In contrast, T cells from synovial fluids of patients with acute crystal arthropathy exhibited marked apoptosis indicating the lack of T-cell apoptosis being a specific feature for RA. These data were of particular interest as it could be shown in this study that T cells at the same time express a certain phenotype (bcl-2^{low}, Bax^{high}, CD45RB^{dull}) which suggests high susceptibility to apoptosis. Intriguingly, it could be demonstrated that the failure of apoptosis was not an intrinsic property of synovial T cells as they rapidly undergo programmed cell death when removed from the joints. However, co-culture experiments of apoptosis-resistant synovial T cells with fibroblast monolayers revealed the preservation of apoptosis resistance in the presence of synovial fibroblasts. The relevant factors preventing synovial T cells from apoptosis appear to be fibroblast-derived rather that lymphocyte dependent. As a consequence of these observations it has been proposed that resolution of inflammation in joints may be promoted most effectively by targeting the fibroblast population rather than T cells themselves [42].

It is also of interest that significant proportions of T cells in RA synovium express granzymes A and B as well as perforin [43,44]. Based on these findings it could be speculated that the production of apoptosis-inducing perforin might be an insufficient attempt of the body to target the activated aggressively growing synovial fibroblasts.

Fibroblasts and macrophages

By analysing large numbers of synovial specimens from RA patients Fassbender found that invasion of cartilage and subchondral bone by synovial lining cells did not require the presence of lymphocyte infiltrates [5]. Moreover, synovial fibroblasts from RA patients were shown to exhibit considerable morphological alterations. They have an abundant cytoplasm, a dense rough endoplasmic reticulum and large pale nuclei with several prominent nucleoli [5]. In the past 10 years considerable efforts have been undertaken to further characterize this 'transformed-appearing' phenotype of synovial fibroblasts and focused on the questions of what characterizes this phenotype on a cellular and molecular level, and what are the mechanisms of activation with respect to their destructive properties.

Expression of certain proto-oncogenes and transcriptional factors in synovial fibroblasts has been described as a major feature indicating the activated nature of these cells [45–47]. The early growth response gene-1 (*egr-1*), a zinc finger protein having DNA binding and transcription regulatory activity, was found constitutively overexpressed in RA synovial fibroblasts [15]. Interestingly, *egr-1* binding sites were found in promoter regions of several genes. Elevated expression of some of these genes such as *sis* and *ras* have been associated with pathogenetic mechanisms of RA [45,47]. The c-*fos* protooncogene which is known to be co-expressed with *egr-1*, has also been found in RA synovium [48]. Interestingly, it encodes for a basic leucin zipper transcription factor and is part of the transcriptional activator AP-1(jun/fos). The proto-oncogene *fos* and *egr-1* have been identified in collagenase-producing rheumatoid synovial fibroblasts [48]. These data suggest *fos*-related proto-oncogenes play an important role in cell activation via AP-1 formation [49,50]. It is noteworthy, as shown in other studies, that proto-oncogenes of the *egr* family are also involved in the activation of the cathepsin L gene [51], a matrix-degrading cysteine proteinase gene which is highly up-regulated in RA synovium [45,52]. These observations are of particular interest, as joint destruction is largely mediated by the action of cathepsins and matrix metalloproteinases (MMPs) [48,52,53].

Attachment of synovial fibroblasts to the joint cartilage is one of the most prominent features involved in rheumatoid joint destruction. This process appears specific for RA as compared with other non-destructive forms of arthritides. Integrins represent a very complex family of adhesion molecules as they contain both an α and a β chain, which combine to form heterodimers. So far, at least 15 different α and eight different β chains have been described [54]. The ligands of the integrins may be either cellular surface molecules or extracellular matrix proteins, and individual adhesion molecules may bind to more than one ligand. For example, CS-1, a spliced isoform of fibronectin, which is highly expressed in RA synovium [55] appears part of a bidirectional adhesion pathway operative in RA as it binds to the integrin very late antigen 4 (VLA-4) (α4β1; CD49d/CD29), which also ligates with VCAM-1 [55]. Most interestingly, the expression of VCAM-1, which is up-regulated in RA activated synovial lining fibroblasts [31], may not only mediate the attachment to cartilage but may also contribute to T-cell anergy [56] and the induction of angiogenesis as described above [32]. Most recently, osteopontin, another extracellular matrix protein that promotes cell attachment, could be demonstrated in synovial fibroblast-like cells [57]. Most notably in the same study, a stimulatory effect of osteopontin on the secretion of collagenase-1/MMP-1 in articular chondrocytes was found. Therefore, it might be hypothesized that osteopontin does not only mediate attachment of synovial cells to cartilage but also contributes to perichondrocytic matrix degradation in RA. Moreover, earlier findings demonstrating that osteopontin stimulates B cells to produce immunoglobulins [58] as well as being chemoattractive for macrophages [59] suggest that osteopontin produced by synovial fibroblasts might play also an important role in stimulating B cells to produce RF in the joint and to attract the influx of large numbers of macrophages to the synovium in RA and therefore potentially explain another hallmark of RA. Therefore, the role of adhesion molecules in RA appears not restricted to the attachment of synovium to cartilage and bone, and the recruitment of inflammatory cells but also to the induction of MMPs.

Research on cytokines has also revealed elevated levels of several chemokines/chemoattractant factors such as MIP-1α, MIP-1β, MCP-1, regulated on activation, normal T cell expressed and secreted (RANTES) and interleukin 8 (IL-8) in synovial fluids from RA patients [60]. These chemokines are produced by synovial fibroblasts and macrophages and mediate chemoattraction of various cells into sites of inflammation using specific chemokine receptors. In this context, the properties of two novel cytokines, IL-15 and IL-16, might be of crucial importance.

McInnes and colleagues demonstrated that IL-15, which attracts CD4+ T cells, induces T-cell proliferation, B-cell maturation and isotype switching, and which may protect T cells from apoptosis, is also produced by fibroblasts in the rheumatoid synovial membrane [61]. Interestingly, the responding migratory T cells are mainly of the CD45RO+ phenotype. Most notably, peripheral blood T cells, activated by IL-15, may induce significant production of TNF-α and IL-1 by macrophages via a cell-contact-dependent mechanism [61]. Even more intriguingly, RA synovial fibroblasts have been identified as the major source for IL-16 within the synovium [62]. In contrast to IL-15 that functions via a heterodimeric receptor, consisting of a unique IL-15 receptor α chain in combination with the IL-2 receptor, IL 16 exerts its biological functions using the CD4 molecule as a receptor [63,64]. In addition to chemoattraction of CD4+ cells, IL-16 induces the expression of IL-2 receptor on resting T cells as well as the expression of MHC class II molecules. In apparent contradiction, IL-16 also has suppressive properties, in so far as it is capable of inducing T-cell anergy [65]. Therefore, it can be hypothesized that IL-16, produced by activated synovial fibroblasts, may attract CD4+ T cells into the synovium, induce the expression of the IL-2 receptor on these T cells and account for the state of anergy found in synovial T cells. Taken together, the intriguing properties of IL-15 and -16 may help to explain the paradox between the abundance of T cells in the rheumatoid synovium and the lack of T-cell-derived cytokines in synovial fluid and tissue.

Lessons from animal models

A major problem in elucidating early events in the pathogenesis of RA as well as the complexity of human disease has been the lack of appropriate animal models for human RA. At present, several different models exist, none of which reflects all features of human RA. However, the detailed characterization of existing as well as the development of novel animal models for human RA in the past years has provided us with important insights into the molecular mechanisms of disease. Generally, animal models of RA can be divided into those in which arthritis is induced artificially and therefore biased by the injection of different agents, and those in which genetic alterations in the animals lead to the spontaneous development of an RA-like disease [66]. The severe combined immunodeficiency (SCID) mouse co-implantation model of RA (see below) constitutes a separate group, because in this model human RA cells are investigated using the mouse as a 'living culture flask'.

T-cell-driven models

Since injection of various antigens can lead to the induction of a relapsing, erosive arthritis, models such as collagen-induced arthritis (CIA) as well as streptococcal wall antigen-induced arthritis (SCW-A) have been proposed and intensively studied as animal models for human RA [67–70]. In fact, they have provided us with important insights into molecular mechanisms of joint inflammation and helped to elucidate key aspects of joint destruction. The SCW-A model in Lewis rats has been of particular interest, because synovial hyperplasia in this model resembles some important features of human RA. There is a tumour-like proliferation of synovial cells which express high levels of several proto-oncogene products, including c-fos and c-myc, MMP-1 and MMP-3 [71,72]. In addition, like RA synovial fibroblasts, these cells do not show contact inhibition and can be grown under anchorage-independent conditions [73]. Most recently, studies on the induction of CIA in stromelysin (MMP-3) knock-out mice showed that stromelysin might not be involved in joint destruction and demonstrated the complexity of cartilage- and bone-degrading enzymes in erosive arthritis [74]. However, as arthritis in all of these animal models is clearly antigen driven, neither of them could satisfactorily answer the aforementioned questions concerning the role of lymphocytes in the induction and perpetuation of human RA [6].

Recently Kouskoff and colleagues described a novel animal model of RA which, although T-cell driven, does not arise from the response to a specific antigen presented in the joint. By crossing the KRN transgenic mouse line carrying the rearranged TCR genes from the R28 T-cell hybridoma with the NOD strain, a mouse strain named KRN×NOD was obtained, which spontaneously developed RA-like disease [75]. According to first characterization of these animals, it appears that the NOD-derived MHC class II molecule A^{g7} is the element responsible for promoting arthritis in KRN×NOD mice. Recognition of this molecule by the transgenic TCR appears to trigger the RA-like disease. Although the induction of organ-specific auto-immunity is a remarkable achievement with this model, there is at present no evidence that a similar pathomechanism may initiate human RA.

The SCID mouse model

After Bosma and colleagues had first described a mutation in mice of the C.B-17 strain that resulted in animals with SCID [76] and Mosier and colleagues could demonstrate that a functionally intact human immune system can survive in SCID mice recipients [77], the SCID mouse model became of wide interest for studying autoimmune diseases. Several studies in which SCID mice were engrafted with human immune cells encouraged investigators to examine the behaviour of RA tissue in SCID mice. First, studies addressing RA pathophysiology showed rheumatoid factor IgM production by SCID mice, which were reconstituted with RA synovial lymphocytes [78]. Based on these experiments, and on a previous observation by Brinckerhoff and Harris, who showed that synovial cells are able to form nodular structures when implanted into nude mice [79], Adams et al. [80] and Rendt et al. [81] implanted rheumatoid synovial tissue under the renal capsule of SCID mice. These experiments demonstrated that lymphocyte infiltrates disappear with time, while lining-layer synoviocytes survive. Moreover, rheumatoid fibroblast-like synoviocytes did not only survive in SCID mice but maintained their characteristic biological features. Based on these results, a novel model for studying molecular mechanisms of rheumatoid joint destruction in vivo was developed—the SCID mouse co-implantation model for RA. To imitate the situation in a rheumatoid joint in this model, human RA synovium was co-implanted with normal human cartilage under the renal capsule of SCID mice [82]. This experimental approach provided us with new insights into the molecular and cellular events leading to destruction of human cartilage mediated by RA synovium. Both RA synovial tissue and normal human cartilage could be successfully implanted into SCID mice for more than 300 days, and implanted RA synovium showed the same invasive growth and progressive cartilage destruction as in human RA joints. Most interestingly, the vast majority of synovial cells found at sites of cartilage invasion resembled activated synovial fibroblasts [82].

To specifically study the molecular properties of these fibroblasts and their contribution to cartilage degradation, we subsequently used normal human cartilage together with isolated synovial fibroblasts from RA patients to analyse the matrix-degrading properties of these cells in the absence of both lymphocytes and macrophages [83]. Utilizing this model, we have been able to show that RA synovial fibroblasts maintain their activated phenotype, especially at sites of invasion. In contrast, osteoarthritis synovial fibroblasts did not exhibit this invasive growth when co-implanted with normal human cartilage. Using *in situ* hybridization techniques to examine the presence of mRNA for matrix-degrading enzymes, a number of cartilage-degrading proteases could be demonstrated. In contrast, none of these matrix-degrading enzymes can be found when normal, skin or osteoarthritis synovial fibroblasts are examined in this model. In addition, RA synovial fibroblasts maintain their ability to express VCAM-1 [83]. Although these studies show that synovial fibroblasts from RA joints maintain their invasive behaviour in the absence of human T cells and macrophages, the contribution of these cells to further stimulate the synovial cells via the production of cytokines such as IL-1 and TNF-α must be emphasized [10].

In this context it is of interest that Mima and colleagues investigated the induction of synovial hyperplasia by injecting synovial mononuclear cells (MNC) from RA patients into the knee joints of SCID mice [84] and showed that synovial hyperplasia could be observed in some animals (25%).

Studies in human disease

In addition to the aforementioned data, some important insights into the pathogenesis of RA have been obtained from the clinical observation of different stages of RA and their histological evaluation.

Most recently, Kraan and colleagues performed a study in which they compared histological features and expression of cell-surface markers in synovial tissues of clinically involved vs. clinically uninvolved knee joints of RA patients [85]. Considerable infiltration of CD68+ macrophage-like cells was found to be present in clinically uninvolved joints of the RA patients, whereas the number of lymphocytes did not significantly differ from that of healthy controls. These results suggest that pathological processes in RA may begin well before clinical signs become obvious and that lymphocytes might be not involved in the early stages of disease.

On the other hand, the progression of RA may also proceed in late stages of the disease in the absence of T cells. Here, the case of a 63-year-old patient with RA who became infected with human immunodeficiency virus (HIV) is of interest. As Müller-Ladner and colleagues reported, HIV infection did improve the clinical symptoms, confirming previous studies.

However, HIV infection did not affect the progression of joint destruction in this patient. Histological evaluation revealed progressive joint destruction with aggressively growing fibroblasts, despite the striking lack of CD4+ T cells [86].

Another intriguing piece of evidence that T-cell-independent mechanisms play a role in rheumatoid joint destruction arises from a recent study showing clinical improvement but radiological deterioration. Analysing serial disease activity measures and hand radiographs in 40 patients with RA over 6 years, Mulherin and colleagues observed a significant improvement in both clinical and laboratory parameters, yet at the same time they found a significant deterioration in articular erosions [87]. These results confirmed previous reports on the dissociation between inflammatory changes and radiological progression in human RA. It was concluded from this study that macrophages and fibroblasts play the critical role in joint destruction.

Lessons from anti-T-cell therapy

In view of the hypothesis that T-cell-mediated immune responses represent the major pathological feature in human RA, several therapeutic approaches have been developed that target T cells. Since antibody-mediated T-cell depletion has been shown to successfully induce long-term disease remission in some animal models of autoimmune diseases [88], several T-cell-specific antibodies have been suggested for the treatment of RA [89]. However, studies performed with such antibodies, in particular with chimeric anti-CD4 monoclonal antibodies, failed to demonstrate a significant and sustained effect [90]. Further investigations revealed the paradoxical feature of persistent T-cell infiltration despite peripheral lymphopenia and a shift of peripheral T-cell repertoire toward the CD45R0+ memory phenotype [37,91]. These results were interpreted as being consistent with a critical role for T cells in the synovial inflammation. However, alternative explanations may be derived from aforementioned data which demonstrate that CD45R0+ memory T cells are selectively attracted to and kept within the rheumatoid synovium by fibroblast- and macrophage-derived factors.

Conclusion

In the past, lymphocytes and in particular T cells have been thought to be the primary driving force in RA. Considerable efforts have been made to identify joint-specific antigens as well as to isolate and characterize disease-specific T-cell populations. However, these attempts have largely failed to confirm antigen-recognition events to dominate the pathogenesis of human RA. Instead, research on lymphocytes has provided several lines of evidence that T-cell-independent mechanisms may play a key role in initiating and perpetuating disease [4,39]. Therefore, it could be shown that attraction of lymphocytes into the joint as well as preservation of T cells from apoptosis depend on fibroblast-derived factors [42]. Moreover, the SCID mouse model has turned out to be a powerful tool for studying the properties of activated fibroblasts and for evaluating the effects of gene transfer to human cells [92]. Thus, important insights can be obtained into the molecular and cellular basis of RA and novel therapeutic approaches are being developed [93], including gene therapy [94].

References

1 O'Sullivan FX, Fassbender HG, Gay S, Koopman WJ. Etiopathogenesis of the rheumatoid arthritis-like disease in MRL/l mice. I. The histomorphologic basis of joint destruction. *Arthritis Rheum* 1985; 28: 529–36.

2 Tanaka A, O'Sullivan FX, Koopman WJ, Gay S. Etiopathogenesis of rheumatoid arthritis-like disease in MRL/1 mice: II. Ultrastructural basis of joint destruction. *J Rheumatol* 1988; 15: 10–6.

3 Gay S, O'Sullivan FX, Gay RE, Koopman WJ. Humoral sensitivity to native collagen types I–VI in the arthritis of MRL/l mice. *Clin Immunol Immunopathol* 1987; 45: 63–9.

4 Gay S, Gay RE. Cellular basis and oncogene expression of rheumatoid joint destruction. *Rheumatol Int* 1989; 9: 105–13.

5 Fassbender HG. Histomorphological basis of articular cartilage destruction in rheumatoid arthritis. *Coll Relat Res* 1983; 3: 141–55.

6 Koopman WJ, Gay S. Do non-immunologically mediated pathways play a role in the pathogenesis of rheumatoid arthritis? *Rheum Dis Clin North Am* 1993; 19: 107–22.

7 Gay S, Gay RE, Koopman WJ. Molecular and cellular mechanisms of joint destruction in rheumatoid arthritis: two cellular mechanisms explain joint destruction? *Ann Rheum Dis* 1993; 52 (Suppl. 1): S39–47.

8 Henderson B, Glynn LE, Chayen J. Cell division in the synovial lining in experimental allergic arthritis: proliferation of cells during the development of chronic arthritis. *Ann Rheum Dis* 1982; 41: 275–81.

9 Kelly PM, Bliss E, Morton JA, Burns J, McGee JO. Monoclonal antibody EBM/11: high cellular specificity for human macrophages. *J Clin Pathol* 1988; 41: 510–5.

10 Burmester GR, Stuhlmuller B, Keyszer G, Kinne RW. Mononuclear phagocytes and rheumatoid synovitis. Mastermind or workhorse in arthritis? *Arthritis Rheum* 1997; 40: 5–18.

11 Firestein GS. Rheumatoid synovitis and pannus. In: Klippel JH, Dieppe PA, eds. *Rheumatology*. London: Mosby, 1998: 5.13.1–5.13.24.

12 Hoyhtya M, Myllyla R, Piuva J, Kivirikko KI, Tryggvason K. Monoclonal antibodies to human prolyl 4-hydroxylase. *Eur J Biochem* 1984; 141: 472–82.

13 Muller Ladner U, Gay RE, Gay S. Cellular pathways of joint destruction. *Curr Opin Rheumatol* 1997; 9: 213–20.

14 Nishioka K, Hasunuma T, Kato T, Sumida T, Kobata T. Apoptosis in rheumatoid arthritis. *Arthritis Rheum* 1998; 41: 1–9.

15 Aicher WK, Heer AH, Trabandt A *et al.* Overexpression of zinc-finger transcription factor Z-225/Egr-1 in synoviocytes from rheumatoid arthritis patients. *J Immunol* 1994; 152: 5940–8.

16 Nykanen P, Bergroth V, Raunio P, Nordstrom D, Konttinen YT. Phenotypic characterization of 3H-thymidine incorporating cells in rheumatoid arthritis synovial

membrane. *Rheumatol Int* 1986;
6: 269–71.

17 Mohr W, Hummler N, Peister B,
Wessinghage D. Proliferation of pannus
tissue cells in rheumatoid arthritis.
Rheumatol Int 1986; 6: 127–32.

18 Petrow P, Theis B, Eckard A *et al.*
Determination of proliferating cells at
sites of cartilage invasion in patients
with rheumatoid arthritis. *Arthritis
Rheum* 1997; 40: S251 (Abstract).

19 Kinne RW, Palombo Kinne E, Emmrich
F. Activation of synovial fibroblasts in
rheumatoid arthritis. *Ann Rheum Dis*
1995; 54: 501–4.

20 Matsumoto S, Muller Ladner U, Gay
RE, Nishioka K, Gay S. Multi-stage
apoptosis and Fas antigen expression
of synovial fibroblasts derived from
patients with rheumatoid arthritis.
J Rheumatol 1996; 23: 1345–52.

21 Nakajima T, Aono H, Hasunuma T
et al. Apoptosis and functional Fas
antigen in rheumatoid arthritis
synoviocytes. *Arthritis Rheum* 1995;
38: 485–91.

22 Matsumoto S, Muller Ladner U, Gay
RE, Nishioka K, Gay S. Ultrastructural
demonstration of apoptosis, Fas and
Bcl-2 expression of rheumatoid synovial
fibroblasts. *J Rheumatol* 1996; 23:
1345–52.

23 Firestein GS, Echeverri F, Yeo M,
Zvaifler NJ, Green DR. Somatic
mutations in the p53 tumor suppressor
gene in rheumatoid arthritis synovium.
Proc Natl Acad Sci USA 1997; 94:
10895–900.

24 Okura T, Gong L, Kamitani T *et al.*
Protection against Fas/APO-1- and
tumor necrosis factor-mediated cell
death by a novel protein, sentrin.
J Immunol 1996; 157: 4277–81.

25 Franz JK, Hummel KM, Aicher WK
et al. Sentrin, a novel anti-apoptotic
molecule is strongly expressed in
synovium of patients with rheumatoid
arthritis (RA). *Arthritis Rheum* 1997;
40: S116 (Abstract).

26 Asahara H, Hasunuma T, Kobata T
et al. In situ expression of
protooncogenes and Fas/Fas ligand
in rheumatoid arthritis synovium.
J Rheumatol 1997; 24: 430–5.

27 Okamoto K, Fujisawa K, Hasunuma T
et al. Selective activation of the

JNK/AP-1 pathway in Fas-mediated
apoptosis of rheumatoid arthritis
synoviocytes. *Arthritis Rheum* 1997;
40: 919–26.

28 Freiberg RA, Spencer DM, Choate KA
et al. Fas signal transduction triggers
either proliferation or apoptosis in
human fibroblasts. *J Invest Dermatol*
1997; 108: 215–19.

29 Aicher WK, Peter HH, Eibel H. Human
synovial fibroblasts are resistant to Fas
induced apoptosis. *Arthritis Rheum*
1996; 39: S75 (Abstract).

30 Koch AE, Robinson PG, Radosevich JA,
Pope RM. Distribution of CD45RA and
CD45RO T-lymphocyte subsets in
rheumatoid arthritis synovial tissue.
J Clin Immunol 1990; 10: 192–9.

31 Kriegsmann J, Keyszer GM, Geiler T
et al. Expression of vascular cell
adhesion molecule-1 mRNA and protein
in rheumatoid synovium demonstrated
by *in situ* hybridization and immunohistochemistry. *Lab Invest* 1995; 72:
209–14.

32 Koch AE, Halloran MM, Haskell CJ,
Shah MR, Polverini PJ. Angiogenesis
mediated by soluble forms of E-selectin
and vascular cell adhesion molecule-1.
Nature 1995; 376: 517–19.

33 Sieper J, Kingsley G. Recent advances
in the pathogenesis of reactive arthritis.
Immunol Today 1996; 17: 160–3.

34 Van Boxel JA, Paget SA. Predominantly
T-cell infiltrate in rheumatoid synovial
membranes. *N Engl J Med* 1975;
293: 517–20.

35 Londei M, Savill CM, Verhoef A *et al.*
Persistence of collagen type II-specific
T-cell clones in the synovial membrane
of a patient with rheumatoid arthritis.
Proc Natl Acad Sci USA 1989; 86:
636–40.

36 Moreland LW, Stewart T, Gay RE *et al.*
Immunohistologic demonstration of
type II collagen in synovial fluid
phagocytes of osteoarthritis and
rheumatoid arthritis patients. *Arthritis
Rheum* 1989; 32: 1458–64.

37 Weyand CM, Goronzy JJ. Pathogenesis
of rheumatoid arthritis. *Med Clin North
Am* 1997; 81: 29–55.

38 Goronzy JJ, Weyand CM. Interplay of
T lymphocytes and HLA-DR molecules
in rheumatoid arthritis. *Curr Opin
Rheumatol* 1993; 5: 169–77.

39 Firestein GS, Wu M, Townsend K *et al.*
Cytokines in chronic inflammatory
arthritis. I. Failure to detect T cell
lymphokines (interleukin 2 and
interleukin 3) and presence of
macrophage colony-stimulating factor
(CSF-1) and a novel mast cell growth
factor in rheumatoid synovitis. *J Exp
Med* 1988; 168: 1573–86.

40 Firestein GS, Zvaifler NJ. How
important are T cells in chronic
rheumatoid synovitis? *Arthritis Rheum*
1990; 33: 768–73.

41 Howell M, Smith J, Cawley M. The
rheumatoid synovium: a model for
T-cell anergy? *Immunol Today* 1992;
13: 191.

42 Salmon M, Scheel Toellner D, Huissoon
AP *et al.* Inhibition of T cell apoptosis
in the rheumatoid synovium. *J Clin
Invest* 1997; 99: 439–46.

43 Müller-Ladner U, Kriegsmann J,
Tschopp J, Gay RE, Gay S.
Demonstration of granzyme A and
perforin messenger RNA in the
synovium of patients with rheumatoid
arthritis. *Arthritis Rheum* 1995;
38: 477–84.

44 Tak PP, Kummer JA, Hack CE *et al.*
Granzyme-positive cytotoxic cells
are specifically increased in early
rheumatoid synovial tissue. *Arthritis
Rheum* 1994; 37: 1735–43.

45 Trabandt A, Gay RE, Gay S. Oncogene
activation in rheumatoid synovium.
APMIS 1992; 100: 861–75.

46 Firestein GS, Zvaifler NJ. Anti-cytokine
therapy in rheumatoid arthritis
[editorial; comment]. *N Engl J Med*
1997; 337: 195–7.

47 Müller-Ladner U, Kriegsmann J, Gay
RE, Gay S. Oncogenes in rheumatoid
arthritis. *Rheum Dis Clin North Am*
1995; 21: 675–90.

48 Trabandt A, Aicher WK, Gay RE
et al. Spontaneous expression of
immediately-early response genes c-fos
and egr-1 in collagenase-producing
rheumatoid synovial fibroblasts.
Rheumatol Int 1992; 12: 53–9.

49 Asahara H, Fujisawa K, Kobata T *et al.*
Direct evidence of high DNA binding
activity of transcription factor AP-1 in
rheumatoid arthritis synovium. *Arthritis
Rheum* 1997; 40: 912–8.

50 Dooley S, Herlitzka I, Hanselmann R

et al. Constitutive expression of c-fos
and c-jun, over-expression of ets-2,
and reduced expression of metastasis
suppressor gene nm23–H1 in
rheumatoid arthritis. *Ann Rheum Dis*
1996; 55: 298–304.

51 Ishidoh K, Taniguchi S, Kominami E.
Egr family member proteins are
involved in the activation of the
cathepsin L gene in v-src-transformed
cells. *Biochem Biophys Res Commun*
1997; 238: 665–9.

52 Müller-Ladner U, Gay RE, Gay S.
Cysteine proteinases in arthritis and
inflammation. *Perspect Drug Disc
Design* 1996; 6: 87–98.

53 Firestein GS, Paine M. Expression
of stromelysin and and TIMP in
rheumatoid arthritis synovium. *Am J
Pathol* 1992; 140: 1309–14.

54 Mojcik CF, Shevach EM. Adhesion
molecules: a rheumatologic perspective.
Arthritis Rheum 1997; 40: 991–1004.

55 Müller-Ladner U, Elices MJ,
Kriegsmann J *et al.* Alternatively
spliced CS-1 fibronectin isoform and
its receptor VLA-4 in rheumatoid
synovium demonstrated by *in
situ* hybridization and immunohistochemistry. *J Rheumatol* 1997;
24: 1873–80.

56 Kitani A, Nakashima N, Matsuda T
et al. T cells bound by vascular cell
adhesion molecule-1/CD106 in synovial
fluid in rheumatoid arthritis: inhibitory
role of soluble vascular cell adhesion
molecule-1 in T cell activation. *J
Immunol* 1996; 156: 2300–8.

57 Petrow P, Franz JK, Müller-Ladner U
et al. Expression of osteopontin mRNA
in synovial tissue of patients with
rheumatoid arthritis (RA) and
osteoarthritis (OA). *Arthritis Rheum*
1997; 39: S36 (Abstract).

58 Lampe MA, Patarca R, Iregui MV,
Cantor H. Polyclonal B cell activation
by Eta-1 cytokine and the development
of systemic autoimmune disease.
J Immunol 1991; 147: 2902–6.

59 Pichler R, Giachelli CM, Lombardi D
et al. Tubulointestinal disease in
glomerulonephritis. Potential role of
osteopontin (uropontin). *Am J Pathol*
1994; 144: 915–26.

60 al Mughales J, Blyth TH, Hunter JA,
Wilkinson PC. The chemoattractant

activity of rheumatoid synovial fluid for human lymphocytes is due to multiple cytokines. *Clin Exp Immunol* 1996; 106: 230–6.

61 McInnes IB, al Mughales J, Field M *et al.* The role of interleukin-15 in T-cell migration and activation in rheumatoid arthritis. *Nat Med* 1996; 2: 175–82.

62 Franz J, Kolb SA, Hummel KM *et al.* Interleukin-16 produced by synovial fibroblasts mediates chemoattractants for CD4+T lymphocytes in rheumatoid arthritis. *Eur J Imm* 1988; 28: 2661–71.

63 Cruikshank WW, Center DM, Nisar N *et al.* Molecular and functional analysis of a lymphocyte chemoattractant factor: association of biologic function with CD4 expression. *Proc Natl Acad Sci USA* 1994; 91: 5109–13.

64 Center DM, Kornfeld H, Cruikshank WW. Interleukin 16 and its function as a CD4 ligand. *Immunol Today* 1996; 17: 476–81.

65 Cruikshank WW, Lim K, Theodore AC *et al.* IL-16 inhibition of CD3-dependent lymphocyte activation and proliferation. *J Immunol* 1996; 157: 5240–8.

66 O'Sullivan FX, Gay RE, Gay S. Spontaneous arthritis models. In: Henderson B, Edwards JCW, Pettipher ER, eds. *Mechanisms and Models in Rheumatoid Arthritis.* London: Academic Press, 1995: 471–83.

67 Trentham DE, Townes AS, Kang AH. Autoimmunity to type II collagen: an experimental model of arthritis. *J Exp Med* 1977; 146: 857–68.

68 Griffiths MM. Immunogenetics of collagen-induced arthritis in rats. *Int Rev Immunol* 1988; 4: 1–15.

69 Holmdahl R, Andersson ME, Goldschmidt TJ *et al.* Collagen induced arthritis as an experimental model for rheumatoid arthritis. Immunogenetics, pathogenesis and autoimmunity. *APMIS* 1989; 97: 575–84.

70 Wilder RL, Case JP, Crofford LJ *et al.* Endothelial cells and the pathogenesis of rheumatoid arthritis in humans and streptococcal cell wall arthritis in Lewis rats. *J Cell Biochem* 1991; 45: 162–6.

71 Case JP, Sano H, Lafyatis R *et al.* Transin/stromelysin expression in the synovium of rats with experimental erosive arthritis. *In situ* localization and kinetics of expression of the transformation-associated metalloproteinase in euthymic and athymic Lewis rats. *J Clin Invest* 1989; 84: 1731–40.

72 Yocum DE, Lafyatis R, Remmers EF, Schumacher HR, Wilder RL. Hyperplastic synoviocytes from rats with streptococcal cell wall-induced arthritis exhibit a transformed phenotype that is thymic-dependent and retinoid inhibitable. *Am J Pathol* 1988; 132: 38–48.

73 Lafyatis R, Remmers EF, Roberts AB *et al.* Anchorage-independent growth of synoviocytes from arthritic and normal joints. Stimulation by exogenous platelet-derived growth factor and inhibition by transforming growth factor-beta and retinoids. *J Clin Invest* 1989; 83: 1267–76.

74 Mudgett JS, Hutchinson NI, Chartrain NA *et al.* Susceptibility of stromelysin 1-deficient mice to collagen-induced arthritis and cartilage destruction. *Arthritis Rheum* 1998; 41: 110–21.

75 Kouskoff V, Korganow AS, Duchatelle V *et al.* Organ-specific disease provoked by systemic autoimmunity. *Cell* 1996; 87: 811–22.

76 Bosma GC, Custer RP, Bosma MJ. A severe combined immunodeficiency mutation in the mouse. *Nature* 1983; 301: 527–30.

77 Mosier DE, Gulizia RJ, Baird SM, Wilson DB. Transfer of a functional human immune system to mice with severe combined immunodeficiency. *Nature* 1988; 335: 256–9.

78 Tighe H, Silverman GJ, Kozin F *et al.* Autoantibody production by severe combined immunodeficient mice reconstituted with synovial cells from rheumatoid arthritis patients. *Eur J Immunol* 1990; 20: 1843–8.

79 Brinckerhoff CE, Harris ED Jr. Survival of rheumatoid synovium implanted into nude mice. *Am J Pathol* 1981; 103: 411–19.

80 Adams CD, Zhou T, Mountz JD. Transplantation of human synovium into a SCID mouse as a model for disease activity. *Arthritis Rheum* 1990; 33: S120 (Abstract).

81 Rendt KE, Barry TS, Jones DM *et al*. Engraftment of human synovium into severe combined immune deficient mice. Migration of human peripheral blood T cells to engrafted human synovium and to mouse lymph nodes. *J Immunol* 1993; 151: 7324–36.

82 Geiler T, Kriegsmann J, Keyszer GM, Gay RE, Gay S. A new model for rheumatoid arthritis generated by engraftment of rheumatoid synovial tissue and normal human cartilage into SCID mice. *Arthritis Rheum* 1994; 37: 1664–71.

83 Müller-Ladner U, Kriegsmann J, Franklin BN *et al*. Synovial fibroblasts of patients with rheumatoid arthritis attach to and invade normal human cartilage when engrafted into SCID mice. *Am J Pathol* 1996; 149: 1607–15.

84 Mima T, Saeki Y, Ohshima S *et al*. Transfer of rheumatoid arthritis into severe combined immunodeficient mice. The pathogenetic implications of T cell populations oligoclonally expanding in the rheumatoid joints. *J Clin Invest* 1995; 96: 1746–58.

85 Kraan MC, Versendaal H, Smeets TJ *et al*. Comparative study on the cellular infiltrate and expression of adhesion molecules in rheumatoid synovial tissue from clinically involved versus clinically uninvolved knee joints. *Arthritis Rheum* 1997; 40: S248 (Abstract).

86 Müller-Ladner U, Kriegsmann J, Gay RE *et al*. Progressive joint destruction in a human immunodeficiency virus-infected patient with rheumatoid arthritis. *Arthritis Rheum* 1995; 38: 1328–32.

87 Mulherin D, Fitzgerald O, Bresnihan B. Clinical improvement and radiological deterioration in rheumatoid arthritis: evidence that the pathogenesis of synovial inflammation and articular erosion may differ. *Br J Rheumatol* 1996; 35: 1263–8.

88 Gutstein NL, Seaman WE, Scott JH, Wofsy D. Induction of immune tolerance by administration of monoclonal antibody to L3T4. *J Immunol* 1986; 137: 1127–32.

89 Cush JJ, Kavanaugh AF. Biologic interventions in rheumatoid arthritis. *Rheum Dis Clin North Am* 1995; 21: 797–816.

90 Moreland LW, Pratt PW, Mayes MD *et al*. Double-blind, placebo-controlled multicenter trial using chimeric monoclonal anti-CD4 antibody, cM-T412, in rheumatoid arthritis patients receiving concomitant methotrexate. *Arthritis Rheum* 1995; 38: 1581–8.

91 Jendro MC, Ganten T, Matteson EL, Weyand CM, Goronzy JJ. Emergence of oligoclonal T cell populations following therapeutic T cell depletion in rheumatoid arthritis. *Arthritis Rheum* 1995; 38: 1242–51.

92 Müller-Ladner U, Roberts CR, Franklin BN *et al*. Human IL-1Ra gene transfer into human synovial fibroblasts is chondroprotective. *J Immunol* 1997; 158: 3492–8.

93 Hummel KM, Gay RE, Gay S. Novel strategies for the therapy of rheumatoid arthritis. *Br J Rheumatol* 1997; 36: 265–7.

94 Jorgensen C, Gay S. Gene therapy in osteoarticular diseases: where are we? *Immunol Today* 1998; 19: 387–91.

5: Are there specific chondrolytic pathways in rheumatoid arthritis?

A.P. Hollander

Introduction

Chondrolysis, a major feature of all arthritic diseases, leads to a loss of articular cartilage thickness which can be observed as joint-space narrowing on
X-rays [1–4]. The proteolytic pathways which may lead to degradation
of cartilage have been studied by many workers in the field and reviewed
extensively [5–8]. However, little direct attention has been paid to the elucidation of enzymatic mechanisms which may be important in rheumatoid
arthritis (RA) but not in osteoarthritis (OA). Any disease-specific mechanisms could be exploited in the development and choice of pharmacological
therapies. The purpose of this chapter is to determine, by reviewing the
available published data, if there is any evidence of such specific pathways.
The discussion will refer, in this chapter, only to RA and OA, since there
are relatively few data available for the other arthritides.

Cartilage

The two major proteins of cartilage are type II collagen and aggrecan.
They provide the tissue with tensile strength and compressive stiffness,
respectively, and degradation of either of them will ultimately lead to loss
of cartilage function [9,10]. There are a variety of less abundant proteins
in cartilage such as decorin, biglycan, collagen types VI, IX and XI, link
protein, fibronectin and cartilage oligomeric matrix protein [9]. Although
these proteins may have very important functions in cartilage, the mechanisms by which they might be degraded are not well understood. Therefore
for the purposes of this chapter, cartilage degradation will be taken to mean
loss of type II collagen and aggrecan from the extracellular matrix.

In mature articular cartilage the only cells resident in the extracellular
matrix are chondrocytes [9], which are capable of synthesizing all the matrix
proteins. In addition, these cells can synthesize and release proteolytic enzymes which may, when activated, degrade aggrecan and type II collagen,

as well as some proteinase inhibitors such as the tissue inhibitors of metalloproteinases (TIMPs) [9,11]. The net effect of resident chondrocytes on extracellular matrix homeostasis is dependent on a balance between synthesis of structural components and their breakdown. This balance between anabolic and catabolic pathways is maintained or perturbed by the actions of a wide variety of cytokines and growth factors [12–14]. In an inflammatory disease such as RA, infiltrating cells may generate high concentrations of interleukin 1α (IL-1α), IL-1β and tumour necrosis factor alpha (TNF-α), all of which are capable of stimulating increased proteinase synthesis by chondrocytes and cartilage degradation [15–17]. However, increased proteolytic activity within the cartilage extracellular matrix is also a feature of OA, despite the relatively low-grade inflammation observed in most OA joints [18]. Identifying the cellular source of proteinases and the role of extra-articular tissues will be critical for the elucidation of disease-specific chondrolytic pathways.

Classes of proteinase involved in chondrolysis

For many years it has been assumed that the matrix metalloproteinases (MMPs) are the major enzymes involved in extracellular matrix breakdown, since they are generally active at neutral pH [19–21]. However, there is increasing evidence of a role for certain cysteine proteinases [22] as well as serine proteinases [23,24] in the proteolytic cascade which results in matrix degradation.

Fibrillar collagen can be damaged by helical cleavage [25,26], resulting in denaturation, or by telopeptide cleavage [27], which may lead to removal of cross-links and depolymerization of the fibrillar network. The extracellular breakdown of fibrillar collagen helices at neutral pH is usually accomplished by the action of a specific collagenase, of which there are at least three: interstitial collagenase (MMP-1; EC 3.4.24.7), neutrophil collagenase (MMP-8; EC 3.4.24.34) and collagenase 3 (MMP-13; EC 3.4.24.–) [26,28]. All the mammalian collagenases initially cleave at a specific Gly–Leu/Ile bond to generate characteristic 1/4 and 3/4 fragments [26] which may then be degraded further by the collagenase itself or by gelatinolytic enzymes such as gelatinase A (MMP-2; EC 3.4.24.24) and B (MMP-9; EC 3.4.24.35) [19], the serine proteinase neutrophil elastase (EC 3.4.21.37) [29] and, at acidic pH, the cysteine proteinases such as cathepsin B (EC 3.4.22.1) [30].

A wide variety of enzymes are capable of cleaving aggrecan in a region of its core protein called the interglobular domain (IGD) [7]. Although there is clear evidence from *ex vivo* tissue culture studies in the presence of selective proteinase inhibitors that the major enzyme that cleaves aggrecan following catabolic stimulation is likely to be a metalloproteinase [31–33], the identity of this enzyme is not yet known. Most of the MMPs can cleave aggrecan at a specific location in the IGD, namely $VDIPEN_{341}$–FFGVG. However, in a ground-breaking study published in 1991, Sandy and colleagues isolated and characterized aggrecan fragments from cultures of bovine articular cartilage stimulated with the catabolic cytokine IL-1α [34]. The sensitive technique of amino-terminal sequencing was used to determine the site at which aggrecan core protein had been cleaved to generate fragments. The derived amino-terminal sequences indicated that the core protein had been cleaved at a location within the IGD that is 32 amino-acid residues C-terminal to the MMP cleavage site, namely $NITEGE_{373}$–ARGSVIL. This cleavage is not normally made by any known proteinase and so the putative enzyme activity which generates these fragments has been called 'aggrecanase' [7]. The neutrophil collagenase MMP-8 has been found, at high concentrations, to cleave aggrecan at the 'aggrecanase' cleavage site as well as the MMP cleavage site [35]. Furthermore there is recent evidence to suggest that chondrocytes can be stimulated to make this enzyme [36]. A role for MMP-8 in aggrecan cleavage cannot be ruled out, although there is no evidence for release of MMP activity in cartilage cultures at the time of aggrecan degradation [33,37].

Cellular source of proteinases

The intra-articular cells most likely to produce enzymes that may contribute to cartilage erosion include chondrocytes, synovial fibroblasts and infiltrating polymorphonuclear leucocytes (PMNs). It is possible that different stimuli will lead to different chondrocyte-mediated proteolytic pathways, one of which might be specifically activated in RA. However, if there are indeed any RA-specific chondrolytic pathways, these are more likely to result from proteinases released by those inflammatory cells which are not usually present in large numbers in the OA joint. It must be remembered, however, that synovial fluid taken from RA patients usually contains a high concentration of proteinase inhibitors as well as the proteinases themselves [38–41] and so the ability of a synovial enzyme to contribute to cartilage matrix destruction will depend on its levels relative to inhibitory activity or on mechanisms by which the enzyme can escape inhibition. It is worth noting that in septic arthritis there may be very little inhibitory activity and so a net excess of proteinases over their inhibitors, leading to uncontrolled proteolysis [42].

Aggrecan degradation

Since degradation of aggrecan may proceed by cleavage at either the

MMP or aggrecanase sites in the IGD, it is clearly important to determine which of these distinct pathways is predominant in an arthritic joint. In two important studies, the aggrecan fragments found in human synovial fluids were isolated and analysed by amino-terminal sequencing. Samples were obtained from patients with traumatic knee injury, primary osteoarthritis, osteochondritis, acute pyrophosphate arthritis, reactive arthritis, psoriatic arthritis and juvenile rheumatoid arthritis. The only major cleavage site detected in all these cases was that due to 'aggrecanase' [43,44]. In a separate study, aggrecan fragments extracted from human normal or OA cartilage specimens were sequenced and found to have been cleaved at the MMP site [45].

Another approach to distinguishing between different cleavage sites is to make 'neoepitope' antibodies, which recognize the new N or C terminus generated at the cleavage site. The method was first used in the field of extracellular matrix biology by Hughes and colleagues to study cleavage of link protein by stromelysin [46] and subsequently for the detection of aggrecanase and stromelysin cleavage sites in aggrecan [47]. Other groups have made similar neoepitope antibodies and used them to study the aggrecan fragments in human cartilage [48] or synovial fluid [49]. Fragments resulting from cleavage at either the MMP or the aggrecanase site were identified in synovial fluids from patients with OA, RA and other arthritic diseases, by immunoassay (MMP site only) and Western immunoblotting [49]. Fragments generated by cleavage at either site were also identified *in situ* by immunostaining of articular cartilage [48]. The neoepitopes were present in normal as well as OA and RA cartilage. The MMP site neoepitope has also been observed in mice with collagen-induced arthritis [50].

In contrast, those fragments of aggrecan detected in cultures of rat chondrosarcoma cells or primary bovine chondrocytes have been shown to be produced entirely by cleavage at the aggrecanase site and not at the MMP site [51]. Similarly, in bovine cartilage explant cultures the degradation of aggrecan occurs before any significant increase in MMP activity can be detected [33,37]. Furthermore the MMPs in human OA cartilage have been found to be present mostly in the inactive proenzyme form [52]. These findings suggest that chondrocyte-mediated aggrecan degradation is a result of the putative enzyme 'aggrecanase' and therefore cleavage at the MMP site of aggrecan in human cartilage is most likely to be a result of MMP release from synovial fibroblasts. If this is indeed the case then the ratio of MMP cleavage to 'aggrecanase' cleavage should be greater in RA, because of the extensive synovial proliferation, than in OA. None of the studies cited above has attempted to directly compare levels of the two different cleavage products in different diseases and so this prediction cannot be tested at present.

Type II collagen degradation

It has been assumed for many years that degradation of cartilage type II collagen is mainly the result of collagenolytic cleavage in the triple helix. This view is based primarily on observations from electron microscopic analysis of RA cartilage [53]. But it can also be inferred from the finding that OA cartilage is often more hydrated than normal tissue, because disruption of the collagen network results in a lower tensile strength and therefore a reduced force to oppose the swelling pressure of hydrated aggrecan [54]. Direct evidence of cartilage collagen denaturation has come from the production and use of antibodies that recognize their epitopes in denatured $\alpha1(II)$ chains, but not in the intact, native molecules. These antibodies to 'hidden epitopes' have been used in both immunohistochemical and immunoassay studies to demonstrate the location and extent of collagen fibril unwinding in human arthritic cartilage and in ageing [55–60].

Ever since the isolation and characterization of MMP-1 from cultures of tadpole tail fins [25] this molecule has been considered to be the key enzyme in extracellular degradation of collagens. Until recently it was the only proteinase synthesized by connective tissue cells known to be capable of cleaving the native triple helix of fibrillar collagens. MMP-8, which is stored in the secondary granules of PMNs, has a similar but not identical substrate selectivity to that of MMP-1 [61] and was recently shown to be synthesized by human articular chondrocytes [36]. MMP-13 is also made by articular chondrocytes and it may be particularly important as it is very efficient at clearing type II collagen [62,63]. At present there is no evidence to suggest that any one of these collagenases is more important than the others in either OA or RA, although the high number of PMNs in RA joints may provide a rich source of MMP-8 which could contribute to cartilage degradation. MMP-13 was shown to produce a secondary cleavage in type II collagen, three amino acid residues C-terminal to the primary cleavage site [63]. However, studies with neoepitope antibodies to both these cleavage sites have since made it clear that MMP-1 can also make the secondary cleavage [64] and it does so most efficiently when acting in combination with either MMP-2 or MMP-3 [65].

An alternative pathway of collagen degradation could involve cleavage of the triple helix by cathepsin K (EC 3.4.22.38), a cysteine proteinase that has also been called cathepsin OC-2 [66] and cathepsin O2 [67]. The mRNA for this enzyme is expressed at high levels by osteoclasts and it is thought to be a major mediator of bone resorption [67,68]. However, it has also been shown to be expressed by mouse hypertrophic chondrocytes [69] and by human RA synovial fibroblasts [70] and so it could play a role in cartilage degradation in the growth plate or in the RA joint. Brömme and colleagues [71] demonstrated that cathepsin K can efficiently degrade type I collagen, even at a pH as high as 6.0, although the mechanism of degradation was not determined. We have found that cathepsin K cleaves both type I and type II collagen in the native triple helix and the identified cleavage sites are close to the amino-terminal end of these molecules [72], thus distinguishing them from those produced by the three collagenases (MMP-1, -8 and -13) which act at a site towards the C-terminal end of the triple helix. These findings, combined with the observation of cathepsin K mRNA expression by RA synovial fibroblasts, raises the intriguing possibility that this enzyme could mediate some of the damage to type II collagen that has been observed at the cartilage–pannus junction in human RA [55,56].

Collagen degradation can, in theory, proceed through cleavage of the telopeptides, without any helical degradation [27,73]. However, there is currently no evidence for such a pathway being of importance in degrading cartilage. Liu and colleagues [73] demonstrated that mutational disruption of the helical collagenase cleavage site in murine type I collagen led to impaired tissue remodelling in adults. However, collagen turnover was not impaired in embryonic and early adult life, when telopeptide cleavage was found to be a dominant pathway of degradation. It may be that the increased cross-linking of collagen molecules with age [74] reduces the availability of telopeptide cleavage sites.

Alternative proteolytic pathways

Although the best described proteolytic pathways in cartilage have been outlined above, a number of other proteinases warrant mention as they could be involved in aspects of cartilage degradation and so could prove to be specific to certain arthritic diseases.

Neutrophil elastase has been investigated widely and numerous studies have demonstrated that it is present in abundance in RA synovial fluid and cartilage, but not in OA specimens [75–80]. However, few studies have attempted to determine if this synovial activity in fact contributes to cartilage erosion. We have found that neutrophil elastase can cleave the triple helix of type I collagen but not type II collagen [81], indicating that it cannot be directly responsible for cartilage collagen degradation. This enzyme can cleave the IGD of aggrecan [7]; however, to date there have been no reports of its cleavage site being detected in naturally occurring aggrecan fragments. If it does play a significant role in cartilage erosion, the exact mechanism by which it does so remains to be established.

Macrophage metalloelastase (MMP-12) has been identified at inflammatory sites, such as in the alveolar macrophages of smokers, as well as in rapidly remodelling tissue such as the full-term placenta [82]. Although its potential role in arthritis has not yet been evaluated, the possibility that it could contribute to degradation of some cartilage proteins in RA cannot be ruled out.

A new subgroup of MMPs has been described consisting of those which have a transmembrane domain and are expressed on the cell membrane. The first of these membrane-type MMPs, MT1-MMP (MMP-14), was described as being on the surface of invading tumour cells [83]. Subsequently, MT2-MMP (MMP-15) MT3-MMP (MMP-16) and MT4-MMP (MMP-17) were identified and characterized [84–87]. Both MMP-14 and MMP-15 have been shown to have the ability to activate pro-MMP-2 [83,88,89]. Furthermore, MMP-14 has been shown to have the capacity to cleave fibrillar collagens at the same 'collagenase' cleavage site as MMP-1 and it may also be able to degrade aggrecan and other extra-cellular matrix proteins [90]. MMP-14 mRNA has been detected in human OA chondrocytes and it is therefore possible that cartilage degradation may proceed by the up-regulation of this and other MT-MMPs in the arthritic joint.

Another class of metalloproteinases thought to be expressed on the cell surface are those with **a d**isintegrin **a**nd a **m**etalloproteinase domain in their structure, called, ADAMs [91,92]. At least three of these complex proteins (ADAM-10, -12 and -15) have been shown at the mRNA level to be expressed by human articular chondrocytes [93] and so they could be involved in the turnover of some extracellular matrix proteins. In addition, one ADAM is responsible for the release of TNF-α from cells, namely TNF-α-converting enzyme (TACE) and so could contribute to cartilage degradation indirectly, by augmenting the catabolic role of TNF-α in joint pathology, particularly in RA [94,95].

Conclusion

The mechanisms leading to cartilage degradation have been intensively studied over many years; however, there is no clear evidence of any pro-teolytic pathways that occur specifically in RA joints. The relative con-tribution of MMP compared with 'aggrecanase' cleavage of aggrecan remains to be established in different pathological states. The degradation of type II collagen by enzymes other than one of the three soluble MMP collagenases could occur in specific diseases; however, once again there is not yet any clinical evidence to demonstrate that this is the case. Future studies will need to focus on these important unanswered questions and uncertainties so that the possibility of tailoring the selectivity of therapeutic proteinase inhibitors can become a reality.

Acknowledgements

I am indebted to the UK Arthritis Research Council for their continued support of work in my laboratory.

References

1 Dieppe P, Brandt KD, Lohmander S, Felson DT. Detecting and measuring disease modification in osteoarthritis. The need for standardized methodology. *J Rheumatol* 1995; 22: 201–3.

2 Akil M, Amos RS. Rheumatoid arthritis—I: Clinical features and diagnosis. *Br Med J* 1995; 310: 587–90.

3 Dougados M. Clinical assessment of osteoarthritis in clinical trials. *Curr Opin Rheumatol* 1995; 7: 87–91.

4 Dieppe PA. Recommended methodology for assessing the progression of osteoarthritis of the hip and knee joints. *Osteoarthritis Cartilage* 1995; 3: 73–7.

5 Poole AR, Alini M, Hollander AP. Cellular biology of cartilage degradation. In: Henderson B, Pettipher ER, Edwards JCW, eds. *Mechanisms and Models in Rheumatoid Arthritis*. London: Academic Press, 1995: 163–204.

6 Buttle DJ, Bramwell H, Hollander AP. Proteolytic mechanisms of cartilage breakdown: a target for arthritis therapy? *J Clin Pathol: Mol Pathol* 1995; 48: M167–M177.

7 Hardingham TE, Fosang AJ. The structure of aggrecan and its turnover in cartilage. *J Rheumatol* 1995; 22 (Suppl. 43): 86–90.

8 Poole AR, Nelson F, Hollander AP *et al*. Collagen II turnover in joint diseases. *Acta Orthop Scand* 1995; 66 (Suppl. 266): 88–91.

9 Poole AR. Cartilage in health and disease. In: McCarty DJ, Koopman WJ, eds. *Arthritis and Allied Conditions: a Textbook of Rheumatology*. Philadelphia: Lea and Febiger, 1993: 279–333.

10 Kempson G. The mechanical properties of articular cartilage. In: Sokoloff L, ed. *The Joints and Synovial Fluid*, Vol 2. New York: Academic Press, 1980: 177–238.

11 Nagase H. Matrix metalloproteinases. In: Hooper NM, ed. *Zinc Metalloproteases in Health and Disease*. London: Taylor and Francis, 1996: 153–204.

12 Lotz M, Blanco FJ, Von Kempis J *et al*. Cytokine regulation of chondrocyte functions. *J Rheumatol* 1995; 22 (Suppl. 43): 104–8.

13 Trippel SB. Growth factor actions on articular cartilage. *J Rheumatol* 1995; 22 (Suppl. 43): 129–32.

14 Hardingham TE, Bayliss MT, Rayan V, Noble DP. Effects of growth factors and cytokines on proteoglycan turnover in articular cartilage. *Br J Rheumatol* 1992; 31 (Suppl. 1): 1–6.

15 Hollander AP, Atkins RM, Eastwood DM, Dieppe PA, Elson CJ. Human cartilage is degraded by rheumatoid arthritis synovial fluid but not by recombinant cytokines *in vitro*. *Clin Exp Immunol* 1991; 83: 52–7.

16 Larbre J-P, Moore AR, Da Silva JAP *et al*. Direct degradation of articular cartilage by rheumatoid synovial fluid: contribution of proteolytic enzymes. *J Rheumatol* 1994; 21: 1796–801.

17 Arend WP, Dayer JM. Inhibition of the production and effects of interleukin-1 and tumor necrosis factor a in rheumatoid arthritis. *Arthritis Rheum* 1995; 38: 151–60.

18 Smith MD, Triantafillou S, Parker A, Youssef PP, Coleman M. Synovial membrane inflammation and cytokine production in patients with early osteoarthritis. *J Rheumatol* 1997; 24: 365–71.

19 Murphy G, Reynolds JJ. Extracellular matrix degradation. In: Royce PM, Steinmann B, eds. *Connective Tissue and its Heritable Disorders: Molecular, Genetic and Medical Aspects*. New York: Wiley-Liss, 1993: 287–316.

20 Birkedal-Hansen H, Moore WGI, Bodden MK *et al*. Matrix

metalloproteinases: a review. *Crit Rev Oral Biol Med* 1993; 4: 197–250.

21 Murphy G. Matrix metalloproteinases and their inhibitors. *Acta Orthop Scand* 1995; 66 (Suppl. 266): 55–60.

22 Buttle DJ, Saklatvala J, Tamai M, Barrett AJ. Inhibition of interleukin 1-stimulated cartilage proteoglycan degradation by a lipophilic inactivator of cysteine endopeptidases. *Biochem J* 1992; 281: 175–7.

23 Treadwell BV, Pavia M, Towle CA, Cooley VJ, Mankin HJ. Cartilage synthesizes the serine protease inhibitor PAI-1: Support for the involvement of serine proteases in cartilage remodeling. *J Orthop Res* 1991; 9: 309–16.

24 Bunning RAD, Crawford A, Richardson HJ *et al.* Interleukin 1 preferentially stimulates the production of tissue-type plasminogen activator by human articular chondrocytes. *Biochem Biophys Acta* 1987; 924: 473–82.

25 Gross J, Nagai Y. Specific degradation of the collagen molecule by tadpole collagenolytic enzyme. *Proc Natl Acad Sci USA* 1965; 54: 1197–204.

26 Gross J, Highberger JH, Johnson-Wint B, Biswas D. Mode of action and regulation of tissue collagenase. In: Woolley DE, Evanson JM, eds. *Collagenase in Normal and Pathological Connective Tissues.* Chichester: Wiley, 1980: 11–35.

27 Wu J-J, Lark MW, Chun LE, Eyre DR. Sites of stromelysin cleavage in collagen types II, IX, X and XI. *J Biol Chem* 1991; 266: 5625–8.

28 Freije JMP, Díez-Itza I, Balbín M *et al.* Molecular cloning and expression of collagenase-3, a novel human matrix metalloproteinase produced by breast carcinomas. *J Biol Chem* 1994; 269: 16766–73.

29 Burleigh MC. Degradation of collagen by non-specific proteinases. In: Barrett AJ, ed. *Proteinases in Mammalian Cells and Tissues.* Amsterdam: Elsevier/North Holland Biomedical Press, 1977: 285–309.

30 Burleigh MC, Barrett AJ, Lazarus GS. Cathepsin B1: A lysosomal enzyme that degrades native collagen. *Biochem J* 1974; 137: 387–98.

31 Mort JS, Dodge GR, Roughley PJ *et al.* Direct evidence for active metalloproteinases mediating matrix degradation in interleukin 1-stimulated human articular cartilage. *Matrix* 1993; 13: 95–102.

32 Buttle DJ, Handley CJ, Ilic MZ *et al.* Inhibition of cartilage proteoglycan release by a specific inactivator of cathepsin B and an inhibitor of matrix metalloproteinases. *Arthritis Rheum* 1993; 36: 1709–17.

33 Brown CJ, Rahman S, Morton AC *et al.* Inhibitors of collagenase but not gelatinase reduce cartilage explant proteoglycan breakdown despite only low levels of matrix metalloproteinases activity. *J Clin Pathol: Mol Pathol* 1996; 49: M331–M339.

34 Sandy JD, Neame PJ, Boynton RE, Flannery CR. Catabolism of aggrecan in cartilage explants. *J Biol Chem* 1991; 266: 8683–5.

35 Fosang AJ, Last K, Neame PJ *et al.* Neutrophil collagenase (MMP-8) cleaves at the aggrecanase site E^{373}-A^{474} in the interglobular domain of cartilage aggrecan. *Biochem J* 1997; 304: 347–51.

36 Cole AA, Chubinskaya S, Schumacher B *et al.* Chondrocyte matrix metallo-proteinase-8. *J Biol Chem* 1996; 271: 11023–6.

37 Kozaci LD, Buttle DJ, Hollander AP. Degradation of type II collagen, but not proteoglycan, correlates with matrix metalloproteinase activity in cartilage explant cultures. *Arthritis Rheum* 1997; 40: 164–74.

38 Brackertz D, Hagmann J, Kueppers F. Proteinase inhibitors in rheumatoid synovial fluid. *Ann Rheum Dis* 1975; 34: 225–30.

39 Borth W, Dunky A, Kleesiek K. Alpha 2-macroglobulin–proteinase complexes as correlated with alpha 1-proteinase inhibitor–elastase complexes in synovial fluids of rheumatoid arthritis patients. *Arthritis Rheum* 1986; 29: 319–25.

40 Mercer E, Cawston TE, De Silva M, Hazleman BL. Purification of a metalloproteinase inhibitor from human rheumatoid synovial fluid. *Biochem J* 1985; 231: 505–10.

41 Cawston TE, Bigg HF, Clark IM, Hazleman BL. Identification of tissue inhibitor of metalloproteinase-2 (TIMP-2)–progelatinase complex as

the third metalloproteinase peak in rheumatoid synovial fluid. *Ann Rheum Dis* 1993; 52: 177–81.

42 Cawston TE, Weaver L, Coughlan RL, Kyle MV, Hazleman BL. Synovial fluids from infected joints contain active metalloproteinases and no inhibitory activity. *Br J Rheumatol* 1989; 28: 386–92.

43 Sandy JD, Flannery CR, Neame PJ, Lohmander LS. The structure of aggrecan fragments in human synovial fluid. *J Clin Invest* 1992; 89: 1512–16.

44 Lohmander LS, Neame PJ, Sandy JD. The structure of aggrecan fragments in human synovial fluid. *Arthritis Rheum* 1993; 36: 1214–22.

45 Flannery CR, Lark MW, Sandy JD. Identification of a stromelysin cleavage site within the interglobulin domain of human aggrecan. *J Biol Chem* 1992; 267: 1008–14.

46 Hughes CE, Caterson B, White RJ, Roughley PJ, Mort JS. Monoclonal antibodies recognizing protease-generated neoepitopes from cartilage proteoglycan degradation. *J Biol Chem* 1992; 267: 16011–14.

47 Hughes CE, Caterson B, Fosang AJ, Roughley PJ, Mort JS. Monoclonal antibodies that specifically recognize neoepitope sequences generated by 'aggrecanase' and matrix metalloproteinase cleavage of aggrecan: application to catabolism *in situ* and *in vitro*. *Biochem J* 1995; 305: 799–804.

48 Lark MW, Bayne EK, Flanagan J *et al*. Aggrecan degradation in human cartilage. Evidence for both matrix metalloproteinase and aggrecanase activity in normal, osteoarthritic and rheumatoid joints. *J Clin Invest* 1997; 100: 93–106.

49 Fosang AJ, Last K, Maciewicz RA. Aggrecan is degraded by matrix metalloproteinases in human arthritis. *J Clin Invest* 1996; 98: 2292–9.

50 Singer II, Kawka DW, Bayne EK *et al*. VDIPEN a metalloproteinase-generated neoepitope, is induced and immunolocalized in articular cartilage during inflammatory arthritis. *J Clin Invest* 1995; 95: 2178–86.

51 Lark M, Gordy JT, Weidner JR *et al*. Cell-mediated catabolism of aggrecan. *J Biol Chem* 1995; 270: 2550–6.

52 Dean DD, Martel-Pelletier J, Pelletier J-P, Howell DS, Woessner JF Jr. Evidence for metalloproteinase and metalloproteinase inhibitor imbalance in human osteoarthritic cartilage. *J Clin Invest* 1989; 84: 678–85.

53 Kobayashi I, Ziff M. Electron microscopic studies of the cartilage–pannus junction in rheumatoid arthritis. *Arthritis Rheum* 1975; 18: 475–83.

54 Venn M, Maroudas A. Chemical composition and swelling of normal and osteoarthritic femoral head cartilage. *Ann Rheum Dis* 1977; 36: 121–9.

55 Dodge GR, Poole AR. Immuno-histochemical detection and immuno-chemical analysis of type II collagen degradation in human normal, rheumatoid, and osteoarthritic articular cartilages and in explants of bovine articular cartilage cultured with interleukin-1. *J Clin Invest* 1989; 83: 647–61.

56 Dodge GR, Pidoux I, Poole AR. The degradation of type II collagen in rheumatoid arthritis: an immuno-electron microscopic study. *Matrix* 1991; 11: 330–8.

57 Hollander AP, Heathfield TF, Webber C *et al*. Increased damage to type II collagen in osteoarthritic articular cartilage detected by a new immuno-assay. *J Clin Invest* 1994; 93: 1722–32.

58 Hollander AP, Pidoux I, Reiner A *et al*. Damage to type II collagen in aging and osteoarthritis starts at the articular surface, originates around chondrocytes, and extends into the cartilage with progressive degeneration. *J Clin Invest* 1995; 96: 2859–69.

59 Hollander AP, Heathfield TF, Liu JJ *et al*. Enhanced denaturation of the a1 (II) chains of type-II collagen in normal adult human intervertebral discs compared with femoral articular cartilage. *J Orthop Res* 1996; 14: 61–6.

60 Antoniou J, Steffen T, Nelson F *et al*. The human lumbar intervertebral disc. Evidence for changes in the biosynthesis and denaturation of the extracellular matrix with growth, maturation, ageing and degeneration. *J Clin Invest* 1996; 98: 996–1003.

61 Netzel-Arnett S, Fields G, Birkedal-Hansen H, Van Wart HE. Sequence specificities of human fibroblast and neutrophil collagenases. *J Biol Chem* 1991; 266: 6747–55.

62 Knäuper V, López-Otín C, Smith B, Knight G, Murphy G. Biochemical characterization of human collagenase-3. *J Biol Chem* 1996; 271: 1544–50.

63 Mitchell PG, Magna HA, Reeves LM *et al.* Cloning, expression and type II collagenolytic activity of matrix metalloproteinase-13 from human osteoarthritic cartilage. *J Clin Invest* 1996; 97: 761–8.

64 Billinghurst RC, Dahlberg L, Reiner A *et al.* Enhanced cleavage of type II collagen by collagenases in osteo-arthritic articular cartilage. *J Clin Invest* 1997; 99: 1534–45.

65 Vankemmelbeke M, Dekeyser PM, Hollander AP, Buttle DJ, Demester J. Characterization of helical cleavages in type II collagen generated by matrixins. *Biochem J* 1998; 330: 633–40.

66 Tezuka K, Tezuka Y, Maejima A *et al.* Molecular cloning of a possible cysteine proteinase predominantly expressed in osteoclasts. *J Biol Chem* 1994; 269: 1106–9.

67 Brömme D, Okamoto K. Human cathepsin O_2, a novel cysteine protease highly expressed in osteoclastomas and ovary. Molecular cloning, sequencing and tissue distribution. *Biol Chem Hoppe-Seyler* 1995; 376: 379–84.

68 Saneshige S, Mano H, Tezuka K *et al.* Retinoic acid directly stimulates osteoclastic bone resorption and gene expression of cathepsin K/OC-2. *Biochem J* 1995; 309: 721–4.

69 Rantakokko J, Aro HT, Savonatus M, Vuorio E. Mouse cathepsin K. cDNA cloning and predominant expression of the gene in osteoclasts, and in some hypertrophying chondrocytes during mouse development. *FEBS Lett* 1996; 393: 307–13.

70 Franz JK, Petrow PK, Hummel KM *et al.* Profile of mRNA expression of cathepsins O_2, S and H in rheumatoid synovial fibroblasts. *Arthritis Rheum* 1996; 39 (Suppl.): S197 (Abstract).

71 Brömme D, Okamoto K, Wang BB, Biroc S. Human cathepsin O_2, a matrix protein-degrading cysteine proteinase expressed in osteoclasts. *J Biol Chem* 1996; 271: 2126–32.

72 Kafienah W, Brömme D, Buttle DJ, Croucher LJ, Hollander AP. Human cathepsin K cleaves native type I and II collagens at the N-terminal end of the triple helix. *Biochem J* 1998; 331: 727–3.

73 Liu X, Wu H, Byrne M *et al.* Targeted mutation at the known collagenase cleavage site in mouse type I collagen impairs tissue remodelling. *J Cell Biol* 1995; 130: 227–37.

74 Eyre DR, Paz MA, Gallop PM. Cross-linking in collagen and elastin. *Annu Rev Biochem* 1984; 53: 717–48.

75 Nakagawa T, Momohara S, Fujita K *et al.* Serine proteinase in articular cartilage, subchondral bone marrow and synovial fluid in human osteoarthritis and rheumatoid arthritis. *Biomed Res* 1995; 16: 11–20.

76 Momohara S, Kashiwazaki S, Inoue K, Saito S, Nakagawa T. Elastase from polymorphonuclear leukocyte in articular cartilage and synovial fluids of patients with rheumatoid arthritis. *Clin Rheumatol* 1997; 16: 133–40.

77 Nordstrom D, Lindy O, Konttinen YT *et al.* Cathepsin G and elastase in synovial fluid and peripheral blood in reactive and rheumatoid arthritis. *Clin Rheumatol* 1996; 15: 35–41.

78 Velvart M, Fehr K, Baici A *et al.* Degradation in vivo of articular cartilage in rheumatoid arthritis by leucocyte elastase from polymorphonuclear leucocytes. *Rheumatol Int* 1981; 1: 121–30.

79 Sandy JD, Sriritana A, Brown HL, Lowther DA. Evidence for polymorphonuclear–leucocyte-derived proteinases in arthritic cartilage. *Biochem J* 1981; 193: 193–202.

80 Huet G, Flipo RM, Richet C *et al.* Measurement of elastase and cysteine proteinases in synovial fluid of patients with rheumatoid arthritis, sero-negative spondyloarthropathies, and osteoarthritis. *Clin Chem* 1992; 38: 1694–7.

81 Kafienah W, Buttle DJ, Burnett D, Hollander AP. Cleavage of native type I collagen by human neutrophil elastase. *Biochem J* 1998; 330: 897–902.

82 Belaaouaj A, Shipley JM, Kobayashi DK *et al.* Human macrophage metal-loelastase. Genomic organization, chromosomal location, gene linkage, and tissue-specific expression. *J Biol Chem* 1995; 270: 14568–75.

83 Sato H, Takino T, Okada Y *et al.* A matrix metalloproteinase expressed on the surface of invasive tumour cells. *Nature* 1994; 370: 61–5.

84 Takino T, Sato H, Shinigawa A, Seiki M. Identification of the second membrane-type matrix metalloproteinase (MT-MMP-2) gene from a human placenta cDNA library. MT-MMPs form a unique membrane-type subclass in the MMP family. *J Biol Chem* 1995; 270: 23013–20.

85 Shofuda K, Yasumitsu H, Nishihashi A, Miki K, Miyazaki K. Expression of three membrane-type matrix metalloproteinases (MT-MMPs) in rat vascular smooth muscle cells and characterization of MT3-MMPs with and without transmembrane domain. *J Biol Chem* 1997; 272: 9749–54.

86 Mattei MG, Roeckel N, Olsen BR, Apte SS. Genes of the membrane-type matrix metalloproteinase (MT-MMP) gene family, MMP14, MMP15 and MMP16, localized to human chromosomes 14, 16 and 8, respectively. *Genomics* 1997; 40: 168–9.

87 Puente XS, Pendás AM, Llano E, Velasco G, López-Otín C. Molecular cloning of a novel membrane-type matrix metalloproteinase from a human breast carcinoma. *Cancer Res* 1996; 56: 944–9.

88 Atkinson SJ, Crabbe T, Cowell S *et al.* Intermolecular autolytic cleavage can contribute to the activation of progelatinase A by cell membranes. *J Biol Chem* 1995; 270: 30479–85.

89 Kolkenbrock H, Hecker-Kia A, Orgel D, Ulbrich N, Will H. Activation of progelatinase A and progelatinase A/TIMP-2 complex by membrane type 2-matrix metalloproteinase. *Biol Chem* 1997; 378: 71–6.

90 Ohuchi E, Imai K, Fujii Y *et al.* Membrane type matrix metalloproteinase digests interstitial collagens and other extracellular matrix macromolecules. *J Biol Chem* 1997; 272: 2446–51.

91 McKie N, Dallas DJ, Edwards T *et al.* Cloning of a novel membrane-linked metalloproteinase from human myeloma cells. *Biochem J* 1996; 318: 459–62.

92 Wolfsberg TG, Primakoff P, Myles DG, White JM. ADAM a novel family of membrane proteins containing a disintegrin and metalloproteinase domain: multipotential functions in cell–cell and cell–matrix interactions. *J Cell Biol* 1995; 131: 275–8.

93 McKie N, Edwards T, Dallas DJ. *et al.* Expression of members of a novel membrane linked metalloproteinase family (ADAM) in human articular chondrocytes. *Biochem Biophys Res Commun* 1997; 230; 335–9.

94 Black RA, Rauch CT, Kozlosky CJ *et al.* A metalloproteinase disintegrin that releases tumour-necrosis factor-α from cells. *Nature* 1997; 385: 729–33.

95 Moss ML, Jin S-LC, Milla ME. *et al.* Cloning of a disintegrin metalloproteinase that processes precursor tumour-necrosis factor-α. *Nature* 1997; 385: 733–6.

Part 2: Disease Progression and Management

6: Are measures of outcome helpful indicators?

P.L.C.M. van Riel and A.M. van Gestel

Introduction

Rheumatoid arthritis (RA) is a chronic systemic inflammatory disease of unknown origin with a highly variable presentation. Its main manifestation is a synovitis of the peripheral joints; however, frequently extra-articular features such as subcutaneous nodules, vasculitis, neurological impairment and internal organ involvement are present. Sometimes this extra-articular involvement may dominate and overshadow the joint manifestations of the disease. This means that the symptoms and signs of RA may vary from joint complaints such as pain, stiffness, swelling and functional impairment, to more constitutional complaints such as fatigue, weight loss and fever, to features relating to organ involvement such as dyspnoea, dry eyes and hepatic failure. This huge variety in disease expression has led in the past decades to the use of an enormous number of variables to monitor the disease course in daily clinical practice and to evaluate interventions in clinical trials. Many of these variables have also been studied for the possibility of predicting course of the disease.

Many efforts have been taken in the past years to standardize the assessment of RA aiming at making study results interchangeable. Consensus has been reached about a minimal set of disease activity variables to be measured in clinical trials. As a following step a start has been made with recommendations for measuring these variables by the European League Against Rheumatism (EULAR) [1], and the American College of Rheumatology (ACR) [2].

In this chapter we will describe the most important variables used in the assessment of RA, discuss the different properties of them and the consequences for their use in clinical trials and daily clinical practice.

Characteristics of assessment variables

Variables to assess disease activity in rheumatoid arthritis are often referred to as outcome measures or endpoint measures ignoring the different properties of these variables. Not taking into account the different characteristics will hamper the interpretation and comparability of clinical trial results, as some of the variables behave differently depending on the amount of destruction that has taken place, which means that in general these variables are dependent on disease duration.

The variables used in the assessment of rheumatoid arthritis can measure process and outcome aspects of the disease. Process can be defined as the instantaneous disease activity and therefore variables measuring process will fluctuate during the course of the disease. Examples of process variables are laboratory measurements such as the acute phase reactants (erythrocyte sedimentation rate (ESR) and C-reactive protein (CRP)) and clinical measurements such as morning stiffness, joint scores, pain scores and global scores of disease activity both by the patient and the assessor. Outcome can be defined as the result of disease activity over a certain period of time as it was originally defined by Fries [3]. An example of such an outcome variable is radiographic damage, this measurement does not reflect actual disease activity at all. However, most of the so-called outcome variables are measuring both process and outcome at the same time, the ratio of which depends at what time-point of the disease course the measurement is used. For instance, grip strength and functional disability may exclusively reflect actual disease activity (process) early in the disease course when no irreversible joint destruction is present; later in the disease if destruction is present these variables will measure a combination of process and outcome.

None of the variables is disease specific; for example, a raised ESR may be caused by many other (for instance, infectious) processes, a joint may be painful due to other causes (for instance, trauma, structural damage) and functional disability measured by a questionnaire might be caused by co-morbidity such as osteoarthritis.

To follow the disease course it is important to use both process variables which reflect instantaneous disease activity as well as outcome variables which reflect a combination of instantaneous disease activity and the resultant of disease activity over a certain period of time. In general, process variables will be measured more frequently to follow the fluctuating course of the disease, while outcome variables will be assessed at larger intervals.

Disease assessment in clinical trials

Clinical trials are designed to evaluate the efficacy of treatments in groups of patients. Measurements are necessary to *indicate* both baseline disease state for patient selection, and treatment efficacy within and between trial groups. Most *helpful* measures are those meeting the following requirements:

- an agreement with international guidelines/consensus;
- valid (construct, criterion, content, discriminant validity);
- reproducible (intra-/interobserver variation);
- well tolerated (patient).

In the past years researchers all over the world have met in several consensus meetings to define a 'core set' of disease activity measures to be assessed in clinical trials. Although consensus has been reached in 'what to assess', no detailed standards are available on 'how to assess', and no agreement exists on how to analyse/define efficacy: treatment groups are compared using change from baseline in single variables and/or indices of disease activity, and by individual improvement criteria. Finally, no agreement exists about the definitions for 'active disease' which are being used as entry criteria in clinical trials.

When developing or choosing variables or indices to measure disease activity the aspects of validity and reproducibility are of major importance. Validity means that a measure will measure what it is supposed to: Does the measure represent the true state (criterion validity)? Does it fit with the theory about the process (construct validity)? Is the measure reasonable (face validity)? Does it comprise all aspects of the feature to be measured (content validity)? Can it detect the smallest important difference between groups or within a group over time (discriminant validity or sensitivity to change)? Criterion validity can be studied by comparing the measure with a gold standard that assesses the true state. Because a gold standard is not always available the performance of the measure might be compared with other methods intending to assess the same aspect (convergent construct validity). Divergent construct validity concerns how well the measurement results reflect expected differences between groups of patients [4].

Reproducibility (precision) means that repeated measurements under the same circumstances give the same results. The same circumstances comprise (among others) the same instrument, the same part of the day, the same place, and the same observer. In trials the most ideal situation will be that measurements are repeated by a single observer (intraobserver variation). The measurement variation between different observers (interobserver variation) will almost always be larger than the intraobserver variation.

It speaks for itself that clinical assessments should be well tolerated by the patient. Any possible risk associated with the measurement should be as small as possible, and within ethical limits.

Assessment variables in clinical trials can be classified in several ways. Below, we classify measures as 'disease activity measures' and as 'criteria'. Criteria are developed to interpret a set of disease activity measures.

Disease activity measures

Disease activity can be assessed by a set of standardized measures covering the variable presentation of the disease, i.e. the 'core set'. A disadvantage of the core set is that the separate components are not combined to give a single value for disease activity. Another approach to assess disease activity is to use an index of disease activity that does combine the different aspects of disease activity into a single value.

Core set

It was recognized by the international community that further standardization of measures in RA clinical trials was necessary. Uniformity of the measures improves the comparability of different studies. Moreover, minimizing the set of required measures decreases the chance of conflicting results and reduces the probability of reaching significance by chance alone (problem of multiple testing). It was agreed upon that potential 'core set' measures should be valid, sensitive to change, reliable and not redundant. During the WHO/ILAR meeting in July 1993 agreement was finally achieved between the different groups on the core set listed in Table 6.1 [5]. It should be stressed that the core set is a minimal requirement for each clinical study, in addition other outcomes such as psychosocial function, patients' preferences, treatment dropouts, side-effects and costs should be considered. Further standardization of measurement techniques is still required.

Joint tenderness and swelling. Several different articular indices have been developed and used in clinical trials. They differ with respect to the number of included joints, the measured (combinations of) abnormalities, grading for tenderness, and weighting for joint surface area. To enhance comparability among trials, one method should be selected. It is obvious that the most valid and least time-consuming measure should be chosen. The 28-joint count, not graded and not weighted, measuring tenderness and swelling separately, satisfies these requirements [6–9]. Tenderness and

---

Joint pain/tenderness
Joint swelling
Acute phase reactants
Pain
Patient global assessment of disease activity
Physician global assessment of disease activity
Physical disability
Radiographs (for studies > 1 year)

Table 6.1 Core set of endpoint measures in rheumatoid arthritis clinical trials. (From [10] with permission.)

swelling are measured separately since they provide different information: tenderness is more sensitive to change and correlates with pain, while swelling correlates with acute-phase reactants and X-ray progression. Grading and weighting are excluded because their advantages (grading: more sensitive to change; weighting: higher correlation with CRP) do not always make up for the lower reproducibility (higher interobserver variability) found with these additions [11]. However, when only one observer is involved, these additions might be very useful. The interobserver variation might also be reduced by a standardization of examination techniques following an 'agreement session'.

Several self-report articular indices have been developed since 1990 [12–16]. These indices are reliable and sensitive to change, and comparable to physicians' assessment with respect to correlations with clinical variables. However, the correlation with the physicians' assessment varies between 0.6 and 0.8, indicating that the measures are not identical. Whether or not the self-report articular indices can replace the rheumatologist's joint count has to be studied further.

Acute-phase reactants. The most frequently used laboratory measures for disease activity are Westergren ESR and CRP. They correlate with other measures of disease activity [17], and are sensitive to change in trials comparing slow-acting anti-rheumatic drugs [18]. There is some evidence that these measures predict X-ray progression [19].

Pain. The most frequently used pain intensity measures in rheumatoid arthritis are numerical rating scales (NRS) and visual analogue scales (VAS). An NRS is an easily performed ordinal scale, grading pain in a number of categories. Some problems arising with this measurement are that it cannot be interpreted as a ratio scale since the meanings of the intervals are unknown, and its sensitivity to change is less than with a continuous scale. A VAS can be interpreted as a ratio scale (i.e. a change from 20 to 10 can be interpreted as a 50% change) and is more sensitive to change. However, it needs more instruction and it is less reliable in illiterate patients. NRS and VAS are associated with one another, but they are not equivalent. The McGill Pain Questionnaire is a multidimensional (sensory, affective, intensity) pain measure with good discriminant validity. It consists of 20 verbal rating scales. The method needs precise instructions and a good knowledge of the used language. It is more time consuming than NRS or VAS.

The ACR and the EULAR recommend the use of either a horizontal VAS of 10 cm with 'no pain' at one end and 'worst possible pain' at the other end without intervening categories, an NRS or a Likert scale (1 = asymptomatic, 2 = mild, 3 = moderate, 4 = severe, 5 = very severe) [1,2].

Global disease activity. Although no validation studies are performed, patients' assessment of global disease activity is generally measured on a VAS using the Arthritis Impact Measurement Scale (AIMS) question: 'Considering all the ways your arthritis affects you, mark "X" on the scale for how well you are doing'. A Likert scale response or an NRS are also acceptable according to ACR and EULAR [1,2]. The same recommendations as for patients' global assessments apply for physicians' (or assessors') global assessment of patients' disease activity.

Physical disability. The most valid assessment of a patient's physical functioning will be obtained by standardized observation of his or her ability to perform specific tasks. A less time-consuming method to assess disability will be to ask for a clinical judgement by the physician. This method is liable to large interobserver variation. Patients' self-reported questionnaires of physical function are the most popular, although there may be discrepancies between actual performance and reported performance of patients. The two most frequently used self-reported questionnaires in arthritis patients, the AIMS [20] and the Stanford Health Assessment Questionnaire (HAQ) [21], are sensitive to clinical changes [22]. The modified HAQ functional disability index predicted increased morbidity and mortality in a study of Wolfe and colleagues [23]. Liang and colleagues compared efficiency and sensitivity of five health status instruments including HAQ and AIMS, and concluded that no single instrument consistently outperformed the others [24]. It would be best to choose *one* of these questionnaires to enhance uniformity among trials.

Radiographs. Joint destruction is an example of an outcome variable that does not reflect actual disease activity at all. Damage measured by radiographs can be seen as the result of disease activity over a certain period of time. The two most frequently used validated radiographic scoring methods were developed by Sharp and colleagues [25] and Larsen [26]. Both methods have been modified several times [27–29]. The Larsen method uses standard radiographs graded from 0 (normal joints) to 5 (completely destroyed joint) and combines joint-space narrowing and erosions. The Sharp method assesses joint-space narrowing in four grades in the hand and scores for erosions in the same areas to a maximum score of 5. A modification of this method has been developed and validated especially for the radiographic evaluation of patients with early rheumatoid arthritis, as it has been shown that in about 30% of the patients who develop erosions, the first erosions appear in the foot joints [30]. Therefore it was decided to include the metatarsophalangeal joints in the modified Sharp method, a maximum score for erosions of 10 was chosen as more separate erosive lesions were seen than in the hands [27]. After about 5 years it becomes more difficult to score the foot joints as the metatarsophalangeal joints become frequently subluxated which makes the evaluation impossible. This might have been the reason why the foot joints were excluded in the original Sharp method. The Sharp method is more time consuming, therefore it was decided to include the Larsen method in the EULAR core set for assessing disease activity in rheumatoid arthritis. A problem using both methods is the so-called 'ceiling effect': when the maximum score in a joint is reached, further damage cannot be quantified. Scoring of radiographs is still very time consuming and subject to large interobserver variation.

Indices

Indices of disease activity are developed to combine disease activity measures into a single expression of disease activity. Some advantages of combined indices of disease activity compared with a set of measures include: no conflicting results, more power, and better comparability between (groups of) patients. Disadvantages of an index are that it cannot be easily re-expressed into its components and that the calculations involved are intricate. Several indices have been developed using a statistical, pseudo-statistical or heuristic approach. The scales of these indices are ordinal or continuous. The advantage of a continuous scale is that no information is lost, which increases sensitivity. The Lansbury systemic index [31] is the oldest measure, although it has not been thoroughly validated. The Disease Activity Score (DAS) [32,33] is a statistically derived index combining tender joints, swollen joints, ESR and general health (Table 6.2). It has been validated in several studies [16,33,34]. The original DAS comprised a graded joint tenderness score, the Ritchie Articular Index, and a 44-swollen-joint count. As a result of new international preferences, the DAS28 was developed which includes the 28-joint counts for tenderness and swelling. The addition of more core-set variables (besides joint counts and ESR) to the DAS formula did not improve the validity of this index.

Table 6.2 The disease activity score (DAS).

$$DAS = 0.53938\sqrt{(RAI)} + 0.06465(S44) + 0.330(lnESR) + 0.00722(GH)$$
$$DAS28 = 0.56\sqrt{(T28)} + 0.28\sqrt{(S28)} + 0.70(lnESR) + 0.014(GH)$$

DAS28, DAS including the 28-joint count; RAI, Ritchie Articular Index, a graded joint tenderness score based on 53 joints; S44, ungraded joint swelling count based on 44 joints; lnESR, natural logarithm of erythrocyte sedimentation rate; GH, general health according to the patient in millimetres on a visual analogue scale of 100 mm; T28, ungraded joint tenderness count based on 28 joints; S28, ungraded joint swelling count based on 28 joints.

≥ 20% improvement in:	**Table 6.3** Preliminary American College of Rheumatology (ACR) improvement criteria.
Tender joint count	
Swollen joint count	
and in 3 of following 5:	
Patient pain assessment	
Patient global assessment	
Physician global assessment	
Patient self-assessed disability	
Acute-phase reactant	

Criteria

Groups of patients can be compared by their measurement 'scores'. A statistically significant difference between or within groups, however, does not automatically imply a clinically relevant difference. Therefore value judgements have to be allocated to the measurement results. Criteria are developed to classify patients according to these value judgements. They are helpful in giving a clinically relevant and standardized interpretation of the assessment scores of individual patients.

Improvement criteria

Improvement criteria are developed to determine the treatment response of individual patients. Individual treatment response is a necessary addition to mean group responses in the evaluation of clinical trials, since it answers the following question: Is the mean group improvement the result of a large group of patients improving moderately, or of a small number of patients with a marked improvement?

Recently, two sets of improvement criteria have been developed following different routes:
1 criteria based upon the core set of disease activity variables (preliminary ACR improvement criteria [35]) (Table 6.3);
2 criteria based upon an index of disease activity (EULAR response criteria [36]) (Table 6.4).
They differ in respect to the way they were developed, the choice of disease activity variables, the implementation of these variables (reached value, absolute/relative change), and the classification of improvement (two vs. three groups). The ACR criteria result from a study investigating ease of use, credibility and discriminant validity (vs. placebo) of improvement criteria. Treatment response is defined as a 20% change from baseline in core-set variables. The EULAR response criteria include not only change in disease activity but also current disease activity. They are based upon

Table 6.4 European League Against Rheumatism (EULAR) response criteria.

Reached DAS (DAS28)	Change in DAS/DAS28 from baseline		
	> 1.2	> 0.6 and ≤ 1.2	≤ 0.6
≤ 2.4 (3.2)	Good	Moderate	Non
2.4 (3.2) to 3.7 (5.1)	Moderate	Moderate	Non
> 3.7 (5.1)	Moderate	Non	Non

DAS, disease activity score.

the DAS. To be classified as responders, patients should have a significant change in DAS and also low current disease activity. Three categories are defined: good, moderate and non-responders.

Future studies should make clear which set of criteria is more valid to be used in clinical trials (or individual patient practice).

Remission criteria

Remission criteria define the absence (or a very low level) of disease activity. Any usable criterion should in addition contain a time component since follow-up for an indefinite period will not be possible in most clinical settings.

The American Rheumatism Association (ARA) developed preliminary criteria for clinical remission in rheumatoid arthritis [37]. The development was based on an optimal discrimination between patients with and without remission according to their rheumatologists. An arbitrary duration of more than 2 months was chosen because 90% of the patients fulfilled this criterion. There are several problems with this definition that obstruct clinical usefulness: no specifications are given as to which measurement technique should be used for the different clinical variables; two out of the six used variables are not included in the presently accepted and validated core set; and finally the outcome is dichotomous which implies that a small change in disease activity may have a great impact on the allocated class.

Another approach would be to define remission with a continuous variable of disease activity such as the DAS and add the time period that the patient was at a certain level or just calculate the cumulative disease activity over a certain time period. A DAS was calculated for patients who were categorized with the ARA criteria as being in remission or not. At a cut-off value of the DAS being 1.6 (DAS28 2.6) the percentage of misclassification for both categories was 10%. The advantage of this method would be that remission can be seen relative to other levels of disease activity [38].

Inclusion criteria

Clinical trials evaluating disease-controlling anti-rheumatic therapy often select patients with 'active' disease. Most studies use different definitions of the minimal required level of disease activity of patients entering the trial. This results in differences between trial populations, which will hamper the comparison of trial results. Standardized inclusion criteria might be based upon the core set or an index of disease activity. An index would provide the advantage of a single figure and a continuous scale, so that (as with remission) 'active' disease can be seen relative to other levels of disease activity.

When using one of the improvement criteria (EULAR or ACR) trial inclusion criteria are required. With the EULAR criteria a DAS > 2.2 at the beginning of the study will be necessary, since a DAS < 1.0 indicates the absence of disease activity, and a change of 1.2 should be possible. With the ACR criteria all included variables should be larger than zero at baseline, since dividing by zero (to calculate relative change) is not possible. Because of this the HAQ score at baseline will be the bottleneck for calculating the ACR improvement criteria.

Disease assessment in daily clinical practice

In daily clinical practice the following are helpful aspects in addition to those mentioned in the clinical trial section:
• face validity;
• ease of use and interpretation;
• low cost.

To guide treatment decisions it is important to follow the fluctuating course of the disease as accurately as possible. For this purpose process variables are needed which can be assessed frequently. This will be dependent on several parameters, namely sensitivity to change, ease of use, tolerability, costs and logistics.

An index expressing disease activity as a single continuous variable will be the most helpful measure to follow the course of the disease. The DAS including two joint counts, an acute-phase reactant and a general health assessment is a valid, easily used tool for this purpose. Although the formula to calculate the DAS is rather complicated, by using a simple programmable calculator (or a personal computer), it only takes a few seconds. Due to its simplicity the DAS including the 28-joint count (DAS28) is easier to use for routine clinical assessments than the DAS with more comprehensive joint counts, and thus will promote its being regularly used to manage the disease. Although in the 28-joint count the foot joints, which are often involved in patients with RA, are not included, we believe that it is still a good choice to give an overview of the disease activity in a patient over time. However, apart from this it is obvious that attention should always be paid to other complaints of a patient—the variables needed for the DAS28 always remain only a minimum requirement.

As outcome variables the HAQ should be performed at 6- or 12-months intervals whereas radiographs of the hands and feet scored either by the Larsen method or the Sharp method can be taken even at longer intervals.

Prognostic factors

Due to the unpredictability of the disease, the impracticability of curing the disease and the potentially toxic therapies, many attempts have been made to find prognostic factors which can correctly identify the course of the disease or the response to treatments. Next to some genetic factors such as HLA-DR4, the amino-acid sequence in the third hypervariable region of the β chain (shared epitope) and a poor sulphoxidation status most of the above-mentioned disease assessment variables have also been used for this purpose.

The most useful variable to predict the disease course seems to be the rheumatoid factor. Patients with a rheumatoid factor-positive RA do in general have a more severe disease course than patients with a rheumatoid factor-negative disease. From all other variables only those which reflect the actual disease activity do have some predictive value. Patients presenting with a more active disease have a more severe disease course than do those presenting with a milder disease. As indices of disease activity such as the DAS do reflect disease activity better than single variables, it is clear that these indices predict a more severe disease course most efficiently. There is still discussion as to whether genetic markers such as the HLA-DR4 locus or the shared epitope do have any prognostic value for the disease course. Nevertheless, it is of no use to guide treatment decisions in daily clinical practice.

Conclusion

Many measures of outcome are being used in the assessment of RA. Core sets of valid outcome measures have been defined to be used in clinical trials. It appears to be important to keep in mind the different aspects of the disease these variables are measuring (process or outcome), as this may differ depending on the disease duration. To follow the disease course it is important to use both variables describing instantaneous disease activity and variables reflecting the result of disease activity over a certain period of time. Next to the different aspects of validity, simplicity and ease of use are important factors which define the usefulness of the outcome measures in daily clinical practice. In the coming years attention should be paid to further standardization of the outcome measures. The exact method of measuring the different variables should be described. In addition criteria to define patients with an active disease to be included in clinical trials as well as criteria to evaluate clinical response must be standardized. This will improve the quality of care given in daily clinical practice and will further increase the possibility of exchanging the results of clinical trials.

References

1 Scott DL, van Riel PL, van der Heijde D, Stunicka Benke A, ESCISIT. Assessing disease activity in rheumatoid arthritis. The *EULAR Handbook of Standard Methods* 1993.
2 Felson DT, Anderson JJ, Boers M *et al.* The American College of Rheumatology preliminary core set of disease activity measures for rheumatoid arthritis clinical trials. *Arthritis Rheum* 1993; 36: 729–40.
3 Fries JF. Toward an understanding of patient outcome measurement. *Arthritis Rheum* 1983; 26: 697–704.
4 Tugwell P, Bombardier CA. Methodological framework for developing and selecting endpoints in clinical trials. *J Rheumatol* 1982; 9: 758–62.
5 Tugwell P, Boers M, Baker PH, Wells G, Snider J. Endpoints in rheumatoid arthritis. *J Rheumatol* 1994; 21 (Suppl. 42): 2–8.
6 Fuchs HA, Brooks RH, Callahan LF, Pincus TA. Simplified twenty-eight-joint quantitative articular index in rheumatoid arthritis. *Arthritis Rheum* 1989; 32: 531–7.
7 Prevoo MLL, van Riel PLCM, van't Hof MA *et al.* Validity and reliability of joint indices. A longitudinal study in patients with recent onset rheumatoid arthritis. *Br J Rheumatol* 1993; 32: 589–94.
8 Fuchs HA, Pincus T. Reduced joint counts in controlled clinical trials in rheumatoid arthritis. *Arthritis Rheum* 1994; 37: 470–5.
9 Smolen JS, Breedveld FC, Eberl G *et al.* Validity and reliability of the twenty-eight-joint count for the assessment of rheumatoid arthritis

activity. *Arthritis Rheum* 1995; 38: 38–43.
10 van Gestel AM, van Riel PLCM. Evaluation of early rheumatoid arthritis disease activity and outcome. *Baillière's Clin Rheum* 1997; 11: 49–63.
11 Thompson PW, Kirwan JR. Joint counts: a review of old and new articular indices of joint inflammation. *Br J Rheumatol* 1995; 34: 1003–8.
12 Stewart MW, Palmer DG, Knight RGA. Self-report articular index measure of arthritic activity: investigations of reliability, validity and sensitivity. *J Rheumatol* 1990; 17: 1011–15.
13 Mason JH, Anderson JJ, Meenan RF *et al.* The rapid assessment of disease activity in rheumatology (radar) questionnaire. Validity and sensitivity to change of a patient self-report measure of joint count and clinical status. *Arthritis Rheum* 1992; 35: 156–62.
14 Stucki G, Liang MH, Stucki S, Bruhlmann P, Michel BAA. Self administered Rheumatoid Arthritis Disease Activity Index (RADAI) for epidemiological research: psychometric properties and correlation with parameters of disease activity. *Arthritis Rheum* 1995; 38: 795–8.
15 Stucki G, Stucki S, Bruhlmann P, Maus S, Michel BA. Comparison of the validity and reliability of self-reported articular indices. *Br J Rheumatol* 1995; 34: 760–6.
16 Prevoo MLL, van Kuper HH, van't Hof MA *et al.* Validity and reproducibility of self-administered joint counts. A large prospective

longitudinal followup study in patients with rheumatoid arthritis. *J Rheumatol* 1996; 23: 841–5.

17 van der Heijde DMFM, van't Hof MA, van Riel PLCM, van de Putte LBA. Validity of single variables and indices to measure disease activity in rheumatoid arthritis. *J Rheumatol* 1993; 20: 538–41.

18 Anderson JJ, Chernoff MC. Sensitivity to change of rheumatoid arthritis clinical trial outcome measures. *J Rheumatol* 1993; 20: 535–7.

19 van Leeuwen MA, van Rijswijk MH, van der Heijde DMFM *et al.* The acute-phase response in relation to radiographic progression in early rheumatoid arthritis: a prospective study during the first three years of the disease. *Br J Rheumatol* 1993; 32: 9–13.

20 Meenan RF, Gertman PM, Mason JM. Measuring health status in arthritis: the arthritis impact measurement scales. *Arthritis Rheum* 1980; 23: 146–52.

21 Fries JF, Spitz P, Kraines RG, Holman HR. Measurement of patient outcome in arthritis. *Arthritis Rheum* 1980; 23: 137–45.

22 Ward MW. Clinical measures in rheumatoid arthritis: which are most useful in assessing patients? *J Rheumatol* 1993; 21: 17–21.

23 Wolfe F, Kleinheksel SM, Cathey MA *et al.* The clinical value of the Stanford Health Assessment Questionnaire Functional Disability Index in patients with rheumatoid arthritis. *J Rheumatol* 1988; 15: 1480–8.

24 Liang MH, Larson MG, Cullen KE, Schwartz JA. Comparative measurement efficiency and sensitivity of five health status instruments for arthritis research. *Arthritis Rheum* 1985; 28: 542–7.

25 Sharp JT, Lidsky MD, Collins LC, Moreland J. Methods of scoring the progression of radiologic changes in rheumatoid arthritis. *Arthritis Rheum* 1971; 14: 206–20.

26 Larsen A. *A radiologic method for grading the severity of rheumatoid arthritis.* PhD Thesis, Oslo University, 1974.

27 van der Heijde DM, van Riel PL, Nuver-Zwart HH *et al.* Effects of hydroxychloroquine and sulphasalazine on progression of joint damage in rheumatoid arthritis. *Lancet* 1989; i: 1036–8.

28 Sharp JT. Assessment of radiographic abnormalities in rheumatoid arthritis: what have we accomplished and where should we go from here? *J Rheumatol* 1995; 22: 1787–91.

29 Larsen A. How to apply Larsen Score in evaluating radiographs of rheumatoid arthritis in longterm studies? *J Rheumatol* 1995; 22: 1974–5.

30 Brook A, Corbett M. Radiographic changes in early RA. *Ann Rheum Dis* 1977; 36: 71–3.

31 Lansbury A. A method for summation of the systemic indices of rheumatoid activity. *Am J Med Sci* 1956; 232: 300–10.

32 van der Heijde DMFM, van't Hof MA, van Riel PLCM, van de Putte LBA. Development of a disease activity score based on judgment in clinical practice by rheumatologists. *J Rheumatol* 1993; 20: 579–81.

33 van Prevoo MLL, van't Hof MA, Kuper HH *et al.* Modified disease activity scores that include twenty-eight-joint counts. *Arthritis Rheum* 1995; 38: 44–8.

34 Fuchs HA. The use of the disease activity score in the analysis of clinical trials in rheumatoid arthritis. *J Rheumatol* 1993; 20: 1863–6.

35 Felson DT, Anderson JJ, Boers M *et al.* American College of Rheumatology preliminary definition of improvement in rheumatoid arthritis. *Arthritis Rheum* 1995; 38: 727–35.

36 van Gestel AM, van Prevoo MLL, van't Hof MA *et al.* Development and validation of the European League Against Rheumatism response criteria for rheumatoid arthritis. *Arthritis Rheum* 1996; 39: 34–40.

37 Pinals RS, Masi AT, Larsen RA. Preliminary criteria for remission in rheumatoid arthritis. *Arthritis Rheum* 1981; 24: 1308–15.

38 Prevoo MLL, van Gestel AM, van't Hof MA *et al.* Remission in a prospective study of patients with rheumatoid arthritis. American Rheumatism Association preliminary remission criteria in relation to the disease activity score. *Br J Rheumatol* 1996; 35: 1101–5.

7: A case for early aggressive therapy

K. Ahmed and P. Emery

Introduction

Rheumatoid arthritis (RA) is probably the commonest cause of treatable disability in the Western world. Despite a better understanding of the pathogenesis of disease specifically and inflammation generally, the long-term outcome has been poor [1,2]. A crucial issue in the management of RA is the timing and extent of pharmacological intervention. In the last 10 years clinical practice has been revolutionized. The traditional 'pyramid' approach to treatment, i.e. requiring the failure of non-steroidal anti-inflammatory drugs (NSAIDs) therapy before the introduction of disease-modifying anti-rheumatic drugs (DMARDs), has been reversed. Many rheumatologists now start early with a single or even a combination of DMARD(s) [3,4].

In this chapter we will review the scientific basis for early and aggressive therapy, usually monotherapy, or combination therapy with DMARDs from the outset.

The progressive nature of RA

In many ways, the synovium in RA behaves like malignant tissue. There is autologous proliferation and local invasion, the disease spreads from one joint to the other and with an increase in the 'bulk' of inflamed tissue, the response to treatment is diminished [5]. Recent study in the department by Devlin and colleagues (unpublished observations) has confirmed that the number of joints involved progressively increases in the first 3 years of the disease. If there is an attempt to achieve remission, therefore, the sooner, the better; indeed, rheumatologists may benefit from strategies developed by the oncologists [6].

The early phase of disease represents a unique window of opportunity for therapeutic intervention. There is good evidence that inflammation/damage is maximum at that time (manifesting as number of swollen joints, high acute-phase response and rate of appearance of erosions) [7–9]. Data from a large monoarthritis study has shown that early definitive treatment results in good outcome [10]. It is possible that early on in the disease, immune mechanisms involved in the pathogenesis may be more vulnerable to suppressive treatment. For example, early intervention may affect the ability of memory T cells [11] to expand, hence reducing the long-term disease mass. Induction of apoptosis by intra-articular corticosteroids may switch off early disease by producing cell death in pathogenetic cells [12].

Persistent inflammation produces damage

Clearly, persistent inflammation is harmful in structural and functional terms. It has previously been shown that the longer the duration of untreated disease, the worse is the disease outcome [13]. Generalized osteoporosis with risk of fractures is a well-known feature of late RA. A study of patients with early arthritis [14] demonstrated that patients who had a disease duration of greater than 6 months at presentation had already lost bone compared with those presenting with disease of shorter duration. In the same study it was also shown that patients with active disease over 3 years lost, on average, 20% of their bone mass from certain sites in the hip. Furthermore it has recently been confirmed that patients with high levels inflammation (as evidenced by a high C-reactive protein (CRP)) deteriorate functionally [15] and that they will predictably develop erosions on X-ray [16]. Van der Heijde and colleagues [17] have reported that joint destruction occurs in the first year of the disease in two-thirds of the patients. Another study [18] showed that hand bone mineral density loss occurs early in the disease and is a marker of poor functional outcome (as measured by the Health Assessment Questionnaire (HAQ)). The effect of treatment on inflammation and functional improvement is not always the same. Inflammation responds to intervention by DMARDs with a steady improvement which is largely independent of the duration of disease whereas final functional outcome is determined by the duration of symptoms before the initiation of therapy [19]. Early treatment is therefore important if long-term disability is to be prevented (Fig. 7.1).

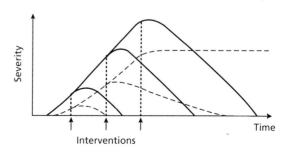

Fig. 7.1 Effect of disease duration of rheumatoid arthritis on inflammation (–) and function (––). (From [19] with permission.)

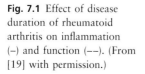

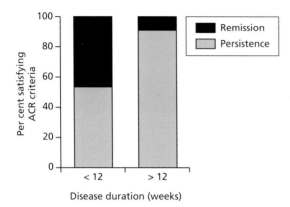

Fig. 7.2 Outcome of intervention in ACR-positive patients.

Early intervention has other advantages. Giving these drugs early results in earlier symptomatic relief with positive psychological implications [20]. Stabilization of function at this stage results in near normality rather than stabilizing in a state of disability. Also, perhaps because of relatively less active acute-phase response due to decreased bulk and localized disease, hepatic handling of drugs may be better with consequently fewer side-effects.

Despite the preceding discussions, early treatment may not be easy. There are problems with early referral by the primary healthcare physicians to the specialist centres. Since initial presentation of RA with symmetrical polyarthritis often responds well to NSAIDs (in short-term), it is important that primary physicians realize that a good response to NSAIDs is all the more reason to refer rather than the contrary. Close collaboration between the specialist clinics and the community is therefore essential. Recent experience in Yorkshire with LEAP (Leeds Early Arthritis Project) is encouraging. Unpublished early data from remission induction regimen (M. Green *et al.* 1997) confirms that ability to induce remission is inversely related to the duration of symptoms at the time of presentation to the specialist centre (Fig. 7.2).

An important aspect of early aggressive treatment is the need to identify those patients who are likely to fare badly later. Clinical features associated with a bad prognosis, such as number of joints involved and the extent of acute-phase response, develop with the evolution of the disease. Clinical features alone therefore are insufficient grounds on which to decide on aggressive treatment. The term PISA (persistent inflammatory symmetrical arthritis), based on important prognostic factors such as presence of shared epitope (3HVR), rheumatoid factor, acute-phase response (CRP) and functional status (as assessed by the HAQ), has been devised (Table 7.1). If the PISA score is 3 or more the current approach is to treat immediately and aggressively. Recent information from a primary care study (NOAR) confirms the consistency of the risk factors [21].

Table 7.1 Predictors of persistent and severe disease: the persistent inflammatory symmetrical arthritis (PISA) score. (With permission of Oxford University Press, from [22].)

Factors in addition to PISA	Score
Abnormal HAQ (HAQ 4–11 scores 1, ≥ 12 scores 2)	1/2
ESR, CRP elevation	1
Rheumatoid factor positive	1
Presence of 3AHVR (disease epitopes)	1
Female sex	1

HAQ, Health Assessment Questionnaire; ESR, erythrocyte sedimentation rate; CRP, C-reactive protein.

Appropriate treatment

Delaying treatment serves no purpose. We know now that almost 90% of patients with RA will receive a second-line drug in the first 3 years. The argument that the associated danger of toxicity should be avoided is not valid, as most patients will eventually require such a drug [23]. It is also possible that the use of NSAIDs may unnecessarily delay the initiation of a DMARD. It is important to keep side-effects of DMARD treatment in mind while not forgetting the side-effects of the disease (RA) itself [1]. The earlier use of DMARDs may reduce the long-term disease load and may be cost effective. Spending more money at an earlier stage with the aim of fundamentally altering the disease at the outset can lead to major savings in the long run.

Earlier DMARDs

Only a few studies have looked at delaying the use of DMARDs in early disease. In a study by Borg and colleagues [24] early treatment with auranofin was compared with an 8-month delayed DMARD treatment during which period patients received placebo. At the end of the second year, the early-treated group showed significantly more improvement in physical function (as measured by Keitel function index and HAQ). The original study was re-analysed at a 5-year follow-up by Egsmose and colleagues [25] and it was shown that there was still a significant difference in Keitel functional index in favour of the early-treated group, although the difference in HAQ did not reach significance. In an open study, 238 patients with recently diagnosed RA were randomized to treatment with NSAID only ('non-DMARD' group) ($n = 57$) or early treatment with a DMARD (hydroxychloroquine 400 mg daily, intramuscular gold 50 mg per week or methotrexate 7.5–15 mg per week) ($n = 181$). In the intention-to-treat analysis, the non-DMARD group included 16 patients who were switched to a DMARD because of insufficient therapeutic response, while the DMARD group included 15 patients who discontinued their drugs, mainly because of adverse effects. After 6 and 12 months, the clinical response was significantly better in those randomized to DMARD, in whom improvement ranged from 54% (for disability) to 78% (joint score) as compared with 28% and 57% for the non-DMARD patients. Radiological progression occurred slowly, and at 1 year did not differ between groups [26].

More aggressive DMARDs

Improvement with early treatment is not just reflected in the functional status. Peltoma and colleagues [27] compared intramuscular gold and sulphasalazine in the treatment of early RA. Significant intragroup improvements were noted with both treatments but no intergroup differences could be seen at 1 year. However, clinical improvement was noted earlier with sulphasalazine. Landewe and colleagues [28] compared cyclosporin with chloroquine in a 24-week trial. Both drugs were effective compared with baseline, with a significant improvement in joint count, morning stiffness and pain (cyclosporin). Intergroup differences, however, were insignificant. In the Finnish inception cohort of 142 early RA patients treated with successive DMARDs, Mottonen and colleagues [29] found a remission percentage of 22% at 2 years. A comparison was made with a Swedish cohort of 99 RA patients with a mean disease duration at entry of 11.2 months. The remission percentage at 2 years appeared to be lower (16%) and disease activity higher (as reflected by the erythrocyte sedimentation rate (ESR)) in the Swedish cohort. The percentage of patients treated with DMARDs in the Finnish cohort was 100% and in the Swedish cohort was less than 50%. At enrolment Swedish patients were older, had longer duration disease, and had higher Larsen scores and HAQ values compared with Finnish patients. There is now evidence therefore that earlier DMARD treatment may reduce joint damage.

Combination DMARDs

The fundamental concept of using combination treatment in any disease is to improve efficacy/toxicity ratio. However, with drugs with immunomodulatory potential, dual or triple therapy could be more effective. In the last few years, combination therapy for RA has been more universally accepted by rheumatologists [30].

Combination therapy in early disease has recently been studied. Nissila and colleagues [31] compared the effect of combination therapy with methotrexate, sulphasalazine, hydroxychloroquine and prednisolone to single-agent treatment with the same DMARDs as single therapy and found combination treatment to be more effective in preventing radiological progression in early RA. It was also shown that combination treatment was more effective in inducing remission compared with single-agent therapy (the respective frequencies of patients in remission in combination and single treatment groups at 3, 6, 12 and 24 months were 10 vs. 4% (NS), 24 vs. 12% ($P = 0.033$), 27 vs. 13% ($P = 0.013$) and 42 vs. 21% ($P = 0.002$)). The combination group was also found to be better at meeting the American College of Rheumatology (ACR) 50% response criteria [32]. Hagasma and colleagues [33] compared combination treatment of sulphasalazine and methotrexate with single agents in a 52-week double-blind randomized study. The dose of methotrexate in this study was 7.5–15 mg per week whereas sulphasalazine was given at the daily dose of 2–3 g. The patients had active arthritis and were rheumatoid factor positive and/or HLA-DR1 and/or DR4 positive. All three treatment groups had a substantial response to therapy and although most efficacy variables improved in favour of combination therapy, there were neither statistically nor clinically significant differences between the three groups. The total number of side-effects did not differ in the three treatment groups although more nausea was noted by patients using two drugs. O'Dell and colleagues [34] have demonstrated that in RA combination therapy with methotrexate, sulphasalazine and hydroxychloroquine is more effective than either methotrexate alone or a combination of sulphasalazine and hydroxychloroquine. Of patients given triple therapy, 77% improved by at least 50%, sustained for 2 years, compared with 40% of those receiving hydroxychloroquine plus sulphasalazine ($P = 0.003$) and 33% of those on methotrexate alone ($P < 0.001$).

'Step-down' approach

With this approach combination therapy is given from the outset (to bring about rapid suppression of active disease), but later tapered to try to maintain disease suppression.

In a recent study Boers and colleagues [35] compared the effects of sulphasalazine alone with a regimen that included an induction phase with high-dose prednisolone plus methotraxate/sulphasalazine, with dose reduction for the first two and maintenance with sulphasalazine. By week 28, 72% patients in the combined treatment group and 49% in the sulphasalazine group improved according to the ACR criteria (ACR 20). Although by the end of the study patients in the combination group had reverted to the same level of disease activity as in the sulphasalazine-alone group, the retardation in hands/feet erosion score continued. There were fewer study withdrawals in the combination group than in the sulphasalazine-alone group.

'Step-up' approach

Here treatment is begun with a single DMARD and a further DMARD is added if the first one fails or ceases to be effective. On similar lines, in one double-blind study 148 patients with advanced RA partially responsive to methotrexate (up to 15 mg per week), were given cyclosporin (2.5–5 mg/kg/day) or placebo as an 'add-on' treatment. By 6 months, the group of patients who received cyclosporin in addition to methotrexate had an improvement of at least 50% in the number of tender joints compared with 27% in the placebo group ($P = 0.02$). The additional benefit was achieved without an increase in toxicity [36].

The preliminary results of a study in our department comparing sulphasalazine treatment with a combination of methotrexate and cyclosprin (remission study) in patients with early RA show benefits at 52 weeks in favour of the combination.

Role of systemic corticosteroids

Corticosteroids have potent anti-inflammatory and immunosuppressive effects and therefore produce rapid improvement in symptoms and signs of synovitis. Although systemic corticosteroids have long been used to treat RA, toxicity has always been a concern.

Controlled studies on their beneficial effects are limited. In a double-blind study, 128 patients with active RA (mean duration 1.3 years) were randomized to treatment with a fixed dose of prednisolone (7.5 mg daily) or placebo for 2 years [37]. Patients could also receive unblinded treatment with a DMARD. Patients given corticosteroids experienced an initially greater reduction in pain, joint swelling and tenderness and in disability, but no sustained improvement in function compared with the placebo group. Progression of radiological damage was slower in the prednisolone-treated group, and fewer of those without erosions of the hand and wrist at study entry developed them during the study. In the study by Boers and colleagues (see above), corticosteroid, given as a high dose at the outset but rapidly tapered, as part of triple therapy regimen, suppressed bony erosions and also improved function over 46 weeks. The study found no significant increase in toxicity, including bone mineral density, but had low power to detect a difference.

The future

The future of early treatment is likely to improve because of developments in imaging. Magnetic resonance imaging (MRI) scanning of joints in early disease with regular follow-up will generate sensitive data to assess response to early intervention. We are currently involved in a study using MRI changes as an outcome measure in patients with early arthritis treated with methotrexate (MEMRI study). Another exciting prospect would be use of biological therapy in early disease. Likely candidates for this approach are anti-tumour necrosis factor (TNF) antibodies and anti-CD4 antibodies alone or in combination with DMARDs. There is evidence now that anti-TNF treatment can suppress inflammation in RA. However, this is often a short-term effect, resulting in the need of repeated infusions which may not be cost effective. Combination with methotrexate has shown a reduction in side-effects and extension in efficacy. TNF ablation at the very beginning of the disease might prove a reasonable approach.

Conclusion

- Inflammation causes damage.
- Early suppression of inflammation avoids damage.
- Early treatment has the potential to provide long-term benefits.

References

1 Pincus T, Callahan LF. The side effects of rheumatoid arthritis: joint destruction, disability and early mortality. *Br J Rheumatol* 1993; 32 (Suppl. 1): 28–37.

2 Gabriel S, Crowson C, O'Fallon M. Mortality in rheumatoid arthritis (RA): Have we made an impact in 3 decades? *Arthritis Rheum* 1997; 1770: S327 (Abstract).

3 Smythe CJ. Therapy of rheumatoid arthritis. A pyramidal plan. *Postgrad Med J* 1972; 51: 31–9.

4 Wilske KR, Healey LA. Remodelling the pyramid. A concept whose time has come. *J Rheumatol* 1989; 16: 565–7.

5 Emery P. The Roche Rheumatology Prize Lecture: The optimal management of early rheumatoid disease: the key to preventing disability. *Br J Rheumatol* 1994; 33: 765–8.

6 Astrow AB. Rethinking cancer. *Lancet* 1994; 343: 494–5.

7 Winfield J, Young A, Williams P, Corbett M. Prospective study of the radiological changes in hands, feet and cervical spine in adult rheumatoid disease. *Ann Rheum Dis* 1983; 42: 613–18.

8 Mottonen TT. Prediction of erosiveness and rate of development of new erosions in early rheumatoid arthritis. *Ann Rheum Dis* 1988; 47: 648–53.

9 Van der Heijde DM, van Riel PL, Nuver-Zwart HH, Gribnau FW, van de Putte LB. Effects of hydroxychloroquine and sulphasalazine on progression of joint damage in rheumatoid arthritis. *Lancet* 1989; i: 1036–8.

10 Devlin J, Gough A, Huissoon A *et al.* Monoarthritis of knee does not progress to rheumatoid arthritis: evidence from 766 referrals to an early arthritis clinic. *Br J Rheumatol* 1994; 32 (Suppl. 2): 5.

11 Matthews N, Emery P, Pilling D, Akbar A, Salmon M. Subpopulations of primed T-helper cells in rheumatoid arthritis. *Arthritis Rheum* 1993; 36: 603–7.

12 Liuz G, Smith SW, McLaughlin KA *et al.* Apoptotic signals delivered through the T-cell receptor of a T-cell hybrid require the immediate early gene Nur 77 N. *Nature* 1994; 367: 281–4.

13 Young A, Cox N, Davis P. *et al.* Early rheumatoid arthritis (RA): clinical patterns and outcome during first 3 years in 207 patients. *Br J Rheumatol* 1993; 31 (Suppl.): 97.

14 Gough AK, Lilley J, Eyre S *et al.* Generalized bone loss in patients with early rheumatoid arthritis occurs early and relates to disease activity. *Lancet* 1994; 344: 23–7.

15 Devlin J, Gough A, Huissoon A *et al.* The acute phase function in early rheumatoid arthritis: C-reactive protein levels correlate with functional outcome. *J Rheumatol* 1997; 24(1): 9–13.

16 Van Leeuwen MA, Van Rijswick MH, Van der Heijde DM *et al.* The acute phase response in relation to radiographic progression in early rheumatoid arthritis: a prospective study during the first three years of the disease. *Br J Rheumatol* 1993; 32 (Suppl. 3): 9–13.

17 Van der Heijde DMFM, Van Riel PLCM, Van Leeuwen MA *et al.* Prognostic factors for radiographic damage and physical disability in early rheumatoid arthritis. *Br J Rheumatol* 1992; 8: 519–26.

18 Devlin J, Lilley J, Gough A *et al.* Clinical associations of dual-energy X-ray absorptiometry measurement of hand bone mass in rheumatoid arthritis. *Br J Rheumatol* 1996; 35: 1256–62.

19 Emery P. Early rheumatoid arthritis: time to aim for remission? *Ann Rheum Dis* 1995; 54: 944–7.

20 Bradley LA. Psychological dimensions of rheumatoid arthritis. In: Wolfe F, Pincus T, eds. *Rheumatoid Arthritis: Pathogenesis, Assessment, Outcome and Treatment.* New York: Marcel Dekker, 1994: 273–95.

21 Symmons DPM, Barrett EM, Bankhead CR *et al.* The incidence of rheumatoid arthritis in United Kingdom: results from Norfolk Arthritis Register. *Br J Rheumatol* 1994; 33: 735–9.

22 Emery P. Therapeutic approaches for early rheumatoid arthritis. How early? How agressive? *Br J Rheumatol* 1995; 34 (Suppl. 2): 87–90.

23 Young A, Cox N, Davis P *et al.* Treatment patterns over 20 years in 577 patients with. *Rheumatoid Arthritis* 1994; 37 (Suppl. 9): S258.

24 Borg G, Allander E, Lund B *et al.* Auranofin improves outcome in early rheumatoid arthritis: results from a 2 year double-blind placebo controlled study. *J Rheumatol* 1988; 15: 1747–54.

25 Egsmose C, Lund B, Borg G *et al.* Patients with rheumatoid arthritis benefit from early second line therapy: 5 year follow-up of a prospective double-blind placebo controlled study. *J Rheumatol* 1995; 22: 2208–13.

26 Van der Heide A, Jacobs JWG, Bijlsma JWJ *et al.* The effectiveness of early treatment with 'second-line' anti-rheumatic drugs: a randomized control trial. *Ann Intern Med* 1996; 124: 699–707.

27 Peltoma R, Paimela L, Helve T *et al.* Comparison of intra-muscular gold and sulphasalazine in the treatment of early rheumatoid arthritis: a one year prospective study. *Scand J Rheumatol* 1995; 24: 330–5.

28 Landewe RB, Goei The HS, Van Rijthoven AW *et al.* A randomized double-blind, 24-week controlled study of low-dose cyclosporin versus chloroquine for early rheumatoid arthritis. *Arthritis Rheum* 1994; 37: 637–43.

29 Mottonen T, Paimela L, Ahonen J *et al.* Outcome in patients treated with early rheumatoid arthritis treated according to the 'saw-tooth' strategy. *Arthritis Rheum* 1996; 39: 996–1005.

30 O'Dell J. Combination DMARD therapy for rheumatoid arthritis: apparent universal acceptance. *Arthritis Rheum* 1997; 119: S50 (Abstract).

31 Nissila M, Laasonen L, Leirisalo-Repo M. Superiority of DMARD. combination therapy to single drug treatment strategy in early rheumatoid arthritis: Progression of structural joint damage. *Arthritis Rheum* 1997; 117: S50 (Abstract).

32 Mottonen T, Hannonen P, Korpela M. Superiority of DMARD. combination to single treatment strategy in early rheumatoid arthritis. *Remissions Arthritis Rheum* 1997; 1128: S212 (Abstract).

33 Hagasma C, Van der Putte L, Van Riel P *et al.* Sulphasalazine, methotrexate: the combination in early RA. A double-blind randomized study. *Arthritis*

Rheum 1995; 38 (Suppl.): S368
(Abstract).

34 O'Dell JR, Haire CE, Erikson N *et al.*
Treatment of rheumatoid arthritis with
methotrexate alone, sulphasalazine and
hydroxychloroquine or a combination
of all three medications. *N Engl J Med*
1996; 334: 1287–91.

35 Boers M, Ver hoeven AC, Markusse
HM *et al.* Randomized comparison
of combined step-down prednisolone,
methotrexate and sulphasalazine with
sulphasalazine alone in early

rheumatoid arthritis. *Lancet* 1997;
350: 309–18.

36 Tugwell P, Pincus T, Yocum D *et al.*
Combination therapy with cyclosporine
and methotrexate in severe rhematoid
arthritis. *N Engl J Med* 1995; 333:
137–41.

37 Kirwan JR. Arthritis and Rheumatism
Council Low-dose Glucocorticoid Study
Group. The effect of glucocorticoids
on joint destruction in rheumatoid
arthritis. *N Engl J Med* 1995;
333: 142–6.

8: The case for conservative treatment in rheumatoid arthritis

H.A. Capell and K. Chaudhuri

Introduction

Rheumatologists have been accused of accepting preliminary and incomplete data on which to base therapeutic decisions. Enthusiasm to help patients with a chronic disabling disease such as rheumatoloid arthritis (RA) is understandable. Unfortunately such enthusiasm may lead to treatments that leave sound evidence-based medicine far behind. For every report of successful combination disease-modifying anti-rheumatic drug (DMARD) therapy there are several negative studies. However, such is the publication bias against negative studies and physician desire to help their patients that the positive studies may assume prominence out of proportion to their true significance. Thus physicians wishing to treat RA patients vigorously must ensure decisions are backed up by carefully scrutinized data, however, difficult this may be [1]. Compared with the large-scale trials in cardiovascular disease and oncology our efforts as rheumatologists appear puny. There are a number of reasons for this discrepancy, not least the lack of an easily identifiable outcome in RA. Death is a readily measured endpoint in other specialties but while premature mortality is a feature of RA [2–5] it is not a useful outcome measure in short- to medium-term studies (except when alarmingly frequent).

Against this background the treatment of RA has evolved agonizingly slowly over the past decade. There has been increasing recognition regarding potential toxicity of non-steroidal anti-inflammatory drugs (NSAIDs) and interest in selective cox II NSAIDs [6]. While the need for additional DMARDs is recognized, a number of experimental compounds have had to be withdrawn [7]. The most valuable 'new' second-line drugs have been sulphasalazine and methotrexate—enthusiasm for sulphasalazine in Europe and for methotrexate in North America has each crossed the Atlantic and both drugs are widely used. There has in addition been reappraisal of other conventional agents and of the potential for combination therapy. Meta-analyses have provided useful pointers but are widely acknowledged as a poor substitute for large, well-conducted, prospective studies [8]. More recently, clinical trials with biological agents have met with variable success [9]. Cost implications for new treatment options are increasingly posing additional hurdles.

The traditional approach to the treatment of RA was the therapeutic pyramid where NSAIDs and simple analgesics were initially tried in addition to general measures, and DMARDs only introduced if these failed after a period of months. Increasing knowledge about the pathogenesis, long-term morbidity and the importance of early treatment in RA has led to calls for a more vigorous approach [10,11]. Wilske and Healy [12] suggested a step-down bridge approach with a vigorous early treatment gradually tapered off and this approach has more recently been used by Boers and colleagues in the COBRA study in the Netherlands [13]. Nevertheless the concept of 'remission induction' as a useful strategy on its own is a fallacy—it is clear that intensive therapy needs to be maintained if beneficial effect is to be sustained and such therapy is associated with unacceptable toxicity. Fries has described a 'saw-tooth' strategy which recognizes the need to modify therapy according to effect and the occurrence of adverse events [14]. While Emery and Salmon [10] and others have proposed early aggressive therapy in the belief that this will reduce long-term morbidity and functional decline, medium- to long-term results from this approach are not yet available.

RA is a notoriously variable [15] and capricious disease and it is clear that any one treatment strategy will not be ideal for all patients. This complex disease has many factors—some known, the majority unknown—affecting pathogenesis, progression and outcome. At present the absence of surrogate markers of disease progression and our lack of knowledge regarding the mechanism of action of most of the commonly used disease modifying agents contribute to difficult therapeutic goals in RA. If we knew which RA patients would pursue a relatively benign disease course, management decisions would be much simpler. These features are further compounded by the fact that the results of short-term clinical trials in a highly selected patient group often cannot be translated into long-term control of disease of patients in a 'true-to-life' out-patient clinic situation [16]. There is also the problem of idiosyncratic adverse reactions to therapies and true drug treatment failures. Thus, the clinical rheumatologist is often obliged to admit that the treatment of RA is more 'art' than science.

What is conservative treatment? (Table 8.1)

The purpose of this chapter is to make a case for 'conservative' treatment for RA. It is essential to emphasize that 'conservative' treatment does *not*

Table 8.1 The conservative approach to management of rheumatoid arthritis.

Multidisciplinary team input
Sustained education and support
Minimal use NSAIDs
Sequential use of single DMARDs
Targeted corticosteroid: preferably intra-articular
Attention to lifestyle factors
Documentation and vigorous treatment of co-morbidity especially sepsis
Appropriate surgical intervention
Aggressive therapy in minority with life-threatening disease

NSAID, non-steroidal anti-inflammatory drug; DMARD, disease-modifying anti-rheumatic drug.

Table 8.2 Why avoid aggressive therapy for the majority?

Uncertainties
    Diagnosis (in some)
    Prognosis (in most)
    Value of multiple treatments
Anxieties
    Patient and family
    Physician and team
Fallacy
    That any Rx reliably induces remission
Toxicities
    Overlapping
    Cumulative
    Late
Efficacy
    Limited
Resources
    May be better targeted more appropriately to sustained approach
Compliance
    More difficult with complex regimen

mean late treatment. Rather, we consider this to be therapy that provides a better efficacy/toxicity ratio and which is more likely to be accepted by the majority of patients and sustained over a prolonged period. We shall try to highlight these advantages but acknowledge that there are shortcomings. We also touch on the evidence that combination therapies may provide better alternatives—this aspect will, however, be addressed in detail in Chapters 13 and 14. A summary of the reasons for avoiding aggressive therapy is shown in Table 8.2.

All RA patients should receive multidisciplinary team input and sustained education and support.

Multidisciplinary team input

The vital role of all the other health professionals involved in looking after patients with chronic debilitating rheumatic diseases should never be neglected. The contribution of physiotherapy, occupational therapy, social work and community support cannot be overemphasized. Therefore, as a part of the holistic 'conservative' approach, it is essential to emphasize the importance of the role of 'kinder and gentler' therapies—pain control, joint-protection principles, exercise therapy and splints. This input, with varying emphasis according to need, should be continued throughout the disease course.

Sustained education and support

All patients should be educated by the multidisciplinary team in connection with what is known about RA and what can be done to modify their prognosis. The recently available literature about the adverse effects of lifestyle factors, e.g. smoking and obesity [17], need to be stressed and support given to change behaviour likely to have an adverse effect on outcome. RA patients have been shown to have high distress scores for emotional reactions (as measured by Nottingham Health Profile) [18]. Avoidance of learned helplessness and allowing patients a feeling of control over their disease, however tenuous, is of great importance [19,20]. Social deprivation has been shown to be associated with poorer function in RA [21] and thus efforts relating to education should be particularly vigorous in disadvantaged patients.

The patient's point of view: avoiding 'learned helplessness'

When managing a chronic, progressive disease such as rheumatoid arthritis an effective working relationship between the patient and the treating physician is of paramount importance. In order to participate in the decision-making process the patient must have access to adequate information regarding their disease and therapeutic options. This aspect of care is integral to the success of the 'conservative' approach. 'Enfranchised' patients are able to take an active role in decisions regarding the initiation and continuation of all therapies. Unless this approach is used there are likely to be problems with compliance in the long term. Patients and physicians who move rapidly through a number of DMARDs without giving each a fair trial rapidly run out of options. Patient helplessness is marked by emotional, motivational and cognitive deficits and is an impediment to effective management of RA. The combination of these factors leads to a non-compliant patient—one who readily tries unproven remedies, has excessive reliance on the healthcare system and has difficulty in coming to terms with the disease. Callaghan and Pincus have indicated that the rheumatology community faces important challenges in endeavouring to understand the complexities and contributions of self care in health studies [20]. These authors have also shown that helplessness is a component of the association between lower formal education level and premature mortality in RA [19].

In her review on patient education in RA, Hill emphasizes this need for adequate patient education [22]. Effective management of RA relies upon the patients' willingness to cooperate and their ability to comply with self-care activities. This can only be achieved if they are able to:

• employ coping techniques;
• tailor their daily exercise programme;
• plan rest/activity periods;
• vary drug usage according to the symptoms.

There is some evidence that health education may reduce costs [23].

Patient choice

The affected individual with RA runs the gauntlet of a protracted disease, discomfort, disability, sometimes loss of income and, in some countries, cost. In addition, medications inevitably have their down side, namely toxicity or lack of efficacy. Clearly, the ideal approach is to practice treatment based on best evidence. However, in the absence of compelling evidence in favour of combination therapy or biological agents, patients should always be given the choice of a conventional approach if they have misgivings about aggressive treatment, about the toxicities of multiple second-line agents, or experimental medication. Many do, however, recognize the importance of research for improved treatment options in the future and willingly agree to participate in studies. In this setting well-designed studies with adequate power are essential, and data should always be reported (negative or positive).

Because second-line medications are associated with significant drop-out rates [24,25] and multiple second-line therapies in combination are likely to produce more side-effects in the longer term (9% in one meta-analysis) [26], it is particularly important to ensure that patients understand the implications of therapy, the adverse events that lead to obligatory cessation of treatment (even if effective) and by contrast, those which can be reduced to acceptable levels by lower doses.

Co-morbidity

Vigorous treatment of co-morbidity, particularly problems such as sepsis, anaemia, osteoporosis, peptic ulcer, hypertension, infections and depression is essential. There is no evidence that aggressive anti-rheumatic treatment improves the well-documented premature mortality [2–5,27–29] of RA, whereas there is abundant evidence to support aggressive treatment of co-morbidity, e.g. hypertension. In almost all series, infection and renal disease are more likely to lead to death than would be expected—this is highly relevant to the potential toxicities of aggressive treatments [2–5].

Optimum use of sequential DMARDs

The term conservative applies to the use of a single DMARD at a time, increased to maximal dose unless: (i) there are compelling reasons in an individual for using a combination; or (ii) a new agent is being introduced in the face of loss of effect of the initial one and both are given in combination for a bridging period. Despite convincing evidence of DMARD effect [30] and the lack of response to placebo [31,32] many patients early on in their disease are resistant to the idea of taking a more powerful drug. It is important to give both verbal and written information to the patient and, if necessary, family and friends, and involve the general practitioner as well as the specialist service in the monitoring and follow-up of such patients. Individual monitoring cards should reflect both safety and efficacy monitoring and patients who are aware of the relevance of the documented findings are more readily able to cooperate with the necessary follow-up, which has to be long-term.

At present the number of DMARDs available is limited and, in a disease which may last 30–40 years, it is essential that a drug should not be discontinued without good cause. It is thus important to try and persuade patients to cope with the temporary discomfort of nitritoid reactions to gold injections, nausea and central nervous system effects from sulphasalazine, gastrointestinal upset from methotrexate, and taste alteration with penicillamine, all of which will reverse if treatment is continued. At the same time it is important to recognize more serious side-effects and adjust the dose of the DMARD promptly or withdraw treatment altogether. It is in this area where combination therapy poses many problems, particularly if drugs with overlapping toxicities are used. It is wasteful of resources and exposes patients to unnecessary potential toxicity to use combination therapy where one drug will suffice.

It is noteworthy that some patients feel that a DMARD is losing effect after they have been on it for a number of years and wish to alter therapy. When they do so, however, sometimes against advice, their disease often flares still further and it is at this time that a bridge of adding a second agent or alternatively using more intra-articular injections may be necessary. Studies of attempted withdrawal of DMARDs have shown a flare in the patients on placebo [33,34] reversed in one study when treatment was reintroduced [35]. Fries and colleagues have shown reduction in long-term disability associated with consistent DMARD use [36].

Influence of psychological outlook

It has recently been shown [37] that patients who are optimistic at the outset of DMARD therapy are more likely to continue treatment. Concentrating on improving psychological well being may be just as important as aggressive therapy. It is essential to encourage patient participation in all therapeutic decisions.

The use of corticosteroids

Judicious use of intra-articular steroid injections is an integral part of the conservative approach. The use of corticosteroids is an emotive topic for many patients, particularly those who have seen friends and neighbours develop Cushingoid side-effects. While Kirwan has suggested that early use of corticosteroids will lead to a reduced number of erosions at 2 years (but no sustained clinical benefit beyond 9 months) [38], Leigh and Fries have documented increased morbidity and mortality in patients who are on long-term steroids [27]. Fries has devised a toxicity index for DMARDs [39] related to symptoms, laboratory abnormalities and hospitalizations attributable to DMARD therapy. Using this system hydroxychloroquine was least toxic (score 1.38) followed by intramuscular gold (score 2.27) whereas prednisolone scored 3.83 (comparable to methotrexate and azathioprine). In addition he considered that the American Rheumatism Association Medical Information System (ARAMIS) might not have captured all events related to prednisolone toxicity. Others have also demonstrated more adverse events with long-term steroid without sustained benefit [27,28,40]. We are thus left with the dilemma of early use which may help erosions (but which does not lead to sustained clinical benefit), and the difficult problem of cumulative toxicity which is often irreversible. A more rational approach within our conservative management framework is to target individual joints with intra-articular steroids—if necessary both large and small joints—while introducing a DMARD or increasing the dose. Intramuscular or oral steroid could be used intermittently at times of particular stress.

What prevents early aggressive treatment of RA?
(see Table 8.2)

Difficulties with diagnosis

The timing of second-line therapy in early rheumatoid arthritis has always been a contentious issue. Some of the problems relate to making a diagnosis of rheumatoid arthritis. The American College of Rheumatology (ACR) criteria originally proposed in 1958 and subsequently revised in 1987 have been extensively used but are essentially tools for epidemiological classification rather than clinical diagnosis of an individual patient [41–43]. Wolfe has shown that RA prognosis depends in part on how RA is defined —'clinical' RA has a worse and epidemiological RA a better prognosis [15]. He also points out that seronegative polyarthritis confounds the assessment of RA since it has a better prognosis.

There is a wide differential diagnosis for an inflammatory polyarthritis. The patient with nodular seropositive erosive disease poses no diagnostic difficulties even if we know that therapy is likely to be challenging. However, in other patients uncertainties arise, e.g. those who have Raynaud's phenomenon, polyarthritis and weakly positive anti-nuclear antibody (ANA) may well evolve into a connective tissue disorder and a suitable choice of a DMARD is vital under these circumstances. Hydroxychloroquine is a valuable option in such patients—antimalarials will often give symptomatic relief while allowing time for other possible manifestations of connective tissue (CT) disease to appear and permit suitable interventions appropriate for that diagnosis.

In addition, a seronegative reactive arthritis to a gut-associated pathogen or a sexually acquired disease may be difficult to differentiate from early RA. Here sulphasalazine may be valuable but a too vigorous approach with multidrug treatment seems inappropriate.

Patients identified in hospital-based clinical rheumatology settings rarely have self-limiting disease, particularly if they have rheumatoid factor in their sera [15,43]. Patients in the clinic setting with uncontrolled synovitis which is thought to be rheumatoid arthritis, usually polyarticular but occasionally oligoarticular, require a decision regarding initiation of second-line therapy.

The earlier patients with synovitis/inflammatory polyarthritis are referred for specialist attention, the more difficult diagnosis will be. Those physicians who see only late severe disease will have little difficulty in diagnosis but will have missed a valuable opportunity to introduce the variety of options noted above which comprise comprehensive conservative therapy.

A rheumatologist who always finds RA easy to diagnose has not noticed the pitfalls!

Difficulties with prognosis

The most common concerns expressed by patients with recently diagnosed RA relate to immediate effect on lifestyle, work and family, and long-term outcome. It remains surprisingly difficult to provide accurate prognostic information in an individual; this is frustrating for patient and physician alike. While seropositivity, high acute-phase measurements [44], involvement of many joints, poor function as measured by initial Health Assessment Questionnaire (HAQ) [45], early erosion on X-ray and the possession of disease-associated alleles are all associated with a worse prognosis, exceptions are frequent, and no single test or combination of tests gives entirely reliable information. Thus, an overall assessment of prognosis is both challenging and notoriously unreliable. Poor educational opportunities [19], poor function (HAQ score) [45] and socio-economic deprivation [21] are certainly associated with a poor outcome but are difficult to modify.

The extent to which some of these factors can be modified will be discussed later; however, clearly at this stage genetic make-up and past deprivation cannot be altered.

Patient perception and acceptance of treatment options

With the introduction of newer drugs and biological agents, rheumatologists have been increasingly inclined to treat patients who are thought to have early RA with DMARDs. However, proponents of delay rightly point out that some cases of inflammatory polyarthritis may remit or become less severe and be quite adequately controlled by supportive measures alone. In the absence of accurate prognostic markers this group of patients would be subjected to unnecessary intensive therapy with allied costs in time, money and exposure to potential side-effects. It is still not clearly known whether DMARDs started within 1–2 months of disease onset or before erosions have occurred will confer any further benefit or even arrest the disease process. Although the principle of early intervention is an attractive one (in an attempt to preserve good function and prevent disability by modifying the course of the disease) we still do not have any agent that is capable of achieving this goal [46]. On the other hand we do know that patients have limited survival time on any given second-line agent which may have to be stopped either due to toxicity or ineffectiveness [24,25]. Therefore one of the problems related to an early aggressive approach is that as patients work their way through second-line agents or slow acting anti-rheumatic drugs (SAARDs), cytotoxic drugs may be invoked earlier in the disease and this is an important point when considering possible late development of neoplasia. What we really need is the ability to reliably identify at an early stage those patients with poor prognosis who can then be singled out for early aggressive therapy.

The popular press often emphasizes drug toxicity without providing a balanced view of potential benefit. This may influence the willingness of RA patients to embark on treatment which they perceive to be hazardous

—whether or not this view is rational. Clinicians vary in their degree of aggression in treating RA, and the timing of treatment has been contentious. Many of these uncertainties percolate through to patients, their friends and relatives.

The vast majority of studies of early aggressive DMARDs or combination therapy report only on those select few included in the study, and provide little or no information about those who refused to participate, nor their reasons for refusal. Such information is vital if the impact of a marginal effect from a combination regimen is to be evaluated in terms of its likely influence on the RA population. Similarly some otherwise well-conducted studies do not account for all patients enrolled—particularly those who dropped out for reasons not clearly related to side-effects or loss of effect. This constitutes a major methodological shortcoming and again has implications for the impact of therapy on RA outcome.

Patients who feel that they are able to cope with their current disease manifestations are not always easily persuaded to undertake intensive treatment regimens—particularly when as noted above prognostic uncertainty is common. In addition, good clinical practice dictates disclosure of potential side-effects. Even if uncommon, these often alarm patients who do not perceive their disease to be life threatening. Progression of disease may seem slow, while occurrence of side-effects may be immediate or only manifest later.

Physician anxieties

The possibility of irreversible side-effects is a major anxiety for all concerned with providing advice to RA patients. Life-threatening adverse effects to DMARDs are rare but are in the main idiosyncratic—the clinician who treats enough patients will inevitably encounter these problems. Thus, a combination of drugs, albeit in lower doses, will expose patients more rapidly to the possibility of severe reactions. In most instances these cannot be foreseen or avoided. The known susceptibilities DR3 [47,48], and poor sulphoxidation status [49,50] in relation to gold and d-penicillamine is not of practical value. Mutations of thiopurine methyltransferase gene in relation to azathioprine [51] may with further research become a practical tool. Being female, older, and with pre-existing lung disease may suggest caution is needed with methotrexate but in practice a fair proportion of patients seen in hospital practice fit in just such a category. In addition there is some evidence that drugs such as methotrexate may be implicated as an associated factor in deaths from infections [52] already a cause of excess morbidity and mortality in RA [5].

Increasing rheumatology services have diluted the experience of each individual clinician. However, the anxiety which arises when an RA patient develops sudden pancytopenia on gold or methotrexate [53,54], leucopenia on sulphasalazine [55], or life-threatening pneumonitis on methotrexate [56] is a difficult area of clinical practice. Feelings of guilt from those who started treatment are inevitable even if inappropriate. How much more of a problem if a newly diagnosed patient with mild disease had been persuaded to embark on aggressive treatment against his or her wishes? Risk/benefit ratios assume a different dimension under these circumstances.

Compliance

RA severity is associated with fewer years of formal education and some patients are illiterate, making delivery of information more difficult [57]. Even a patient who has a thorough understanding of goals of treatments may fail to take medication as directed—the Royal Pharmaceutical Society has estimated that up to 50% of patients with chronic disease do not take their medication in fully therapeutic doses [58] leading to increased costs and wasted resources. Patients who are taking a complicated dose regimen or feel they have been persuaded to take multiple treatments against their wishes, are less likely to comply.

Patients readily turn to alternative remedies rather than brave what they perceive as less compassionate care with multiple 'dangerous' drug therapies on offer—66% of Canadian rheumatic patients resort to this alternative approach [59]. While it has been pointed out that 'the battle for the minds of our patients must be fought more aggressively' [60] rheumatologists need to be sure that the ground on which such battles are fought is sound—a difficult task!

Cornerstones of conservative treatment of RA

Radiological progression: the fallacy that all damage is early

Rheumatologists have been criticized for failure to demonstrate an effect of therapies on radiological progression of disease [61]. To some extent the symptomatic benefit of DMARDs precludes sustained placebo groups [62], although interestingly Kirwan was able to perform a placebo-controlled study of oral low-dose steroid [38]. However, his patients were all also on a DMARD and the symptomatic benefit of prednisolone was short lived, unlike that of DMARDs which, if tolerated, usually provide sustained benefit for prolonged periods. Van der Heidje [63] used hydroxychloroquine, a relatively 'weak' DMARD but one with undoubted symptomatic benefit as a comparative treatment in a study with sulphasalazine and showed slowing of erosions with sulphasalazine. Nevertheless no therapy has been shown to halt the progress of RA whether given singly or in combination, early or late.

It has been claimed that most radiological progression occurs in the first 2 years of RA [64] but clinical experience as well as some well-conducted studies [65–67] contradict this claim. Any clinician who treats RA over the long term is only too aware of the succession of joints that show radiological damage over the years. Thus, therapeutic strategies need to be consistently maintained over many years.

What can be achieved with single DMARDs?

In pursuing the conservative approach it is essential to be aware of what can be achieved with individual DMARDs given singly, and compare these results with 'successful' combinations.

First, individual DMARDs can be given to patients of all ages, disease duration and either sex with a reasonable expectation of success [68]. Secondly, all have a high drop-out rate over the medium term although methotrexate may be slightly better tolerated [69].

The effectiveness of early treatment with DMARDs was evaluated in 238 recently diagnosed patients [70]. Those receiving immediate treatment were significantly better at 12 months in terms of disability, pain, joint score and erythrocyte sedimentation rate (ESR). The case for early use of a DMARD is not disputed.

Felson's meta-analysis has shown what can be expected of individual DMARDs in a study setting and that intramuscular gold, sulphasalazine, methotrexate and d-penicillamine have broadly similar effects when given singly [60]. Changes in articular index of joint tenderness and ESR from his analysis and comparable figures from Glasgow collected analysis [25] are shown in Table 8.3. These changes are mirrored by improvements in pain, morning stiffness, and global assessment made by patients and physicians and functional outcomes. However, it must be noted that there have been no trials performed with sufficient statistical power to prove unequivocally that there are no differences in efficacy between individual agents. Fries and colleagues [36] have shown an association between consistent DMARD use and improvement in long-term functional outcome. What no one has been able to show to date is that more aggressive early therapy gives long-term better outcome, although Boers [13] has some preliminary short-term results favouring this approach (unfortunately with a therapeutic regimen that could not be sustained in the long term). Combination therapy might work because it selects some patients who respond to one drug while others respond to another drug. It might be argued that rheumatologists could use single agents

Table 8.3 Efficacy of disease-modifying anti-rheumatic drugs (DMARDs) given singly. Decrease in (a) articular index of joint tenderness (AI) and (b) erythrocyte sedimentation rate (ESR) during DMARD therapy.

	Felson meta-analysis n = 5343	Glasgow collected analysis n = 1140	
	Mean change	Median change	Mean change
(a) *Articular index*			
Placebo	5		
Auranofin	8	10	
Methotrexate	12	8	
d-penicillamine	9	15†	
Sulphasalazine	12*	10	9
IM gold	9	9	8
(b) *Erythrocyte sedimentation rate*			
Placebo	1	2	
Auranofin	9	19	
Methotrexate	12	22	
d-penicillamine	22	29	
Sulphasalazine	24*	31	28
IM gold	19	31	30

* 3/7 studies from Glasgow.
† High initial AI.

sequentially to establish the same endpoint and avoid unnecessary over-lapping toxicities. True additional benefit from more than one DMARD would of course be highly beneficial so an open mind in this respect is essential.

How can DMARD therapy be enhanced?

As noted above all DMARDs are associated with many side-effects, some of which are common and minor, and others potentially serious. Treatment terminations are common, especially with long-term follow-up. Felson's meta-analysis [71] showed that methotrexate was slightly less toxic than gold, d-penicillamine and sulphasalazine, but had higher rates of discontinuation of therapy for 'other' reasons.

Treating early is easier—fewer co-morbidities intervene. The Early RA Study (ERAS) looked at second-line therapy in early rheumatoid arthritis and showed continuation rates of 78% on sulphasalazine (SASP) and intramuscular gold and 75% on d-penicillamine at the end of 2 years [72]. SASP was the first-choice second-line agent in all the ERAS centres and had a better risk/benefit profile. The Dutch inception cohort study [73] which looked at survival on SASP and methotrexate by rank order concluded that SASP was used for longer periods compared with hydroxychloroquine and intramuscular gold whether it was used as a first or second SAARD. There was also no difference in survival time between SASP and methotrexate. The SASP group had a mild toxicity profile compared with methotrexate and the drop-out due to lack of efficacy was lowest in the SASP and methotrexate groups. Fries has compared the relative toxicity of DMARDs [39] and assigned toxicity scores of 1.38 to hydroxychloroquine, 2.27 to intramuscular gold, 3.38 to d-penicillamine, 3.82 to methotrexate and 3.92 to azathioprine (lowest score = least toxicity). ARAMIS data did not include sulphasalazine which was not extensively used in the USA at that time. Thus, there is some evidence to support a hierarchy amongst available options but in practice most patients will require a number of DMARDs over the decades of their disease and many will exhaust currently available options.

Long-term studies [69,74] show still higher drop-out rates. Thus, the likelihood of patients staying on aggressive combination in the long term seems remote. Clearly research into new therapies is vital.

Pitfalls of combination therapy

For the purposes of this section of our discussion, combination therapy refers to the use of more than one DMARD at any given time. Combinations of second-line drugs with NSAIDs and either oral or intra-articular steroids are routine practice and need not be considered further. The concept of combining two immunomodulating drugs which might have different sites of action is logical and attractive conceptually. However, as we do not know the exact modes of action of second-line agents, the design of different combinations has largely been empirical and in most reported studies disappointing.

Rheumatologists have long realized that all DMARDs had limitations and sought to enhance their effect. Combination therapy for rheumatoid arthritis has been used for decades [75]. McCarty and Carrera published a series of 17 patients treated with a combination of cyclophosphamide, azathioprine and hydroxychloroquine in 1982 and sparked off a renewed interest in reassessment of combinations [75]. Most combination studies yielded negative results until relatively recently when two studies [76,77] proved positive.

What, however, is the degree of response to single agents compared with combinations? O'Dell and colleagues [76] studied 102 RA patients over 2 years and randomly allocated them to methotrexate alone, a combination of sulphasalazine and hydroxychloroquine, or all three drugs. Using a composite index 33% of methotrexate alone, 40% of sulphasalazine +

hydroxychloroquine and 77% (24/31) of three-drug combination had 50% improvement. The numbers of patients in each group were, however, small, raising the possibility of a type I error. If one compares his results with 200 RA patients randomly allocated to sulphasalazine or d-penicillamine given singly [78] 69% of sulphasalazine- and 72% of d-penicillamine-treated patients achieved 50% or more improvement in morning stiffness over 2 years and 42% sulphasalazine, and 56% of d-penicillamine, 50% or more improvement in ESR. Basing far-reaching conclusions on either study alone (particularly since numbers are small in each) seems misguided. Meta-analyses have obvious disadvantages: nevertheless, that of Felson [26] clearly showed minimal benefit from combination therapy. When endeavouring to study hydroxychloroquine (HCQ)/placebo as step-up therapy in 190/440 patients with an incomplete response to gold [79] 48/190 (25%) patients who had a suboptimal response at 6 months refused to take part in an additional treatment arm despite physician advice to the contrary. The patients' perception of response to intramuscular gold was such that at that stage further treatment was not warranted (in any event the study was to provide negative results—the combination provided unhelpful).

In addition to problems associated with small patient numbers the use of composite indices of effect may give an inflated idea of efficacy of therapy. Our brief is not to discuss the pros and cons of combination therapy *per se* but to raise a few cautionary points which we feel are important in the present climate of early aggressive therapy for RA. Most studies related to combination therapy in RA are either too small or inexact. Tugwell [80] in his review of the methodological issues relevant to the assessment of combination therapy makes a number of valid points. Sample sizes in excess of 3000 patients are needed to achieve the appropriate statistical power to detect a minimal clinically important difference between combination therapy and single drugs. The cost of designing and executing a single trial of this magnitude in RA with its inherent variability in prognosis is probably prohibitive. Tugwell and others have also argued that there is a need to standardize data that can be compared in a meaningful meta-analysis. So far such trials have not been done. The most widely quoted meta-analysis is Felson's study [26]. He and his colleagues could only identify five studies out of 214 which met the inclusion criteria for their analysis related to the efficacy and toxicity of combination therapy. In total 719 patients entered and 516 of these completed the trials. There was a very modest advantage in favour of combination therapy in terms of tender joints and ESR. Overall toxicity was 9% more with the combinations. While toxicity was not increased over 6 months in patients treated with a combination of cyclosporin and methotrexate [77] this study duration is too short for meaningful comment. Late side-effects are a feature of both drugs.

In clinical practice, rheumatologists base their decisions regarding DMARD on the published evidence as well as on personal experience with individual drugs. Both are limited. The limitations of extrapolating conclusions of short-term controlled clinical trials in the evaluation of long-term chronic diseases like RA have been highlighted by Pincus and colleagues [16]. These are particularly true for combination treatment trials. These trials are not entirely 'true to life' and have a number of intrinsic shortcomings, namely relatively short observation period, patient selection bias as a result of exclusion criteria, inflexible dosage schedules, and concomitant therapies, inadequate surrogate markers for joint damage, the fact that statistically significant results are not necessarily clinically important and the lack of capacity to detect rare side-effects. This aspect is also addressed by Wolfe [81] who observed that observational studies following controlled clinical trials may yield important information not available from controlled trials alone.

The data available from published combination trials to date at best show a marginal benefit in clinical terms. These results are over relatively short periods (6 months to 2 years) and medium- to long-term data, some observational, are urgently needed.

Using inappropriate combinations may exhaust the limited options we have at present sooner than if we use them in a sequential manner. Patients may be exposed to multiple and overlapping side-effects—which may manifest in the longer- rather than in the short-term trial period. Decisions regarding discontinuation of second-line medications, when used in combination, are often difficult when faced with side-effects which could be due to either agent.

Limited resources

In the current economic climate virtually all healthcare systems are experiencing major constraints. Therefore the issue of cost needs to be addressed as well as efficacy/toxicity ratios. One might speculate that combination of second-line drugs over a longer term could add to the cost because of increments in monitoring costs and those related to complications which may require increased frequency of out-patient visits and/or hospitalization. Yelin [82] has suggested that DMARDs add little to the overall medical costs of RA. Whether the cost of using multiple second-line agents will be offset by compensatory improvement in health status still remains to be determined. To date additional benefit in the few studies with a positive outcome have been modest.

In the UK shared care protocols are widespread and the onus of monitoring second-line therapy is primarily on the general practitioners. We have yet to evaluate whether these family practices would be willing to take on the extra burden of closer monitoring of patients on combination therapy. If not, additional resources would have to be allocated for hospital monitoring of these patients.

As noted in the discussion above, patients themselves are often reluctant to try combinations of what they perceive to be potentially toxic drugs. This can lead to difficulties with compliance in the longer term. Therefore until we can have clinically superior combinations with acceptable toxicity profiles and are able to target patients with poorer outcome selectively the general principle of *primum non nocere* should be followed. Clinicians should aim for moderate reduction in disease activity which can be sustained in the long term in the majority of patients rather than brief intensive therapy in an unrepresentative minority. We are already using DMARDs in milder disease [83] in the knowledge that very few patients with established disease remit spontaneously [84].

Funding bodies should, however, remain willing to support well-designed prospective studies. Only in this way can we hope to answer the many aspects of RA which are unclear and ameliorate a disease which leads to much suffering.

The need for breadth of vision in treating RA

The excess mortality of RA

It has long been recognized that there is an excess premature mortality in RA. In various series the standardized mortality rates for RA patients vary from 1.98 (Wichita) to 3.08 (Stanford) [5]: in Glasgow [85] in a recent series it was 2.78. Excess deaths have been shown across all causes (except cancer) with a large excess of deaths from cardiovascular and cerebrovascular causes [4]. 'Conservative' broad-based management of RA which addresses issues such as poor diet, lack of exercise, obesity, hyperlipidaemia and hypertension is more likely to have a major impact on these causes of morbidity and mortality than aggressive multiple DMARD therapy. Indeed, since the other causes of premature mortality include infection and lymphoproliferative disorders the early use of multiple cytotoxic agents and the cumulative problems of systemic corticosteroids can only be possible adverse influences. Leigh and Fries have shown an increased mortality with corticosteroid use [27]. Other experimental treatments such as total lymphoid irradiation have subsequently been shown to have an unacceptable outcome at 10 years [86]. Only the small numbers of excess deaths attributable to amyloid and to RA itself including vasculitis might be amenable to aggressive therapy. It is of course possible that RA might be an indirect contributory cause to other causes of deaths.

Effect of social deprivation on disease severity and outcome in RA

It is recognized that patients with poorer functional status (e.g. as measured by HAQ) have poorer long-term outcome and excess premature mortality [19]. McEntegart and colleagues [21] have shown that patients from more deprived areas in the west of Scotland have poorer function which is associated with greater need. In this respect there is an indication for a more aggressive approach but here the aims are political and social rather than pharmacological or biological.

Conclusion

There is at present no cure for RA and it is misleading to suggest evidence points to the contrary. Overall morbidity and mortality in RA is comparable to a delicate ecological system. Some therapeutic measures appear to have a straightforward and easily measured effect while other interventions may have far-reaching consequences—not all of which are fully understood. There is evidence that patient education, supportive care, and addressing co-morbidity, social disadvantage and depression make a substantial impact on outcome in RA. Attention to these aspects of 'conservative care' may necessitate additional resources but should not be neglected.

If it could be clearly shown that suppressing disease activity in the first few months of disease prevented later disease progression then early aggressive therapy would undoubtedly be worthwhile and could be presented to the patient in that way. Similarly if it could be shown that an intensive albeit highly toxic regimen would induce sustained remission the toxicity of the therapy might be justified to an apprehensive patient. As it is there is no cure, nor indeed has there been a recent dramatic advance in the management of RA. There remains a need for individualized broad-ranging sustained care—a considerable intellectual and professional challenge for rheumatologists and their multidisciplinary teams.

References

1 Knottnerus JA, Dinant GJ. Medicine based evidence, a prerequisite for evidence based medicine. *Br Med J* 1997; 315: 1109–10.

2 Pincus T, Callaghan LF, Sale WG *et al.* Severe functional declines, work disability, and increased mortality in seventy-five rheumatoid arthritis patients studied over nine years. *Arthritis Rheum* 1984; 27(8): 864–72.

3 Mitchell DM, Spitz PW, Young DY *et al.* Survival, prognosis, and causes of death in rheumatoid arthritis. *Arthritis Rheum* 1986; 29(6): 706–12.

4 Symmons DPM. Mortality in rheumatoid arthritis. *Br J Rheumatol* 1988; 27 (Suppl.): 44–54.

5 Wolfe F, Mitchell DM, Sibley JT *et al.* The mortality of rheumatoid arthritis. *Arthritis Rheum* 1994; 37(4): 481–94.

6 Hayllar J, Bjarnason I. NSAIDs, Cox-2 inhibitors, and the gut. *Lancet* 1995; 346: 1629.

7 Capell HA, Brzeski M. Slow drugs: slow progress? Use of slow acting antirheumatic drugs (SAARDs) in rheumatoid arthritis. *Ann Rheum Dis* 1992; 51: 424–9.

8 LeLorier J, Gregori G, Benhaddad A *et al.* Discrepancies between meta-analysis and subsequent large randomised controlled trials. *N Engl J Med* 1997; 338: 536–42.

9 Moreland L, Heck LW Jr, Koopman WJ. Biological agents for treating rheumatoid arthritis. *Arthritis Rheum* 1997; 40: 397–409.

10 Emery P, Solmon M. Early rheumatoid arthritis—time to aim for remission. *Ann Rheum Dis* 1995; 54(12): 944–7.

11 Weinblatt M. Rheumatoid arthritis: Treat now, not later. *Ann Intern Med* 1996; 124: 773–5.

12 Wilske KR, Healey LA. Challenging the therapeutic pyramid: a new look at the treatment strategies for rheumatoid arthritis. *J Rheumatol* 1990; 17 (Suppl. 25): 4–7.

13 Boers M, Verhoeven AC, Markusse HM *et al.* Randomised comparison of combined step-down prednisolone, methotrexate, and sulphasalazine with sulphasalazine alone in early rheumatoid arthritis. *Lancet* 1997; 350: 309–18.

14 Fries JF. Re-evaluating the therapeutic approach to rheumatoid arthritis: the 'sawtooth' strategy. *J Rheumatol* 1990; 17 (Suppl. 22): 12.

15 Wolfe F. The natural history of rheumatoid arthritis. *J Rheumatol* 1996; 23 (Suppl. 44): 13–22.

16 Pincus T, Stein CM. Why randomised controlled clinical trials do not depict accurately long-term outcomes in rheumatoid arthritis. Some explanations and suggestions for future studies. *Clin Exp Rheum* 1997; 15 (Suppl. 17): S27–S38.

17 Symmons DP, Bankhead CR, Harrison BJ *et al.* Blood transfusion, smoking and obesity as risk factors for the development of rheumatoid arthritis. *Arthritis Rheum* 1997; 40(11): 1955–61.

18 Houssien DA, McKenna SP, Scott DL.

The Nottingham health profile as a measure of disease activity and outcome in rheumatoid arthritis. *Br J Rheumatol* 1997; 36: 69–73.

19 Callaghan LF, Cordray DS, Walls G, Pincus T. Formal education and five-year mortality in rheumatoid arthritis: mediation by helplessness scale scores. *Arthritis Care Res* 1996; 9(6): 463–72.

20 Callahan LF, Pincus T. Education, self-care, and outcomes of rheumatic diseases: further challenges to the 'Biomedical Model' paradigm. *Arthritis Care Res* 1997; 10(5): 283–8.

21 McEntegart A, Morrison E, Capell HA *et al.* Effect of social deprivation on disease severity and outcome in patients with rheumatoid arthritis. *Ann Rheum Dis* 1997; 56: 410–13.

22 Hill J. A practical guide to patient education and information giving. *Ballière's Clin Rheumatol* 1997; 11(1): 109–27.

23 Lorig KR, Mazonon PD, Holman DR. Evidence suggesting that health education for self-management in patients with chronic arthritis has sustained health benefits while reducing health costs. *Arthritis Rheum* 1993; 36: 439–46.

24 Situnayake RD, Grindulis KA, McConkey B. Long term treatment of rheumatoid arthritis with sulphasalazine, gold, or penicillamine: a comparison using life-table methods. *Ann Rheum Dis* 1987; 46: 177–83.

25 Porter DR, McInnes I, Hunter J, Capell HA. Outcome of second line therapy in rheumatoid arthritis. *Ann Rheum Dis* 1994; 53: 812–15.

26 Felson DT, Anderson JJ, Meenan RF. The efficacy and toxicity of combination therapy in rheumatoid arthritis. *Arthritis Rheum* 1994; 37(10): 1487–91.

27 Leigh JP, Fries JF. Mortality predictors among 263 patients with rheumatoid arthritis. *J Rheumatol* 1991; 18: 1307–12.

28 Capell HA, Murphy EA, Hunter JA. Rheumatoid arthritis: workload and outcome over 10 years. *Q J Med* 1991; 79: 461–76.

29 Pincus T, Brooks RH, Callahan LF. Prediction of long term mortality in patients with rheumatoid arthritis

according to simple questionnaire and joint count measures. *Ann Intern Med* 1994; 120: 26–34.

30 Felson DT, Anderson JJ, Meenan RF. The comparative efficacy and toxicity of second-line drugs in rheumatoid arthritis. Results of two metaanalyses. *Arthritis Rheum* 1990; 33(10): 1449.

31 Paulus HE, Egger MJ, Ward JR *et al.* Analysis of improvement in individual rheumatoid arthritis patients treated with disease-modifying antirheumatoid drugs, based on the findings in patients treated with placebo. *Arthritis Rheum* 1990; 33(4): 477–84.

32 Porter DR, Capell HA. The 'natural' history of active rheumatoid arthritis over 3–6 months—an analysis of patients enrolled into trials of potential disease-modifying anti-rheumatic drugs, and treated with placebo. *Br J Rheumatol* 1993; 32: 463–6.

33 Getzsche PC, Hansen M, Stoltenberg M *et al.* Randomized, placebo controlled trial of withdrawal of slow-acting antirheumatic drugs and of observer bias in rheumatoid arthritis. *Scand J Rheumatol* 1996; 25: 194–9.

34 ten Wolde S, Breedveld FC, Hermans J *et al.* Randomized placebo controlled study of stopping second-line drugs in rheumatoid arthritis. *Lancet* 1996; 347: 347–52.

35 ten Wolde S, Hermans J, Breedveld FC, Dijkmans BAC. Effect of resumption of second line drugs in patients with rheumatoid arthritis that flared up after treatment discontinuation. *Ann Rheum Dis* 1997; 56: 235–9.

36 Fries JF, Williams CA, Morfeld D *et al.* Reduction in long-term disability in patients with rheumatoid arthritis by disease-modifying antirheumatic drug-based treated strategies. *Arthritis Rheum* 1994; 39(4): 616–22.

37 Listing J, Alten R, Brauer D *et al.* Importance of psychological well being and disease activity in termination of an initial DMARD therapy. *J Rheumatol* 1997; 24: 2097–105.

38 Kirwan JR and the Arthritis and Rheumatism Council Low-Dose Glucocorticoid Study Group. The effect of glucocorticoids on joint destruction in rheumatoid arthritis. *N Engl J Med* 1995; 333(3): 142–6.

39 Fries JF, Williams CA, Ramey D, Bloch DA. The relative toxicity of disease-modifying antirheumatic drugs. *Arthritis Rheum* 1993; 36(3): 297.

40 McDougall R, Sibley J, Haga M *et al.* Outcome in patients with rheumatoid arthritis receiving prednisone compared to matched controls. *J Rheumatol* 1994; 21: 1207–13.

41 Felson DT, Anderson JJ. Methodological and statistical approaches to criteria development in rheumatoid diseases. *Ballière's Clin Rheumatol* 1995; 9: 253–66.

42 Emery P, Symmons DPM. What is early rheumatoid arthritis? Definition and diagnosis. *Ballière's Clin Rheumatol* 1997; 11: 13–26.

43 Wolfe AD, Hall ND, Goulding NJ *et al.* Predictors of the long-term outcome of early synovitis: a 5 year follow-up study. *Br J Rheumatol* 1991; 30: 251–4.

44 Devlin J, Gough A, Huissoon A *et al.* The acute phase and function in early rheumatoid arthritis. C-reactive protein levels correlate with functional outcome. *J Rheumatol* 1997; 24: 9–13.

45 Leigh JP, Fries JF. Predictors of disability in a longitudinal sample of patients with rheumatoid arthritis. *Ann Rheum Dis* 1992; 51: 581–7.

46 Emery P, Salmon M. Early rheumatoid arthritis: time to aim for remission? *Ann Rheum Dis* 1995; 54: 944–7.

47 Madhok R, Pullar T, Capell HA *et al.* Chrysotherapy and thrombocytopenia. *Ann Rheum Dis* 1985; 44: 589–91.

48 Singal DP, Reid B, Green D *et al.* Polymorphism of major histocompatibility complex extended haplotypes bearing HLS-DR3 in patients with rheumatoid arthritis with gold induced thrombocytopenia or proteinuria. *Ann Rheum Dis* 1990; 49: 582–6.

49 Madhok R, Capell HA, Waring R. Does sulphoxidation state predict gold toxicity in rheumatoid arthritis? *Br Med J* 1987; 294: 483.

50 Emery P, Bradley H, Gough A *et al.* Increased prevalence of poor sulphoxidation in patients with rheumatoid arthritis: effect of changes in the acute phase response and second line drug treatment. *Ann Rheum Dis* 1992; 51: 318–20.

51 Black AJ, McLeod HL, Capell HA *et al.*
Thiopurine methyltransferase genotype
predicts therapy-limiting severe toxicity
from azathioprine. *Ann Int Med* 1998;
129: 716–18.

52 Alarcon GS, Tracy IC, Strand GM
et al. Survival and drug discontinuation
analyses in a large cohort of methotrexate treated rheumatoid arthritis
patients. *Ann Rheum Dis* 1995; 54:
708–12.

53 Yan A, Davis P. Gold induced marrow
suppression: a review of 10 cases.
J Rheumatol 1990; 17: 47–51.

54 Gutierrex-Urena S, Molina JF, Garvia
CO *et al.* Pancytopenia secondary to
methotrexate therapy in rheumatoid
arthritis. *Arthritis Rheum* 1996; 39(2):
272–6.

55 Marabani M, Madhok R, Capell HA,
Hunter JA. Leucopenia during
sulphasalazine treatment for rheumatoid
arthritis. *Ann Rheum Dis* 1989;
48: 505–7.

56 Ohosone Y, Okano Y, Kameda H *et al.*
Clinical characteristics of patients with
rheumatoid arthritis and methotrexate
induced pneumonitis. *J Rheumatol*
1997; 24: 2299–303.

57 Callaghan LF, Pincus T. Formal
education level as a significant marker
of clinical status in RA. *Arthritis
Rheum* 1988; 31: 1346–57.

58 Holland M. Compliance helps keep
kidneys. *Medical Interface* November,
1997; 915–16.

59 Boisset M, Fitzcharles MA. Alternative
medicine use by rheumatology patients
in a universal health care setting.
J Rheumatol 1994; 21: 148–52.

60 Ames BN, Gold LS. Alternative
therapies—medicine, magic, or
quackery. Who is winning the battle?
J Rheumatol 1997; 24(12): 2276–7.

61 Iannuzzi L, Dawson N, Zein N *et al.*
Does drug therapy slow radiographic
deterioration in rheumatoid arthritis?
N Engl J Med 1983; 309(17): 10234–7.

62 Pullar T, Capell HA. A rheumatological
dilemma: is it possible to modify the
course of rheumatoid arthritis? Can we
answer the question? *Ann Rheum Dis*
1985; 44: 134–40.

63 van der Heidje DM, van Riel PL,
Nuver-Zwart IH *et al.* Effects of
hydroxychloroquine and sulphasalazine

on progress of joint damage in
rheumatoid arthritis. *Lancet* 1989;
i: 1036–8.

64 Fuchs HA, Kaye JJ, Callahan LF *et al.*
Evidence of significant radiographic
damage in rheumatoid arthritis within
the first 2 years of disease. *J Rheumatol*
1989; 16: 585–91.

65 Scott DL, Coulton BL, Popert AJ. Long
term progression of joint damage in
rheumatoid arthritis. *Ann Rheum Dis*
1986; 45: 373–8.

66 Sharp JT, Wolfe F, Mitchell DM, Bloch
DA. The progression of erosion and
joint space narrowing scores in
rheumatoid arthritis during the first
twenty-five years of disease. *Arthritis
Rheum* 1991; 34(6): 660–8.

67 Kaarela K, Kautiainen H. Continuous
progression of radiological destruction
in seropositive rheumatoid arthritis.
J Rheumatol 1997; 24L: 1285–7.

68 Capell HA, Porter DR, Madhok R,
Hunter JA. Second line (disease
modifying) treatment in rheumatoid
arthritis: which drug for which patient?
Ann Rheum Dis 1993; 52: 423–8.

69 Wolfe F, Hawley DJ, Cathey MA.
Termination of slow acting antirheumatic therapy in rheumatoid arthritis: a
14-year prospective evaluation of 1017
consecutive starts. *J Rheumatol* 1990;
17(8): 994–1002.

70 van der Heide A, Jacobs JWG, Bijlsma
JWJ *et al.* The effectiveness of early
treatment with 'second line' anti-
rheumatic drugs. A randomized,
controlled trial. *Ann Intern Med* 1996;
124: 699–707.

71 Felson DT, Anderson JJ, Menan RF.
The comparative efficacy and toxicity
of second line drugs in rheumatoid
arthritis. *Arthritis Rheum* 1990;
33: 1449–61.

72 Young A. Short term outcomes in
recent-onset rheumatoid arthritis. *Br J
Rheumatol* 1995; 34 (Suppl. 2): 79–86.

73 van Gestel AM, Haagsma CJ, Furst DE,
van Riel PLCM. Treatment of early
rheumatoid arthritis patients with
slow-acting anti-rheumatic drugs
(SAARDs). *Baillière's Clin Rheumatol*
1997; 11(1): 65–81.

74 Capell HA, Maiden N, Madhok R,
Hampson R, Thomson EA. Outcome in
200 RA patients 12 years after random

allocation to either sulphasalazine or penicillamine. *Arthritis Rheum* 1997; 40 (Suppl. 9): S192.

75 McCarty DJ, Carrera GF. Intractable rheumatoid arthritis. Treatment with combined cyclophosphamide, azathioprine and hydroxychloroquine. *JAMA* 1982; 248: 1718–23.

76 O'Dell JR, Haire CE, Erikson N *et al.* Treatment of rheumatoid arthritis with methotrexate alone, sulfasalazine and hydroxychloroquine or a combination of all three medications. *N Engl J Med* 1996; 334: 1287–91.

77 Tugwell P, Pincus T, Yocum D *et al.* Combination therapy with cyclosporine and methotrexate in severe rheumatoid arthritis. *N Engl J Med* 1995; 333(3): 137–41.

78 Capell HA, Marabani M, Madhok R *et al.* Degree and extent of response to sulphasalazine or penicillamine therapy for rheumatoid arthritis: Results from a routine clinical environment over a two-year period. *Q J Med* 1990, 75(276): 335–44.

79 Porter DR, Capell HA, Hunter J. Combination therapy in rheumatoid arthritis—no benefit of addition of hydroxychloroquine to patient with suboptimal response to intramuscular gold therapy. *J Rheumatol* 1993; 20: 645–9.

80 Tugwell P. Combination therapy in rheumatoid arthritis: metaanalysis.

J Rheumatol 1996; 23 (Suppl. 44): 43–6.

81 Hawley DJ, Wolfe F. Are the results of controlled clinical trials and observational studies of second line therapy in rheumatoid arthritis valid and generalizable as measures of rheumatoid arthritis outcome: analysis of 122 studies. *J Rheumatol* 1991; 18(7): 1008–14.

82 Yelin E. The costs of rheumatoid arthritis: absolute, incremental and marginal estimates. *J Rheumatol* 1996; 23 (Suppl. 44): 47–51.

83 Porter DR, Capell HA, McInnes I *et al.* Is rheumatoid arthritis becoming a milder disease or are we starting second-line therapy in patients with milder disease? *Br J Rheumatol* 1996; 35: 1305–8.

84 Harrison BJ, Symmons DPM, Brennan P *et al.* Natural remission in inflammatory polyarthritis: issues of definition and prediction. *Br J Rheumatol* 1996; 35: 1094–100.

85 Maiden N, Capell HA, Madhok R, Thomson EA, Hampson R. The influence of relative poverty on mortality in RA. A study of 200 patients over 12 years. *Arthritis Rheum* 1997; 40 (Suppl. 9): S115.

86 Westhovens R, Verwilghen J, Dequeker J. Total lymphoid irradiation in rheumatoid arthritis. *Arthritis Rheum* 1997; 40(3): 426–9.

9: Does histology at arthroscopy predict outcome?

P.P. Tak and F.C. Breedveld

Introduction

The synovium lines the non-cartilaginous surfaces of the synovial joints and provides nutrients to avascular structures, such as cartilage. In the chronic stages of rheumatoid arthritis (RA), the synovium is hypertrophic and oedematous. Villous projections of synovial tissue protrude into the joint cavity, overgrowing and invading the underlying cartilage and bone. Proliferating synovial tissue near the synovium–cartilage junction is often referred to as pannus.

The availability of new methods of synovial biopsy and the advent of immunohistological methods has stimulated studies on the pathological changes of synovial tissue from patients with RA. At present synovial biopsy specimens of rheumatoid synovium are obtained mainly by two methods: the blind needle biopsy technique and needle arthroscopy. The blind needle biopsy technique is a safe, well-tolerated and technically simple method to acquire synovial tissue in a high percentage of patients with RA [1,2]. A limitation of this method is that it provides access only to the suprapatellar pouch. Moreover, in clinical practice it is restricted to the knee joint. Arthroscopic sampling of synovial tissue under direct vision is a similarly safe and well-tolerated procedure, but more complicated and expensive [3–5]. However, tissue in adequate amounts can always be obtained, and arthroscopy allows access to most joints and to most areas within the joint, including the cartilage–pannus junction.

Preliminary findings suggest that the synovial tissue volume, which can be assessed by arthroscopy or magnetic resonance imaging, may be a predictor of disease activity and treatment outcome in RA [6]. Since there are at present no systematic studies available on the relationship between macroscopic evaluation of the rheumatoid joint and outcome, this chapter will only focus on the analysis of synovial biopsy specimens.

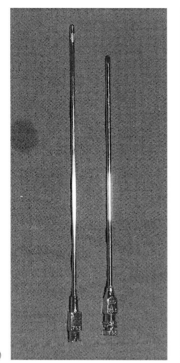
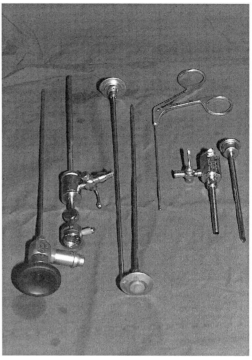

(a)   (b)

Fig. 9.1 (a) Parker–Pearson synovial biopsy needle, consisting of a thin-walled needle with matching stylet and an aspirating needle, and (b) 2.7-mm needle arthroscope (Storz).

Synovial biopsy specimens selected at arthroscopy compared with samples taken blindly by needle biopsy

In some studies on the relationship between features of synovial inflammation and clinical parameters, synovial tissue was obtained by needle arthroscopy, whereas in other studies blind needle biopsy was performed (Fig. 9.1). A crucial question for the interpretation of these studies as well as for clinical practice is whether these two techniques reveal identical tissue characteristics. Recently, a study was undertaken to compare measures of inflammation in synovial tissue samples selected under direct vision at arthroscopy with those taken blindly from the suprapatellar pouch by blind needle biopsy at the same time from the same joint [7]. It was shown that it is not useful to know the macroscopic appearance of the rheumatoid synovium in order to predict the microscopic features [7,8]. Moreover, most measures of inflammation in needle biopsies were similar to those selected at arthroscopy. Infiltration of macrophages was lower, particularly in samples taken from the suprapatellar pouch when compared with the samples selected from areas adjacent to the cartilage–pannus junction.

Thus, samples which are obtained by blind needle biopsy are generally similar to those selected at arthroscopy, but the intensity of macrophage infiltration may be underestimated in some patients when blind needle biopsies are used.

Evaluation of synovial inflammation

Adequate analysis of synovial inflammation is essential when examining synovial biopsy specimens. There are essentially three methods to quantify the features of synovial inflammation: semiquantitative analysis, quantitative analysis and computer-assisted analysis [9,10]. Semiquantitative analysis involves assigning one of a limited number of scores, quantitative analysis involves counting of cells, and image analysis uses computerized digital image processing techniques to extract numerical information from visual images.

Semiquantitative analysis is widely used by pathologists. The grading systems take relatively little time and therefore offer the opportunity to evaluate sections from many biopsy specimens and from many patients, minimizing sampling error. This is a major advantage due to the variation of synovial inflammation that can be found within the joint [3,8,11–14] and between individuals within one diagnostic group [15,16]. Semiquantitative analysis has been used in relatively large studies and has been shown to be a sensitive and reproducible tool for assessing differences between patient groups as well as the effects of therapeutic interventions [17–25]. Moreover, it is possible to find highly significant correlations between semi quantitative scores for immunohistological features of synovial tissue and scores for local disease activity [15,26] (Fig. 9.2).

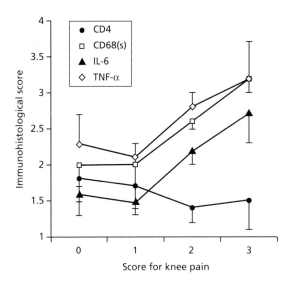

Fig. 9.2 Mean semiquantitative scores ± SEM for the number of CD4+ T cells and CD68+ sublining macrophages and the expression of interleukin 6 (IL-6) and TNF-α in synovial tissue of 62 patients with rheumatoid arthritis in relation to the scores for knee pain. (From [15] with permission.)

Quantitative analysis is an accurate, but laborious method. A recent study suggests that analysis of a limited number of microscopic fields is sufficient, rendering the technique somewhat more practical [27]. Still, a complete evaluation of one patient with limited quantitative analysis takes about four times longer than with semiquantitative methods. A recent cross-sectional comparison between semiquantitative and quantitative analysis showed a highly significant correlation for evaluation of macrophages and T cells [9], suggesting that both methods can be used. In some patients, demonstrating a decrease in serum levels of C-reactive protein and global subjective scores, reduced numbers of cells were found by quantitative analysis, whereas the semiquantitative scores remained unchanged [9]. Since there are no examples of studies showing a significant beneficial effect of treatment without a concomitant decrease in semiquantitative scores, it is too early to determine whether quantitative analysis is superior to semiquantitative analysis. The fact that a strong reduction in synovial inflammation is not necessarily associated with clinical improvement [20] cautions against systems that are too sensitive.

The major advantage of computer-assisted image analysis is the ability to quantify the concentration of the cell or molecule of interest, which may be important especially in the detection of cytokines, and the potential to minimize observer variability [10]. This method requires specialized expensive equipment. The ultimate role of digital techniques in synovial tissue analysis has, as yet, not been determined. At present, there are no studies showing that this method produces data in a more objective or efficient way than the previously described methods. It can be anticipated, however, that image analysis will be increasingly important with the advent of more sophisticated computer systems.

Rheumatoid synovial tissue and differential diagnosis

The synovial lining layer, which comprises normally only one to three cell layers without an underlying basal membrane, consists mainly of macrophages and fibroblast-like synoviocytes. On the other hand, the rheumatoid synovium is characterized by marked synovial lining hyperplasia and by the accumulation of T cells, plasma cells, macrophages, B cells and a relatively low number of other cell types, such as neutrophils, mast cells and natural killer cells in the synovial sublining [15] (Fig. 9.3). Synovial inflammation is quite variable between individual patients in both early and long-standing RA. Surprisingly, systematic comparison of synovial tissue obtained from patients with so-called early RA, which is preceded by asymptomatic synovitis [26], and long-standing RA shows on average similar immunohistological features [15,28,29].

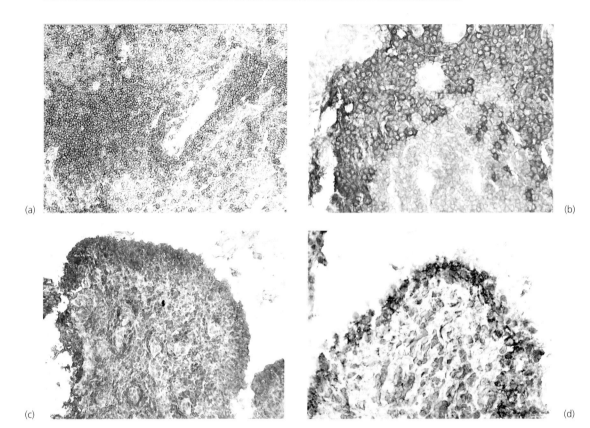

Fig. 9.3 Rheumatoid synovial tissue showing (a) CD3+ T cells in a lymphocytic aggregate; (b) CD38+ plasma cells surrounding a lymphocytic aggregate; (c) CD68+ macrophages in the synovial lining layer and synovial sublining; and (d) CD55+ fibroblast-like synoviocytes in the synovial lining layer. Original magnification (a),(c): ×200; (b),(d): ×400.

Obtaining a definite diagnosis early in the disease process may have important therapeutic consequences and makes it possible to provide information about the prognosis. The question arises whether analysis of synovial biopsy specimens can be used to differentiate between different diseases at the early stage. It is clear that examination of synovial tissue may help to make a diagnosis in some relatively rare infectious, infiltrative, and deposition diseases of joints. Moreover, it has been shown that it is possible to assess differences in the synovial cellular infiltrate as well as in the expression of adhesion molecules, cytokines and metalloproteinases in biopsy specimens when different diagnostic groups are compared [17–19,30,31].

To use synovial biopsy as a diagnostic tool for RA, appropriate markers must be recognized. Unfortunately, many of the pathological changes in the rheumatoid synovium, such as vascular congestion, synovial lining hyperplasia, mononuclear cell infiltration and fibrin depositions commonly occur in disorders other than RA [17–19,24,32–39]. In a recent study the pathological changes of synovial tissue from 95 patients with early arthritis were analysed in relation to the definite diagnosis after follow-up [16]. Logistic regression analysis revealed that a high number of plasma cells, the presence of lymphocytic aggregates, and a high number of macrophages in the synovial sublining are the best discriminating features to differentiate RA patients from patients with other forms of arthritis (Fig. 9.3). Thus, examination of synovial biopsies may help to make a diagnosis when these characteristics are present, although there is not a single pathological feature that is pathognomonic for RA. Conceivably, examination of synovial biopsy specimens will play a more important role as a diagnostic tool when more data become available on the sensitivity and specificity of particular characteristics of the cellular infiltrate in relation to the differential diagnosis.

Rheumatoid synovial tissue and disease activity

Some studies on the relationship between pathological changes of rheumatoid synovium and clinical signs of arthritis at the time of the biopsy reported a positive correlation between the histological features and disease activity [40,41]. Others have failed to confirm such a relationship [42]. It has been described in some longitudinal studies that clinical improvement may be accompanied by a decrease in the lymphocytic infiltrate [43–45]. However, marked clinical improvement may occur with a striking lack of change in the degree of lymphocytic infiltration [46] and, conversely, a strong reduction of the number of synovial lymphocytes has been observed without concomitant clinical amelioration [20,47].

A number of caveats should be recognized when interpreting studies on the correlation between synovial tissue characteristics and disease activity. It is important to restrict the number of immunohistological and clinical variables involved in the analysis to decrease the chance of erroneously reporting statistically significant effects. Moreover, multivariate analysis should be used, since the numbers of the different inflammatory cells in the synovial biopsies are highly correlated to each other and therefore not independent variables. In a study on synovial biopsies from 62 RA patients, regression analysis showed that the number of macrophages and the expression of macrophage-derived cytokines, such as tumour necrosis factor alpha (TNF-α), correlate positively with local disease activity [15] (see Fig. 9.2).

Rheumatoid synovial tissue response to therapy

Examination of serial synovial biopsies has recently been proposed as a screening method for predicting the effects of anti-rheumatic treatment [48]. Such studies may not be immediately relevant to the clinician. However, they may yield insights into the relationship between pathological changes in the synovium and clinical signs of the disease. In previous studies, changes in the synovial tissue after treatment with gold [43,44,49,50], methotrexate [25,51], intra-articular steroids [22,31,52], tenidap [23], Campath-1H [53], anti-CD4 monoclonal antibodies [20] and anti-TNF-α antibodies [21] have been reported.

These studies indicate the association between changes in the synovial tissue, especially reduced numbers of macrophages as well as decreased expression of macrophage-derived cytokines, and clinical improvement. Moreover, the studies suggest that serial analysis of synovial biopsies may provide useful surrogate endpoints for clinical studies, which may offer a rapid screening method requiring relatively low numbers of patients for predicting the effects of novel anti-rheumatic drugs.

Does synovial tissue analysis predict outcome?

The positive correlation between the changes in the synovium, diagnosis, disease activity, and the effects of treatment suggest there may also be a relationship between synovial tissue characteristics and outcome. In light of the observation that a notable percentage of RA patients have signs of joint destruction at the time of initial diagnosis, it is conceivable that examination of synovial biopsy specimens may lead to the determination of markers of outcome that are in fact superior to clinical markers. Signs of joint destruction can even be observed in the absence of clinical signs of inflammation in a particular joint [54], when synovial inflammation is already present [26]. In line with this notion, the progression of joint destruction in RA patients who are in clinical remission [55] could be explained by infiltration by inflammatory cells in the synovium in quiescent joints [26,56].

Studies that examined the relationship between histological charac-teristics of rheumatoid synovial tissue obtained in early RA and outcome after long-term follow-up have as yet not been published. One pioneering study describes the correlation between different synovial tissue mononuclear cell populations in synovial biopsies obtained at a mean disease duration of 2.5 years and articular destruction in 27 RA patients, who were followed up for a mean of almost 6 years [57]. Synovial lining layer depth and cell counts for sublining macrophages, but not for lymphocytes, correlated significantly with articular destruction, determined by radiographs. However, the correlations between the counts for various inflammatory cell types and disease activity after follow-up are difficult to interpret because multivariate analysis was not applied. Several groups have now started long-term follow-up studies after a synovial biopsy procedure early in the disease to identify synovial features that may be used as predictors of outcome and of clinical remission.

Conclusion

Interest in the pathological changes of synovial tissue from patients with arthritis has increased recently because of the advent of novel research tools and the availability of new methods to obtain biopsy specimens. Synovial biopsy specimens, which are obtained by blind needle biopsy, are generally similar to those selected at arthroscopy, but the intensity of macrophage infiltration may be underestimated in some patients when blind needle biopsies are used. The characteristics of synovial tissue can be evaluated by quantitative analysis, semiquantitative analysis and computer-assisted analysis. The correlation between quantitative and semiquantitative analysis is highly significant, but the former may be more sensitive to change after treatment. Whether this is actually an advantage remains to be proven. Computer-assisted image analysis will be increasingly important, in particular to quantify the concentration of antigen per cell. For studies on the relationship between synovial tissue features and clinical parameters, it is more important to include sufficient patients than to use an ultrasensitive scoring system because of the large variation between RA patients.

A high number of plasma cells, the presence of lymphocytic aggregates, and a high number of macrophages in the synovial sublining are the best discriminating features to differentiate RA patients from patients with other forms of arthritis. However, a single pathological feature that is pathognomonic for RA has not been found. Measurements of local disease activity correlate with the number of macrophages and expression of macrophage-derived cytokines in the synovium. Furthermore, analysis of synovial biopsies before and after anti-rheumatic therapy indicates an association between a reduction in the numbers of macrophages and the expression of serial macrophage-derived cytokines on the one hand and clinical improvement on the other. Synovial lining layer hyperplasia and infiltration of the synovial sublining by macrophages are also associated with articular destruction after long-term follow-up. More extensive studies to identify markers of outcome are now in progress.

References

1 Parker RH, Pearson CM. A simplified synovial biopsy needle. *Arthritis Rheum* 1963; 6: 172–6.
2 Tak PP, Lindblad S, Klareskog L, Breedveld FC. Synovial biopsies for analysis of the synovial membrane: new perspectives. *Newslett Eur Rheumatol Res* 1994; 2: 27–9.
3 Lindblad S, Hedfors E. Intraarticular variation in synovitis. Local macroscopic and microscopic signs of inflammatory activity are significantly correlated. *Arthritis Rheum* 1985; 28: 977–86.
4 Reece R, Emery P. Needle arthroscopy. *Br J Rheumatol* 1995; 34: 1102–4.
5 Ike RW. Diagnostic arthroscopy. *Baillière's Clin Rheumatol* 1996; 10: 495–517.
6 Ostergaard M, Stoltenberg M, Lovgreennielsen P *et al.* Magnetic resonance imaging-determined synovial membrane and joint effusion volumes in rheumatoid arthritis and osteoarthritis: Comparison with the macroscopic and microscopic appearance of the synovium. *Arthritis Rheum* 1997; 40: 1856–67.
7 Youssef PP, Kraan MC, Bresnihan B *et al.* Quantitative microscopic analysis of inflammation in rheumatoid synovial membrane samples selected at arthroscopy compared with samples taken blindly by needle biopsy. *Arthritis Rheum* 1998; 41(4): 663–9.
8 Rooney M, Condell D, Daly L *et al.* Analysis of the histologic variation of synovitis in rheumatoid arthritis. *Arthritis Rheum* 1988; 31: 956–63.
9 Youssef PP, Smeets TJM, Bresnihan B *et al.* Microscopic measurement of cellular inflammation in the rheumatoid arthritis synovial membrane: a comparison of semiquantitative and quantitative analysis. *Br J Rheumatol* 1998; 37: 1003–7.
10 Youssef PP, Triantafillou S, Parker A *et al.* Variability in cytokine and cell adhesion molecule staining in arthroscopic synovial biopsies: quantification using color video image analysis. *J Rheumatol* 1997; 24: 2291–8.
11 Cruickshank B. Interpretation of multiple biopsies of synovial tissue in rheumatic diseases. *Ann Rheum Dis* 1951; 11: 137–45.
12 Hutton CW, Hinton C, Dieppe PA. Intra-articular variation of synovial changes in knee arthritis: biopsy study comparing changes in patellofemoral synovium and the medial tibiofemoral synovium. *Br J Rheumatol* 1987; 26: 5–8.
13 Parker F, Keefer CS. Gross and histologic changes in the knee joint in rheumatoid arthritis. *Arch Pathol* 1935; 20: 507–22.
14 Miyasaka N, Sato K, Goto M *et al.* Augmented interleukin-1 production and HLA-DR expression in the synovium of rheumatoid arthritis patients. Possible involvement in joint destruction. *Arthritis Rheum* 1988; 31: 480–6.
15 Tak PP, Smeets TJM, Daha MR *et al.* Analysis of the synovial cellular infiltrate in early rheumatoid synovial tissue in relation to local disease activity. *Arthritis Rheum* 1997; 40: 217–25.
16 Kraan MC, Haringman JJ, Post WJ *et al.* Immunohistologic analysis of synovial tissue for differential diagnosis of early arthritis. *Arthritis Rheum* 1998; 41: S238.
17 Tak PP, Thurkow EW, Daha MR *et al.* Expression of adhesion molecules in early rheumatoid synovial tissue. *Clin Immunol Immunopathol* 1995; 77: 236–42.
18 Tak PP, Kummer JA, Hack CE *et al.* Granzyme positive cytotoxic cells are specifically increased in early rheumatoid synovial tissue. *Arthritis Rheum* 1994; 37: 1735–43.
19 Thurkow EW, Van der Heijden IM, Breedveld FC *et al.* Increased expression of IL-15 in the synovium of patients with rheumatoid arthritis compared to patients with *Yersinia*-induced arthritis and osteoarthritis. *J Pathol* 1997; 181: 444–50.
20 Tak PP, Van der Lubbe PA, Cauli A *et al.* Reduction of synovial inflammation after anti-CD4 monoclonal

antibody treatment in early rheumatoid arthritis. *Arthritis Rheum* 1995; 38: 1457–65.

21 Tak PP, Taylor PC, Breedveld FC *et al.* Decreases in cellularity and expression of adhesion molecules by anti-tumor necrosis factor alpha treatment in patients with rheumatoid arthritis. *Arthritis Rheum* 1996; 39: 1077–81.

22 De Bois MHW, Arndt JW, Tak PP *et al.* 99Tcm-labelled polyclonal human immunoglobulin G scintigraphy before and after intra-articular knee injection of triamcinolone hexacetonide in patients with rheumatoid arthritis. *Nucl Med Commun* 1993; 14: 883–7.

23 Littman BH, Schumacher HR Jr, Boyle DL, Weisman MH, Firestein GS. Effect of tenidap on metalloproteinase gene expression in rheumatoid arthritis: a synovial biopsy study. *J Clin Rheumatol* 1997; 3: 194–202.

24 Smeets TJM, Dolhain RJEM, Breedveld FC, Tak PP. Analysis of the cellular infiltrates and expression of cytokines in synovial tissue from patients with rheumatoid arthritis and reactive arthritis. *J Pathol* 1998; 186: 75–81.

25 Dolhain RJEM, Tak PP, Dijkmans BAC *et al.* Methotrexate (MTX) treatment reduces inflammatory cell numbers, expression of monokines and of adhesion molecules in synovial tissue of patients with rheumatoid arthritis (RA). *Br J Rheumatol* 1998; 37: 502–8.

26 Kraan MC, Versendaal H, Jonker M *et al.* Asymptomatic synovitis precedes clinically manifest arthritis. *Arthritis Rheum* 1998; 41(8): 1481–8.

27 Bresnihan B, Cunnane G, Youssef PP *et al.* Microscopic measurement of synovial membrane inflammation in rheumatoid arthritis—proposals for the evaluation of tissue samples by quantitative analysis. *Br J Rheumatol* 1980; 37(6): 636–42.

28 Schumacher HR Jr, Kitridou RC. Synovitis of recent onset. A clinico-pathologic study during the first month of disease. *Arthritis Rheum* 1972; 15: 465–85.

29 Konttinen YT, Bergroth V, Nordstrom D *et al.* Cellular immunohistopathology of acute, subacute, and chronic synovitis in rheumatoid arthritis. *Ann Rheum Dis* 1985; 44: 549–55.

30 Dolhain RJEM, Ter Haar NT, Hoefakker S *et al.* Increased expression of interferon (IFN)-gamma together with IFN-gamma receptor in the rheumatoid synovial membrane compared with synovium of patients with osteoarthritis. *Br J Rheumatol* 1996; 35: 24–32.

31 Firestein GS, Paine MM, Littman BH. Gene expression (collagenase, tissue inhibitor of metalloproteinases, complement, and HLA-DR) in rheumatoid arthritis and osteoarthritis synovium. Quantitative analysis and effect of intraarticular corticosteroids. *Arthritis Rheum* 1991; 34: 1094–105.

32 Goldenberg DL, Cohen AS. Synovial membrane histopathology in the differential diagnosis of rheumatoid arthritis, gout, pseudogout, systemic lupus erythematosus, infectious arthritis and degenerative joint disease. *Medicine (Baltimore)* 1978; 57: 239–52.

33 Cooper NS, Soren A, McEwen C, Rosenberger JL. Diagnostic specificity of synovial lesions. *Hum Pathol* 1981; 12: 314–28.

34 Lindblad S, Klareskog L, Hedfors E, Forsum U, Sundstrom C. Phenotypic characterization of synovial tissue cells in situ in different types of synovitis. *Arthritis Rheum* 1983; 26: 1321–32.

35 Schulte E, Fisselereckhoff A, Muller KM. Differential diagnosis of synovialitis—correlation between the histomorphological findings of arthro-scopically obtained biopsies and clinical signs. *Pathologe* 1994; 15: 22–7.

36 Iguchi T, Matsubara T, Kawai K, Hirohata K. Clinical and histologic observations of monoarthritis. *Clin Orthop* 1990; 250: 241–9.

37 Cush JJ, Lipsky PE. Cellular basis for rheumatoid inflammation. *Clin Orthop* 1991; 265: 9–22.

38 Veale D, Yanni G, Rogers S *et al.* Reduced synovial membrane macrophage numbers, ELAM-1 expression, and lining layer hyperplasia in psoriatic arthritis as compared with rheumatoid arthritis. *Arthritis Rheum* 1993; 36: 893–900.

39 Cunnane G, Bresnihan B, FitzGerald O. Immunohistologic analysis of peripheral joint disease in ankylosing spondylitis. *Arthritis Rheum* 1998; 41: 180–2.

40 Waxman BA, Sledge CB. Correlation of histochemical, histologic and biochemical evaluations of human synovium with clinical activity. *Arthritis Rheum* 1973; 16: 376–82.

41 Rooney M, Whelan A, Feighery C, Bresnihan B. The immunohistologic features of synovitis, disease activity and *in vitro* IgM rheumatoid factor synthesis by blood mononuclear cells in rheumatoid arthritis. *J Rheumatol* 1989; 16: 459–67.

42 Henderson DR, Jayson MI, Tribe CR. Lack of correlation of synovial histology with joint damage in rheumatoid arthritis. *Ann Rheum Dis* 1975; 34: 7–11.

43 Walters MT, Smith JL, Moore K, Evans PR, Cawley MI. An investigation of the action of disease modifying antirheumatic drugs on the rheumatoid synovial membrane: reduction in T lymphocyte subpopulations and HLA-DP and DQ antigen expression after gold or penicillamine therapy. *Ann Rheum Dis* 1987; 46: 7–16.

44 Rooney M, Whelan A, Feighery C, Bresnihan B. Changes in lymphocyte infiltration of the synovial membrane and the clinical course of rheumatoid arthritis. *Arthritis Rheum* 1989; 32: 361–9.

45 Paus AC, Mellbye OJ, Forre O. Immunohistopathologic findings in synovial biopsies before and after synovectomy in patients with chronic inflammatory joint diseases and their relation to clinical evaluation. A prospective study of biopsies taken from areas selected by arthroscopy. *Scand J Rheumatol* 1990; 19: 269–79.

46 Corkill MM, Kirkham BW, Haskard DO *et al.* Gold treatment of rheumatoid arthritis decreases synovial expression of the endothelial leukocyte adhesion receptor ELAM-1. *J Rheumatol* 1991; 18: 1453–60.

47 Muller-Ladner U, Kriegsmann J, Gay RE *et al.* Progressive joint destruction in a human immunodeficiency virus-infected patient with rheumatoid arthritis. *Arthritis Rheum* 1995; 38: 1328–32.

48 Tak PP, Breedveld FC. Analysis of serial synovial biopsies as a screening method for predicting the effects of therapeutic interventions. *J Clin Rheumatol* 1997; 3: 186–7.

49 Yanni G, Farahat MNMR, Poston RN, Panayi GS. Intramuscular gold decreases cytokine expression and macrophage numbers in the rheumatoid synovial membrane. *Ann Rheum Dis* 1994; 53: 315–22.

50 Kirkham BW, Navarro FJ, Corkill MM, Panayi GS. *In vivo* analysis of disease modifying drug therapy activity in rheumatoid arthritis by sequential immunohistological analysis of synovial membrane interleukin 1 beta. *J Rheumatol* 1994; 21: 1615–19.

51 Firestein GS, Paine MM, Boyle DL. Mechanisms of methotrexate action in rheumatoid arthritis—selective decrease in synovial collagenase gene expression. *Arthritis Rheum* 1994; 37: 193–200.

52 Youssef PP, Triantafillou S, Parker A *et al.* Effect of pulse methylprednisolone on cell adhesion molecules in the synovial membrane in rheumatoid arthritis. *Arthritis Rheum* 1997; 39: 1970–9.

53 Ruderman EM, Weinblatt ME, Thurmond LM, Pinkus GS, Gravallese EM. Synovial tissue response to treatment with Campath-1H. *Arthritis Rheum* 1995; 38: 254–8.

54 van der Heijde DM. Joint erosions and patients with early rheumatoid arthritis. *Br J Rheumatol* 1995; 34 (Suppl. 2): 74–8.

55 Kirwan JR. The relationship between synovitis and erosions in rheumatoid arthritis. *Br J Rheumatol* 1997; 36: 225–8.

56 Soden M, Rooney M, Cullen A *et al.* Immunohistological features in the synovium obtained from clinically uninvolved knee joints of patients with rheumatoid arthritis. *Br J Rheumatol* 1989; 28: 287–92.

57 Mulherin D, FitzGerald O, Bresnihan B. Synovial tissue macrophage populations and articular damage in rheumatoid arthritis. *Arthritis Rheum* 1996; 39: 115–24.

10: How valuable is imaging?

W.P. Butt and M.F.R. Martin

Clinical rheumatology

In clinical rheumatology, imaging must make a significant contribution to management or to prognosis or it is an irrelevance; imaging in the majority of patients with rheumatoid arthritis (RA) is unnecessary. If most of the patients currently imaged were not, a different approach could be made to the few who remain. Patients who meet the criteria in Table 10.1a require high-quality precision radiography almost certainly more extensive than that currently offered. It is preferable if the one patient in 10 with RA who needs imaging receives a high-quality investigation rather than all 10 receiving mediocre studies.

If plain films are to be used to confirm a diagnosis of RA they must include those images likely to provide the information required—

Table 10.1 Use of imaging for rheumatoid arthritis (RA).

---

1 DIAGNOSIS
   (a) *Of the presence of RA*
      Early in unknown with clinical findings suggesting RA
      Early in unknown with clinical findings not suggesting RA
      In transferred patient who has had disease altering drugs to the point that clinical
         findings are no longer diagnostic
   (b) *Of the extent of RA*
      For example in this patient known to have RA, is the left hip involved?
        And with what?
   (c) *Of the severity of RA*
      For example in this patient known to have RA is involvement of joint X to the
        degree that function Y is interfered with?
   (d) *Of complications of RA*
      Presence, extent and clinical signifiance of complications known or suspected

2 MANAGEMENT
   (a) *Guiding physical interference*
      For example synovectomy, biopsy, injection
   (b) *Guiding the care of complications*

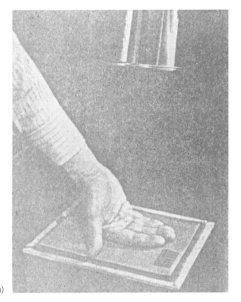
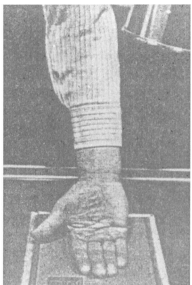

(a)

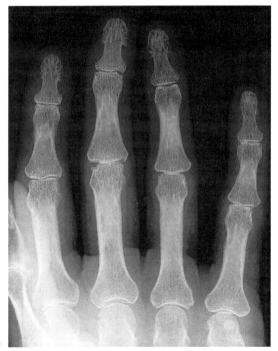

(b)

Fig. 10.1 The Brewerton view (a) is every bit as useful today as it was decades ago when first described. It permits the joints of the fingers to be seen in proper antero-posterior projection (b).

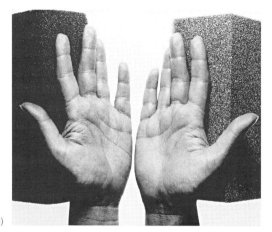

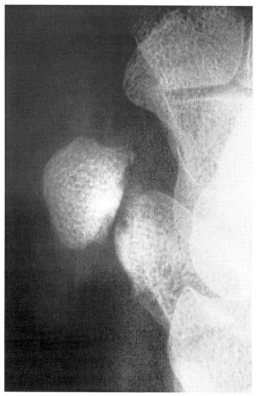

Fig. 10.2 The reverse oblique of the wrist
(a) is the only projection which will show the
joint between the pisiform and the triquetrum.
(b) This joint is frequently involved early in
rheumatoid arthritis.

(a)

(b)

Brewerton's views of the fingers (Fig. 10.1), reverse oblique views of the
wrist to show the pisiform–triquetral joint (Fig. 10.2), lateral films of
the os calcis to show both the plantar fascia and the Achilles tendon
bursa (Fig. 10.3) and films of the sacro-iliac (SI) joints. Frontal films of
the hands and feet, oblique views of the hands and a film of the suspicious
joint are also useful. Early in RA, the diagnostic changes may not be appreciable on unmagnified radiographs and magnification of standard radiographs
is often unrewarding. Therefore it is preferable that routine arthritis surveys
be performed as often as possible on mammographic apparatus with mammographic film because of the high-contrast, high-resolution capability of
the apparatus (Fig. 10.4). We have not been convinced that digital radiographs are sufficiently detailed to register the subtle changes of early RA
although others differ [1]. Although the necessary equipment, technical ex-
pertise, space and time are available in every hospital, few if any provide
a high-quality arthritic survey. The reason is simply a lack of appropriate
patient selection. Both patients with minimal joint symptoms, perhaps just
a little arthralgia, and, the other extreme, patients with severe rheumatoid
arthritis of at least 20 years' duration, are unlikely to provide subtle change
on plain films. The message is clear; patients require selection!

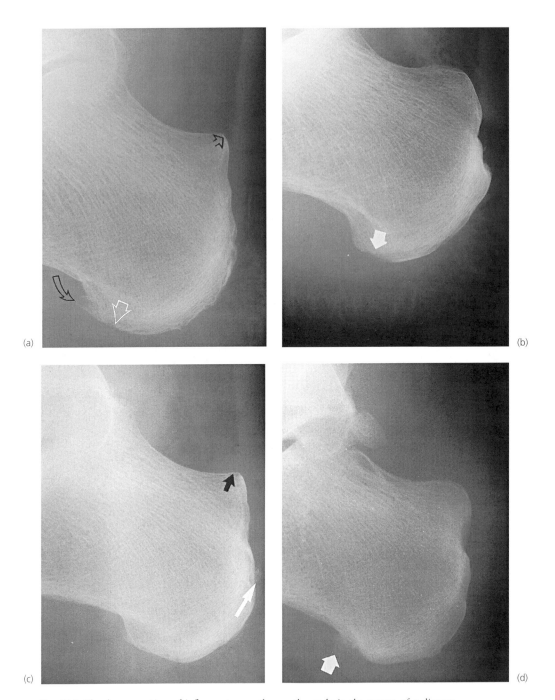

(a)

(b)

(c)

(d)

Fig. 10.3 The demonstration of inflammatory enthesopathy early in the course of a disease excludes rheumatoid arthritis. The earliest radiological sign of inflammatory enthesopathy is loss of the subperiosteal cortical continuity at the insertion of the fibrous tissue (b) cf. normal (a) (ultrasound, scintigraphy and MRI will all be positive at this stage). Later the inflamed fibrous tissue shows new bone formation (c, d, white arrows). Mature enthesophytes (a, curved arrow) have no differentiating value, are not significant, and do not indicate systemic disease. The normal Achilles tendon is separated from the superior posterior corner of the os calcis by a pad of fat (open black arrow). With swelling of the Achilles tendon bursa the triangle of fat is obliterated and elevated (black arrow).

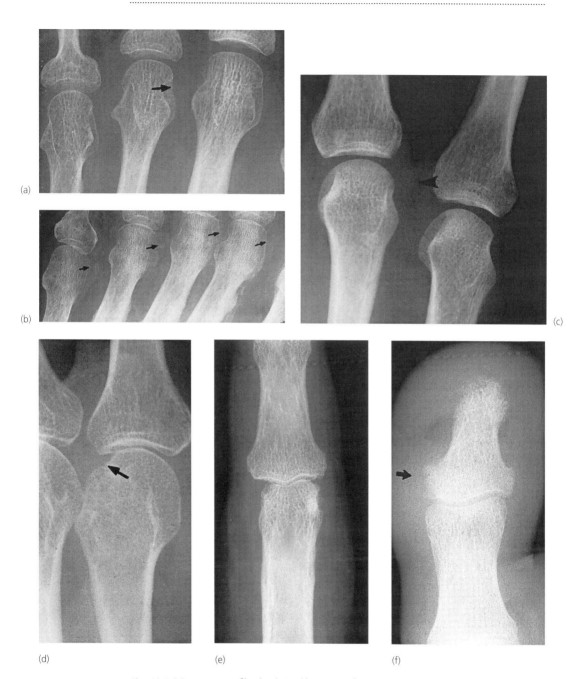

Fig. 10.4 Mammogram film lends itself to magnification. Compare (a) which shows loss of subchondral cortical integrity and therefore indicates joint disease with (b) where the subchondral cortical bone is preserved indicating there is no joint disease despite the marked bone atrophy and prolonged symptoms; (c) shows synovial swelling before proteolysis or loss of subchondral cortical integrity is appreciable; (d) shows the unequivocal sign of the presence of pannus—the focal erosion of subchondral cortical bone; (e) demonstrates that peripheral (i.e. synovial) disease can be differentiated from surface disease (osteoarthritis) in the phalanges; (f) shows early enthesopathy.

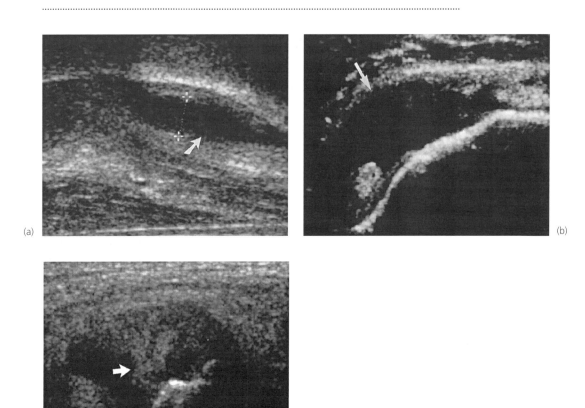

(a)

(b)

(c)

Fig. 10.5 Ultrasound readily shows collections of fluid as areas of poor echogenicity (black) within the deep joints such as the hip (a) or the shoulder (b). Not uncommonly, ultrasound will detect synovial proliferation projecting into the fluid (c).

Ultrasound is an extension of the examining hand and should be available for all to use just as a stethoscope and an ophthalmoscope are. Ultrasound can confirm joint disease in the joints that are inaccessible to palpation such as the shoulder and hip (Figs 10.5 & 10.6) and can differentiate joint swelling from soft tissue swelling and from tendon sheath swelling (Fig. 10.7). Differentiation of synovial proliferation from synovial effusion can be difficult and there is no face lost by asking for expert help in this circumstance. It seems odd that one should need to request expert help for the easy demonstration of joint effusion or tendonitis. Joint scintigraphy is underused but is an ideal tool in assessing the patient with monoarticular synovitis in whom a biopsy is not an urgent consideration. Its main virtue lies in demonstrating polyarticular disease in a patient who has only one symptomatic joint. High-definition scintigraphy such as that obtained with a pin-hole collimator [2] is capable of differentiating synovial from

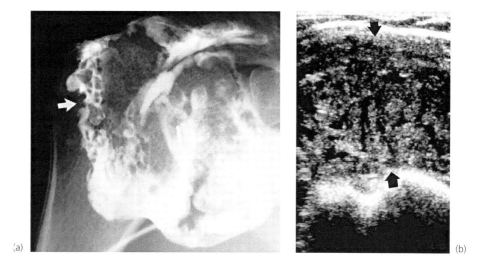

(a)

(b)

Fig. 10.6 Rheumatoid pannus shown by arthrography (a) may be easier to appreciate than when it is shown by ultrasound (b) but it is no more believable. Arthrography is certainly not faster, easier, cheaper or less painful than ultrasound.

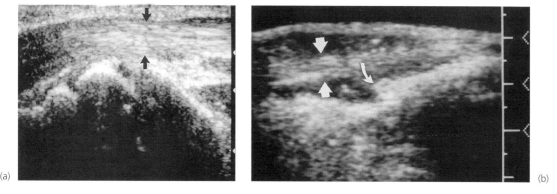

(a)

(b)

Fig. 10.7 The straight arrows in (a) enclose a normal tendon whereas in (b) they enclose an abnormal tendon in a tendon sheath which contains fluid (black) and masses of pannus (curved arrow). This is the appearance of rheumatoid tendonitis.

adjacent osseous abnormality and distinguishing articular surface disorder (osteoarthritis) from synovial disorder (e.g. RA) (Fig. 10.8). It is as accurate as any other method of imaging in diagnosing avascular necrosis. It is also useful in establishing that a patient with multicentric joint symptomatology does or does not have multicentred joint disease. We are very reluctant to accept the diagnosis of RA in a patient whose joint scintigraphy is still negative after 6 months of disease.

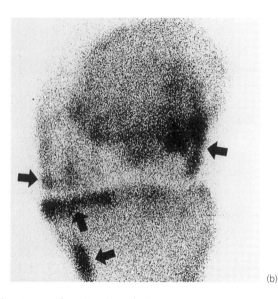

(a)   (b)

Fig. 10.8 Pin-hole collimation bone scintigraphy can differentiate surface disorders of joints (osteoarthritis) (a) from peripheral synovial disease of joints (rheumatoid arthritis) (b). (Cases courtesy of Yong Whee Bahk [2] with permission.)

Computed tomography (CT) scanning is particularly useful for assessing deformities because of its three-dimensional capability (Fig. 10.9). It is the standard way of imaging the sacrum and should precede plain films here (Fig. 10.10)

Magnetic resonance imaging (MRI) can and does show 'everything better' but it takes some getting used to. We have noted how difficult it is to make a diagnosis of ankylosing spondylitis on the MRI but once the diagnosis has been made from the plain films the MRI shows the extent of the involvement much better. Similarly once the CT scan has shown sacroiliitis the MRI will show its extent and, perhaps, give an idea of its severity better than other forms of imaging (Table 10.2). MRI comes into

Table 10.2 Imaging diagnosis of rheumatoid arthritis.

Step 1	Establish that the joint is abnormal, i.e. effusion, by ultrasound or high-contrast radiography
Step 2	That the joint is diseased, i.e. synovial thickening by high-definition radiography, ultrasound, isotopes or magnetic resonance imaging
Step 3	That the disease is proteolytic and pannus forming, i.e. loss of articular cartilage and subchondral cortical invasive destruction, by high-resolution radiography
Step 4	That the disease is rheumatoid arthritis, i.e. is a proteolytic pannus-forming arthritis showing joint-for-joint symmetry on bone scintigraphy and/or high-definition radiography. No enthesopathy

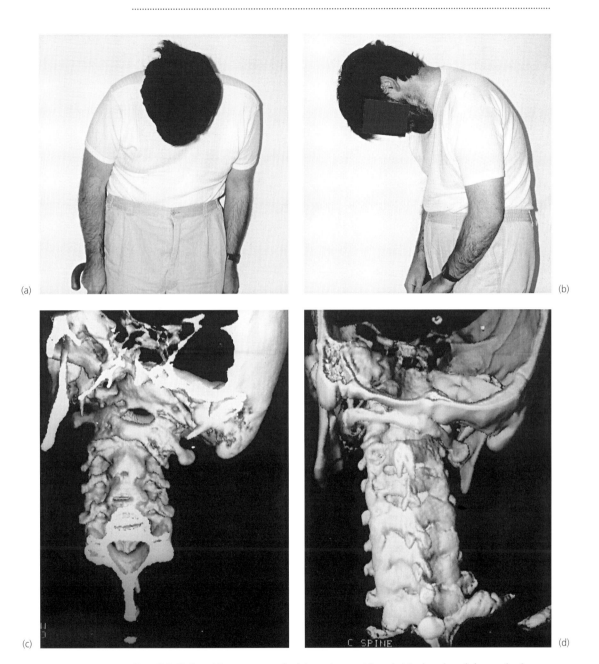

(a)

(b)

(c)

(d)

Fig. 10.9 Deformities can get so bad in patients with arthritis that they defy standard radiological investigation (a, b). This is the place for reformatted CT and three-dimensional reconstruction of the spine from the front (c) and from the back (d) showing that the patient has a rotational dislocation of C1 on C2.

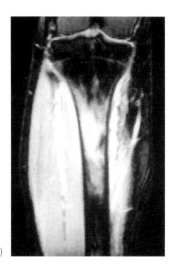
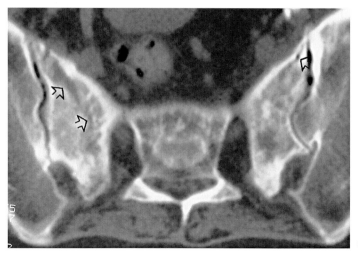

(a)   (b)

Fig. 10.10 CT scanning is still the best way to show stress fractures or insufficiency fractures although MRI certainly indicates something is altered. Stress injuries are frequently extremely high-signal on STIR (a) or T2 weighted images to the point that one has difficulty believing that it is simply stress. CT is best for demonstrating bone disruption (b) and should be the first examination of any suspected disorder of the sacrum such as insufficiency fractures. Plain films are insensitive to the point of being misleading in investigating sacral abnormalities.

its own in the investigation of the complications of RA whether it be avascular necrosis, amyloidosis, cord compression or sepsis (Fig. 10.11). A cautionary note—remember there are no imaging signals that allow one to differentiate inflammation, tumour and trauma even if gadolinium is used. If gadolinium is not used, cysts and abscesses cannot be differentiated from tumours. When the newer MRIs that permit surgical intervention become more widespread, MRI will really take over.

It is our opinion that insufficient use is made of imaging to guide injection and biopsy. No one disputes that it is possible to put a needle where you want to put it without looking, but it is a lot more difficult and less certain. The hip and subtalar joints as well as the subacromial bursa are not easy to inject clinically particularly if one wishes to be certain of the needle site. To the intrepid, no joint is unapproachable; lateral C1/2 injections are routine and even the odontoid/C1 joint can be approached through the spinal canal (Fig. 10.12). The epidural space is a particular minefield. It should not happen, but it is entirely possible for injections to enter the subarachnoid space even when the needle is nowhere near that structure (Fig. 10.13). It has been our experience that injected material can enter the subarachnoid space even though there is no fluid returned by aspiration and, similarly, the injected material can enter the epidural

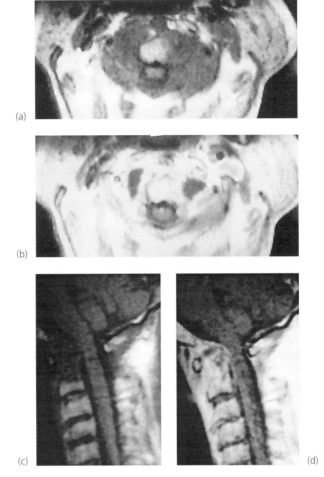

Fig. 10.11 T1 weighted spine echo (T1 WSE) sagittal and axial before and after intravenous Magnevist show extensive pannus about the odontoid and in both lateral C1/C2 articulations. This pannus is compressing the cervical spinal cord. MRI is the only method of proving that cord compression is due to pannus.

(a)

(b)

(c)

(d)

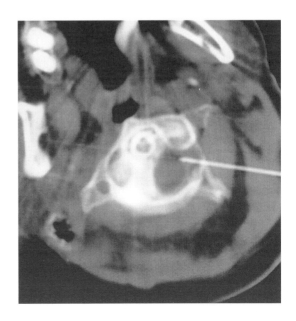

Fig. 10.12 No joint is safe any longer. The axial CT scan shows the articulation between the odontoid and C1 being punctured by a posterior trans-spinal approach. The spinal cord and dural sac are displaced away from the needle tip by saline. These injections are remarkably effective in long-term relief of headache. (Case courtesy of Dr P.J. O'Connor, Leeds General Infirmary.)

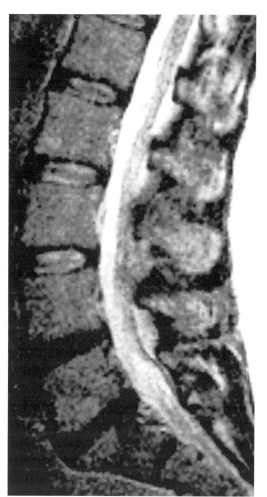

(a)

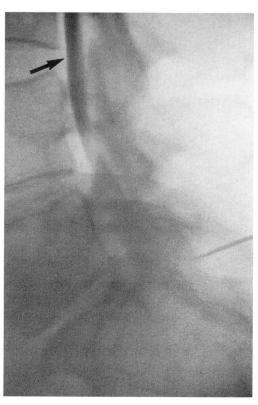

(b)

Fig. 10.13 Needling of the epidural space can result in filling of the subarachnoid space even though apparently anatomically impossible. The needle in this 22-stone female patient never passed into the bony spinal canal and no significant pseudomeningocele is demonstrable by MRI (a) yet contrast medium injected through the needle entered the subarachnoid space (b, arrow). No cerebrospinal fluid could be aspirated before or after the injection.

venous plexus even though no blood is aspirated. If small needles are used for epidural injections pressure changes are not a reliable indicator of the localization of the needle tip. Previous surgery makes things even more difficult.

The use of imaging to predict the course and outcome of a patient with RA is imprecise and is no more accurate than the general advice 'patients with severe disease do badly'.

Academic rheumatology

Should academic rheumatology use imaging differently? Should every assessment of management have radiological controls? The answer to both questions should be 'no' but in practice is almost universally 'yes'. There are approximately 250 papers per year on some aspect of the imaging of RA and it is very common to find that the authors have ignored critical previous work which shows that variations in radiographic technique can produce a greater change in the patients' grading than does an alteration in management. It is really quite remarkable that many studies which note a difference in the radiological progression of the disease from the clinical and laboratory progression assume that the clinical findings and laboratory findings are incorrect and the radiology is the true observation; at least one paper goes so far as to say that there are two different processes occurring in patients with RA, one that affects the clinical findings, and another which affects the X-rays and laboratory findings [3]. It is well known in other inflammatory diseases of bone such as osteomyelitis that X-ray changes lag so far behind clinical progress that they are of little use in assessing that progress. In our opinion, none of these recent papers includes enough patients from a sufficiently wide spectrum of the population to be of specific clinical use. It is surprising to us that papers describing management of 50 or 100 patients with RA are published. That number is reasonable for a pilot study but a study for publication requires confirmation with patients numbered in the thousands.

Studies that assess the validity of imaging are uncommon and currently MRI is receiving virtually all the attention. It is being used to look at basic processes in RA and perhaps this in combination with molecular biology and nuclear magnetic resonance (NMR) assay will lead to an understanding of basic pathological processes, but as yet there is little of use which has emerged.

References

1 Swee RG, Gray JE, Beabout JW *et al.* Screen film versus computed radiography imaging of the hand: a direct comparison. *Am J Roentgenol* 1997; 168(2): 539–42.

2 Yong Whee Bahk. *Combined Scintigraphic and Radiographic Diagnosis of Bone and Joint Diseases*. Berlin: Springer-Verlag, 1994.

3 Coste J, Spira A, Clerc D, Paolaggi JB. Prediction of articular destruction in rheumatoid arthritis: Disease activity markers revisited. *J Rheumatol* 1997; 24(1): 28–34.

Part 3: Drug Treatment of Rheumatoid Arthritis

11: Do early systemic glucocorticoids prevent disease progression?

J.R. Kirwan and M. Byron

Introduction

Glucocorticoids were first used to treat rheumatoid arthritis (RA) in 1947 [1]. The immediate anti-inflammatory effect of hydrocortisone was dramatic and glucocorticoids became a popular treatment. The recognition of serious toxicity [2] from the doses then employed was a factor contributing to their relative decline. Many rheumatologists in the UK profess a disinclination to prescribe glucocorticoids, preferring to reserve them for elderly people or late in the course of the disease [3]. In the same survey, however, 24 of 100 consecutive out-patients with RA were taking glucocorticoids of which nine were under 50 years of age and 13 had a disease duration of less than 5 years.

Systemic glucocorticoids have numerous and widespread effects on the immune system and other body systems [4]. About 80% of serum glucocorticoid is bound to transcortin. Free cortisol, the active moiety, diffuses into cells and combines with specific receptors in the cytoplasm. This steroid–receptor complex enters the nucleus and binds reversibly at specific chromatin sites, thereby stimulating a variety of gene transcription promoters and inhibitors. It has been known for many years that glucocorticoid effects on the immune system include alteration in cytokine expression, down-regulation of immune function, inhibition of cell-mediated immunity, reduced cellular accumulation at inflammatory sites and reduced vascular responses during inflammation [5–7]. Patients with RA might also have a defect in the regulation of corticosteroid-releasing factor (CRF) by the hypothalamus [8]. In active inflammatory RA, such cortisol levels are reduced and the cortisol response during surgical stress is dampened [9]. This raises the possibility that alterations in glucocorticoid action or control may play a more fundamental role in the development and progress of RA than previously thought.

Whatever the potential effects of glucocorticoid, the rationale for their use to control RA should be informed by the results of randomized

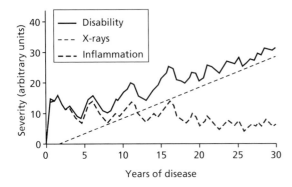

Fig. 11.1 Schematic representation of course of RA.

controlled trials. Some of the first such trials published in rheumatology concerned the use of glucocorticoids. They, together with more recent studies, provide the evidence (reviewed below) on which conclusions about efficacy can be drawn.

Whether glucocorticoids can prevent the progression of RA depends upon the definition of 'progression' (Fig. 11.1). This can be viewed in several ways: the symptoms and signs of inflammation may be reduced or abolished; the slow progression of disability may be reduced; or the onset of structural change may be delayed or abolished. Evidence is mounting that these may be independent processes [10]. The stage of the disease may also determine the outcome of intervention with glucocorticoids. As 70–75% of patients develop erosions within the first 3 years of disease, and very few do so thereafter [11], 'early' could be defined as within 3 years of onset of symptoms.

The effect of glucocorticoids on symptoms

Large doses of glucocorticoids can rapidly suppress the symptoms of inflammation in the very short term [12–16]. In RA there have been a number of longer-term randomized controlled trials of glucocorticoids which have focused on symptom control. The Empire Rheumatism Council (ERC) trial [17] compared cortisone treatment with aspirin for 3 years in patients with established RA (average disease duration 7 years). The results are illustrated in Fig. 11.2. It can be seen that even at the end of the first year of treatment there was no symptomatic benefit from glucocorticoids compared with aspirin. Similar results have been obtained for a number of studies (Table 11.1).

Our conclusion therefore is that oral glucocorticoids clearly offer short-term relief of pain and may reduce symptoms of RA for 6–12 months, but that the benefit is then lost.

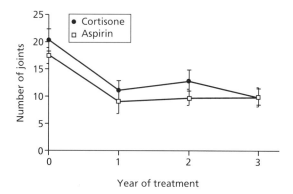

Fig. 11.2 Data from Empire Rheumatism Council Study (1957) comparing cortisone and aspirin in RA. The number of joints involved is similar throughout for both groups of patients.

Table 11.1 Clinical outcome in studies comparing corticosteroids with anti-inflammatories.

Study	Year	Ref.	No. of patients (No. remaining at end of study)	Treatment (mg/day)	Comparator	Duration (months)	Clinical result
MRC	1957	30	61 (53)	Cortisone (80)	Aspirin (4.5 g/day)	36	Cortisone did not maintain well-being more than aspirin; withdrawal flares noted on both medications
ERC	1957	17	100 (53)	Cortisone (69)	Aspirin (4 g/day)	36	No clinical differences but ESR reduced in first few months in cortisone group
MRC	1960	20	84 (77)	Prednisolone (17–12 year 1, 12–10 year 2)	Aspirin (6 g/day initially, slowly reducing)	36	Prednisolone group better in first year
Harris	1983	31	34 (34)	Prednisolone (5)	Placebo and crossover at 24/52	8	Improved function and sense of well-being at 6 months, lost on changing to placebo
Kirwan	1995	21	128 (106)	Prednisolone (7.5)	Placebo	24	Clinical benefit for 3–9 months, functional benefit for up to 15 months
Boers	1997	22	155 (126)	Sulphasalazine Prednisolone Methotrexate	Sulphasalazine	20	Early clinical benefit in combined therapy group; benefit lost as prednisolone withdrawn

ESR, erythrocyte sedimentation rate; ERC, Empire Rheumatism Council; MRC, Medical Research Council.

	Prednisolone		Aspirin	
Time	Hands	Feet	Hands	Feet
1 year*	17	12	49	44
2 years*	41	10	72	71
4 years†			94	
5 years†		23		

Table 11.2 Proportion (%) of patients showing X-ray progression after different periods of treatment. (From MRC study [20] and follow-up by West [23].)

* Radiograph taken after 1 and 2 years in a randomized controlled trial of prednisolone vs. aspirin.
† Most of the prednisolone-treated patients from the original study continued to take prednisolone, and most of the placebo patients were not prescribed prednisolone.

The effect of glucocorticoids on radiographic changes

For some time it has been recognized in retrospective observational studies that patients who take glucocorticoids may have progressive disease [18,19]. However, this association could easily result from a tendency to treat patients with more severe disease with glucocorticoids. A more rational approach to this issue is to directly assess the effect of glucocorticoids on radiological progression in randomized controlled trials. Three such studies are available in the literature [20–22] and deserve review.

The Joint Committee of the Medical Research Council (MRC) and Nuffield Foundation study found a benefit on the X-rays which was not fully appreciated within the original trial report [20]. These data together with the follow-up review by West [23] have since been highlighted [24] and are shown in Table 11.2. The method used to score the radiographs was an overall grading of X-ray severity in the hands and feet. The initial dose of prednisolone in this study was 20 mg daily reducing to 12 mg over 1 year and to 10 mg at the end of year 2. These data, relatively ignored until recently, provide prima facie evidence that glucocorticoids may suppress the progression of erosive disease.

The Arthritis and Rheumatism Council (ARC) Low Dose Glucocorticoid Study [21] admitted patients with active inflammatory disease within 2 years of diagnosis and prescribed 7.5 mg prednisolone or placebo as a fixed daily dose given in addition to all other medications. Treatment was taken for 2 years and a 1-year blind follow-up study was also undertaken [25]. The primary outcome measures were the progression of erosions in the hands using the Larsen score [26] and the proportion of hands which had no erosions at entry but went on to develop erosions during the study. (Secondary outcomes included clinical symptoms as reported in Table 11.1.) Figure 11.3 illustrates the radiographic outcome. Prednisolone substantially reduced the progression of erosions during the

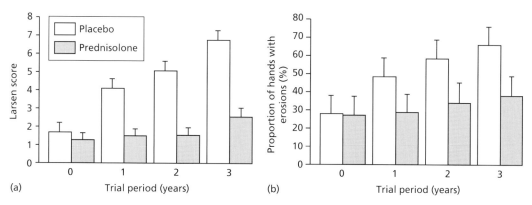

Fig. 11.3 Radiological assessment in the Arthritis and Rheumatism Council Study (1995) comparing prednisolone (7.5 mg/day) with placebo in early RA. Prednisolone therapy was discontinued after 2 years. (a) Larsen scores. (b) Proportion of hand X-rays showing erosions.

time it was taken. Furthermore, the proportion of hands which had not yet developed erosions was also unchanged during the treatment period, showing that both the onset of erosions and their progression was inhibited by the prednisolone.

One year after the treatment was terminated erosive progression had resumed at a rate roughly parallel to the control group [25]. The proportion of hands which were erosive also increased during the follow-up year after treatment withdrawal, but not to such an extent. This raises the possibility that some patients are still being protected from developing erosive disease even after the treatment has stopped.

It should be noted that most patients in this study were also treated with non-steroidal anti-inflammatory drugs (NSAIDs) and specific anti-rheumatoid drugs (SARDs). No restrictions were placed on the use of such treatment and it was used with equal frequency in the prednisolone and placebo-treated patients. Overall 89% took an NSAID while 8% were treated with intramuscular gold, 30% with penicillamine, 26% with sulphasalazine, 4% with methotrexate and 3% with other agents.

In the Dutch COBRA study [22], 76 test and 79 control patients received continuous sulphasalazine. The test subjects were also treated with methotrexate for 40 weeks and prednisolone for 28 weeks. The daily prednisolone dose was 60 mg in week 1, 40 mg in week 2, 25 mg in week 3, 20 mg in week 4, 15 mg in week 5, 10 mg in week 6 and 7.5 mg thereafter. Both methotrexate and prednisolone were discontinued gradually. The radiographic results are illustrated in Fig. 11.4. Hand and feet radiographs were included in this study and were assessed using an erosion score devised for the study [22]. Erosive progression was prevented during the period of treatment with prednisolone and methotrexate in addition to sulphasalazine. In this study the benefits of the prednisolone seemed to persist for several

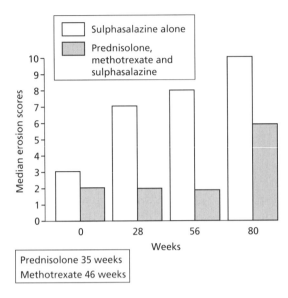

Fig. 11.4 Radiographic progression in the Dutch Collaborative Study comparing sulphasalazine alone with sulphasalazine, methotrexate and prednisolone.

weeks after treatment was discontinued, but erosive progression resumed between 56 and 80 weeks.

The effect of glucocorticoids on disablity

Disability is notoriously difficult to measure [27] and early studies had only the Steinbrocker grading system for its assessment. It is likely that in early RA, disability relates to the degree of inflammation present, whereas later in the disease it relates more to structural damage of joints (see Fig. 11.1). However, this remains a likelihood from sensible extrapolation, rather than a certainty from direct observation. If true, it implies that in the medium term the suppression of joint destruction will result in improved functional outcome. On the other hand, there may be other influences of long-term glucocorticoid therapy, such as loosening of ligaments and joint capsules, which may contribute in a different way to reduced joint function. Only longer-term observational and controlled studies will provide definitive answers.

The development of the Health Assessment Questionnaire (HAQ) [28] has provided an instrument which is much more sensitive to changes in function [29]. The ERC trial [17] measured the 'sense of well-being' of the study patients and reported a benefit from glucocorticoids lasting up to 3 years. In the ARC study [21] the HAQ in the prednisolone group showed a statistically significant improvement compared with the placebo group for 15 months but not thereafter. There may be an effect of glucocorticoids on quality of life over and above improvement in function caused by the suppression of inflammatory symptoms, but this aspect has not so far been well captured in investigations.

Conclusion

The data from randomized controlled clinical trials consistently show that, in doses arguably acceptable to long-term use, there is an improvement in the signs and symptoms of inflammation. The onset of this benefit is rapid but it lasts for only 6–12 months. By this criterion glucocorticoids do not prevent disease progression. In three well-conducted studies of the radiographic progression of disease, glucocorticoid treatment was associated with a substantial suppression of joint destruction. In general, this effect lasted for the duration of treatment, but some data raise the possibility that there may be a more long-lasting effect. Thus, a low dose of glucocorticoid (7.5 mg/day prednisolone) does prevent the progression of joint destruction revealed by radiographs. At present it remains an assumption that this will result in a lessening of long-term pain and disability. Extrapolation of the results from the UK and Dutch studies [21,22] suggest that continuing treatment may continue to prevent joint destruction. Although there were few adverse effects of low-dose glucocorticoids taken for 2 years, whether longer-term treatment would indeed continue to protect joints and remain free of adverse effects remains to be evaluated.

It is reasonable to conclude that a fixed low dose of 7.5 mg prednisolone daily given in addition to standard treatment in patients with early, active RA will improve symptoms for about 6 months and prevent joint destruction for 2 years or more. Discontinuation of therapy after 2–4 years would be wise in view of the potential for longer-term adverse effects such as osteoporosis or cardiovascular disease. A proposed policy for selecting and treating appropriately is given in Table 11.3.

Table 11.3 Policy for selecting and treating patients with prednisolone 7.5 mg/day. Patients should have active inflammatory disease and all other treatment modalities should be used as clinically indicated.

Erosion status	Disease duration (years)		
	1–2	3–4	> 4
Erosive	Treat for 2–4 years then stop	Probably treat for 2 years then stop	Do not treat as risk–benefit ratio is unknown
Non-erosive	Treat for 2–4 years then stop	Do not treat as probably will never be erosive	

Discontinuation of therapy should be by rapid tapering off. One suitable regimen is alternate-day treatment for 2 weeks then every third day for 2 weeks, then stop [21,25].

References

1 Hench PS, Kendall EC, Slocumb CH et al. Effects of a hormone of the adrenal cortex (17-hydroxy-11 dehydrocorticosterone: compound E) and of pituitary adrenocorticotrophic hormone on rheumatoid arthritis. Preliminary report. *Proc Staff Meet Mayo Clin* 1949; 24: 181–97.

2 Cooper C, Kirwan JR. The risk of local and systemic corticosteroid administration. *Baillière's Clin Rheumatol* 1990; 4: 305–32.

3 Byron MA, Mowat AG. Corticosteroid prescribing in rheumatoid arthritis—the fiction and the fact. *Br J Rheumatol* 1985; 24: 164–6.

4 George E, Kirwan JR. Cortiscosteroid therapy in rheumatoid arthritis. *Baillière's Clin Rheumatol* 1990; 4: 621–47.

5 Dinarello CA. Interleukin 1. *Rev Infect Dis* 1984; 6(1): 51–95.

6 Grabstein K, Dower S, Gillis S et al. Expression of interleukin 2, interferon-gamma and the IL-2 receptor by human peripheral blood lymphocytes. *J Immunol* 1986; 15: 136(12): 4503–8.

7 Beutler B, Krochen N, Milsark IW et al. Control of cachectin (TNF) synthesis mechanisms of endotoxin resistance. *Science* 1986; 232: 977–80.

8 Panayi GS. Heberden Oration, 1992. The pathogenesis of rheumatoid arthritis: from molecules to the whole patient. *Br J Rheumatol* 1993; 32(7): 533–6.

9 Chikanza IC, Petrou P, Kingsley G, Chrousos G, Panayi GS. Defective hypothalamic response to immune and inflammatory stimuli in patients with rheumatoid arthritis. *Arthritis Rheum* 1992; 35(11): 1281–8.

10 Mulherin D, FitzGerald O, Bresnihan B. Synovial tissue macrophage populations and articular damage in rheumatoid arthritis. *Arthritis Rheum* 1996; 39: 115–24.

11 Brook A, Corbett M. Radiographic change in early rheumatoid disease. *Ann Rheum Dis* 1977; 36: 71–3.

12 Berry H, Huskisson EC. Isotopic indices as a measure of inflammation in rheumatoid arthritis. *Ann Rheum Dis* 1974; 33: 523–5.

13 Boardman PL, Dudley Hart F. Clinical measurement of the anti-inflammatory effects of salicilates in rheumatoid arthritis. *Br Med J* 1967; 4: 264–8.

14 Jasani MK, Downie WW, Samuels BM, Buchanan WW. Ibuprofen in rheumatoid arthritis. *Scand J Rheumatol* 1973; 2: 71–7.

15 Lee P, Webb J, Anderson J, Buchanan WW. Evaluation of analgesic action and efficacy of antirheumatic drugs. *J Rheumatol* 1976; 3: 283–94.

16 Dick WC, Nuki G, Whaley K, Deodhar S, Buchanan WW. Some aspects in the quantitation of inflammation in joints of patients suffering from rheumatoid arthritis. *Rheumatol Phys Med* 1970; 10 (Suppl.): 40–7.

17 Empire Rheumatism Council. Multi-centre controlled trial comparing cortisone acetate and acetyl salicylic in the long term treatment of rheumatoid arthritis. *Ann Rheum Dis* 1957; 16: 277–89.

18 Pincus T. Rheumatoid arthritis: disappointing long-term outcomes despite successful short-term clinical trials. *J Clin Epidemiol* 1988; 41: 1037–41.

19 Scott DL, Spector TD, Pullar T, McConkey B. What should we hope to achieve when treating rheumatoid arthritis? *Ann Rheum Dis* 1989; 48: 256–61.

20 Joint Committee of the Medical Research Council and Nuffield Foundation. A comparison of prednisolone with aspirin or other analgesics in the treatment of rheumatoid arthritis. *Ann Rheum Dis* 1960; 19: 331–7.

21 Kirwan JR and the Arthritis and Rheumatism Council Low Dose Glucocorticoid Study Group. The effect of glucocorticoids on joint destruction in rheumatoid arthritis. *N Engl J Med* 1995; 333: 142–6.

22 Boers M, Verhoeven AC, Markusse HM et al. Randomised comparison of combined step down prednisolone, methotrexate and sulphasalazine with sulphasalazine alone in early rheumatoid arthritis. *Lancet* 1997; 350: 309–18.

23 West HF. Rheumatoid arthritis: the relevance of clinical knowledge to research activities. *Abstracts World Med* 1967; 41: 401–17.

24 Byron MA, Kirwan JR. Corticosteroids in rheumatoid arthritis: is a trial of their 'disease modifying' potential feasible? *Ann Rheum Dis* 1986; 46: 171–3.

25 Hickling P, Jacoby RK, Kirwan JR. Joint destruction recommences after glucocorticoids are withdrawn in early rheumatoid arthritis. *Br J Rheumatol* 1996; 35 (Suppl. 2): 22.

26 Larsen A, Dale K, Eek M. Radiographic evaluation of rheumatoid arthritis and related conditions by standard reference films. *Acta Radiol* 1977; 18: 481–91.

27 Steinbrocker O, Traegar CH, Batterman RC. Therapeutic criteria in rheumatoid arthritis. *JAMA* 1949; 140: 659–62.

28 Fries JF, Spitz P, Kraines RG, Holman HR. Measurement of patient outcome in arthritis. *Arthritis Rheum* 1980; 23(2): 137–45.

29 Kirwan JR, Reeback JS. Stanford Health Assessment Questionnaire modified to assess disability in British patients with rheumatoid arthritis. *Br J Rheumatol* 1986; 25: 206–9.

30 Joint Committee of the Medical Research Council and Nuffield Foundation. Long term results in early cases of rheumatoid arthritis treated with either cortisone or aspirin. *Br Med J* 1957; 1: 847–50.

31 Harris ED, Emkey RD, Nichols JE, Newberg A. Low dose prednisolone therapy in rheumatoid arthritis: a double blind study. *J Rheumatol* 1983; 10: 713–21.

12: Are intra-articular steroids as effective?

S. Brady, R.O. Day and G.G. Graham

Introduction

Since their introduction in 1950 intra-articular injections of corticosteroids have been used widely in the treatment of rheumatoid arthritis (RA) and other arthritic conditions. Their apparent efficacy is predominantly supported by uncontrolled data. Widespread differences exist in methods of administration and choice of corticosteroid for injection [1,2], reflecting the relative lack of experimental and comparative data and the empirical nature of their use. Corticosteroids have not been considered as disease-modifying anti-rheumatic drugs, such as d-penicillamine and gold, but as highly effective anti-inflammatory agents. A recent placebo-controlled trial in early RA revealed, however, a significantly reduced rate of joint destruction which was demonstrated radiologically in patients treated orally with prednisolone for 2 years [3]. Given the proximity of the pathological lesion of RA to the joint, this result raises the question about whether judicious use of intra-articular corticosteroids may have disease-modifying properties which are as yet unrecognized.

Mechanism of action

The corticosteroid receptor is activated by binding with steroid and the activated receptor then binds to specific DNA sequences known as corticosteroid response elements. The binding to the response elements either induces or represses particular genes. Binding to a response element which is in the promoter region of a gene initiates transcription. An example is the transcription of the anti-inflammatory protein, lipocortin, which decreases the activity of phospholipase A_2. Lesser activity of phospholipase A_2 leads to reduced migration of leucocytes [4] and decreased synthesis of the pro-inflammatory prostaglandins and leucotrienes [5].

Most of the critical mediators of inflammation are proteins coded by genes with promoter sites for the important transcription factors, NF-κB and AP-1. Activated glucocorticosteroid receptors inhibit NF-κB- and AP-1-mediated transcription directly, thus bypassing the corticosteroid response element mechanism [6]. Several mechanisms for this effect have been proposed. This action on NF-κB and AP-1 is probably the major mechanism of the anti-inflammatory and anti-rheumatic properties of the glucocorticosteroids. Thus, they inhibit the AP-1-mediated expression of collagenases I and IV and the NF-κB-mediated expression of the cytokines, interleukin 2 (IL-2), IL-6 and IL-8, intercellular adhesion molecule 1 (ICAM-1) and E-selectin (ELAM-1) and pro-inflammatory enzymes, nitric oxide synthase and cyclo-oxygenase 2.

Can intra-articular corticosteroids achieve these effects when placed in high and continuing concentrations in inflamed joints? Should we explore protocols of the appropriate, regular administration of the corticosteroids by the intra-articular route to achieve better long-term outcomes for inflamed joints?

Development of intra-articular corticosteroids

Soon after their isolation and synthesis, corticosteroids were administered by intra-articular injection in rheumatological practice [7]. Cortisone was ineffective [8] because it requires systemic reductive metabolism to hydrocortisone to be active. Intra-articular injections of hydrocortisone were demonstrated to be effective but the perceived rapid loss from synovial fluid and a variable duration of action led to a search for longer-acting corticosteroids for intra-articular use. This was achieved with the formulation of less soluble steroids [9]. Subsequently a number of longer-acting steroid ester preparations have been developed and marketed. Methylprednisolone acetate, triamcinolone acetonide and triamcinolone hexacetonide are the intra-articular steroids preferred by the majority of American rheumatologists [2].

Both methylprednisolone acetate and triamcinolone hexacetonide are prodrugs and require hydrolysis to methylprednisolone and triamcinolone acetonide (Fig. 12.1), respectively, before they have pharmacological activity. Triamcinolone acetonide is an active corticosteroid. It is closely related to the active steroid, triamcinolone, but only small amounts of the acetonide are metabolized to triamcinolone [10].

Pharmacokinetics

The major factor controlling the clearance of the corticosteroids from the joint is their rate of dissolution. In early studies, it was found that hydrocortisone (cortisol) and cortisone and their acetate esters disappear from

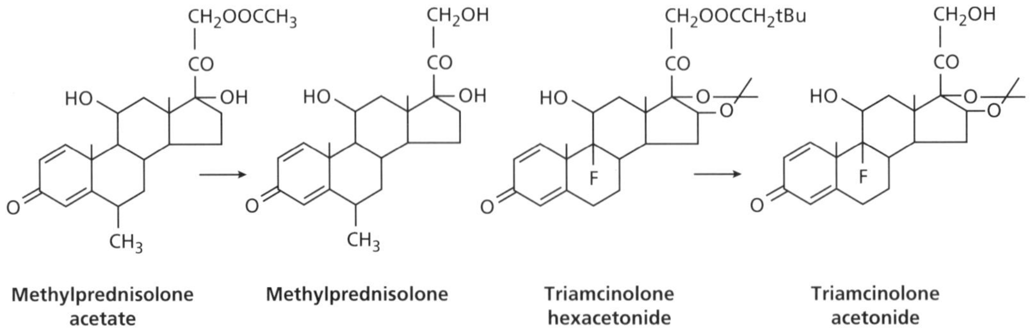

Fig. 12.1 Structures and hydrolysis of the ester corticosteroids and their metabolites which are commonly used by intra-articular injection.

synovial fluid very quickly [11–13]. For example, it was reported that there was a 40% loss of hydrocortisone acetate within 5 min [12]. Hydrocortisone acetate is administered as a suspension and the apparent rapid loss is almost certainly the result of the crystalline material settling onto the surface of the synovium and not to extremely rapid diffusion out of the synovial compartment.

The most complete studies on the synovial pharmacokinetics of corticosteroids have been obtained with the now widely used preparations of methylprednisolone acetate, triamcinolone acetonide and triamcinolone hexacetonide. Although several conclusions about the pharmacokinetics of the intra-articular corticosteroids are based on limited information, present conclusions on their pharmacokinetics and some supporting data include the following.

Corticosteroid suspensions dissolve slowly in synovial fluid with prolonged local anti-inflammatory effects

Kinetic analysis of the plasma concentrations of triamcinolone acetonide indicates that both triamcinolone acetonide and hexacetonide are absorbed slowly with half-lives of absorption of 3–6 days. Triamcinolone hexacetonide is absorbed more slowly than triamcinolone acetonide [14]. The total absorption takes 2–3 weeks (Fig. 12.2). Suppression of inflammation, as assessed by thermography, is reported to last for about 4 days after methylprednisolone acetate and for at least 6 weeks with triamcinolone hexacetonide [15], although such a large difference is surprising in view of the similar duration of inhibition of cortisol secretion produced by the two steroids (see below).

The slow rate of absorption of the corticosteroids from the synovial cavity is not just due to the corticosteroid dissolving slowly from a free

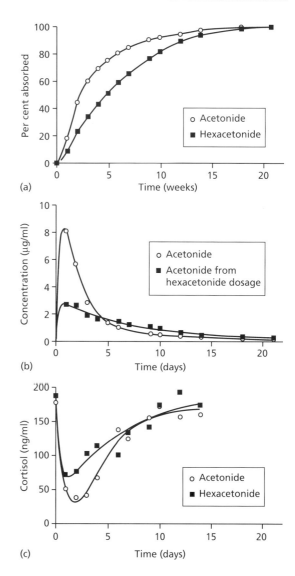

Fig. 12.2 Pharmacokinetics and systemic effects of triaminolone acetonide and hexacetonide following the intra-articular injections of 40 mg of triamcinolone acetonide and triamcinolone hexacetonide. (a) Fractions of triamcinolone acetonide and triamcinolone hexacetonide remaining to be absorbed. (b) Plasma concentrations of triamcinolone acetonide following intra-articular injections. Note that the hexacetonide is hydrolysed to triamcinolone acetonide (see Fig. 12.1). (c) Endogenous cortisol concentrations in plasma. (From [14].)

suspension in synovial fluid. In cows, methylprednisolone acetate becomes incorporated in a fibrin-like mass which is considered to decrease the dissolution of the corticosteroid [16]. It is likely that a similar effect in humans slows the absorption of the intra-articular corticosteroids.

It should be noted that the intra-articular corticosteroids may have actions which outlast their presence in the joint. For example, intra-articular injections of triamcinolone hexacetonide produced benefit which lasted for at least 6 months in ≈ 60% of injected knees and for 12 months in 45% of injected knees [17]. This duration of action is far longer than the 3 weeks required for complete absorption from the knee and indicates that at least temporary remission is obtained in many patients. The prolonged decrease in the thermographic index in inflamed joints after intra-articular triamcinolone hexacetonide may similarly be due to the development of remission (see above).

Intra-articular corticosteroid suspensions lead to sustained plasma concentrations and systemic effects

Following an intra-articular injection of methylprednisolone acetate, peak plasma concentrations of methylprednisolone are achieved between 2 and 16 h with no significant difference between patients with RA and osteoarthritis (OA) [18,19]. The hypertrophied synovium in RA is quite different to the synovium in OA but the rate of absorption is, on average, very much the same. This result indicates that the rate of absorption is controlled by the rate of dissolution. The plasma concentrations of methylprednisolone decline with a half-life of 18 h [18,19], in contrast to a half-life of about 2.6 h after oral administration of methylprednisolone itself [20], a further indication of very slow release from the synovial compartment.

The plasma concentrations of triamcinolone acetonide are also sustained after the administration of both the parent acetonide and the hexacetonide. The terminal half-life of triamcinolone acetonide in plasma is 3–6 days [14], compared with a terminal half-life of about 1.5 h after systemic dosage [10], again consistent with slow release due to slow dissolution in the synovial compartment. For the same doses of the two preparations, the peak plasma concentrations of triamcinolone acetonide are lower but the concentrations are slightly more sustained after the administration of triamcinolone hexacetonide (see Fig. 12.2) [14]. This result is consistent with the lower water solubility of the hexacetonide and its consequent slower dissolution and absorption from the synovial compartment.

Large doses of all the intra-articular corticosteroids suppress the hypothalamic–pituitary–adrenal axis, a clear indicator of substantial levels of exogenous corticosteroids in the circulation. The plasma concentrations of cortisol are suppressed for about a week after single doses of 20–40 mg methylprednisolone acetate [15] or either triamcinolone preparation [14]. The prodrug, triamcinolone hexacetonide, tends to produce a lower maximum effect but more prolonged suppression of cortisol than triamcinolone acetonide itself although detailed statistical analysis was not reported. The suppression of cortisol secretion does not coincide with the pattern of release of the triamcinolone preparations. Thus, cortisol secretion is inhibited for about a week despite the total release taking 2–3 weeks (see Fig. 12.2) [14]. The discrepancy probably lies in the plasma levels of triamcinolone acetonide. After 6–8 days, detectable levels of triamcinolone acetonide are still in the circulation but are too low to inhibit the secretion of cortisol (see Fig. 12.2).

The hypothalamic–pituitary–adrenal axis is inhibited by the intra-articular steroids but the period of this effect is still short in comparison to the suppression time caused by continuous treatment with oral corticosteroids. The clinical significance is, correspondingly, greater with the oral corticosteroids. Although there is clear suppression of the hypothalamic–pituitary–adrenal axis, the intra-articular corticosteroids do not produce an overall improvement in patients with RA. Some patients may, however, show modest improvement [15], and many patients report temporary improvement in joints that have not been injected. Intra-articular injections of 20–40 mg of methylprednisolone or either triamcinolone preparation also lead to ≈ 50% decreases in the markers of inflammation, erythrocyte sedimentation rate and C-reactive protein [21].

There is considerable intersubject variation in the rate of dissolution and systemic effects of intra-articular injections of corticosteroid suspensions

There are large interpatient variations in the plasma concentrations of methylprednisolone following intra-articular injection [18,19]. The suppression of the hypothalamic–pituitary–adrenal axis may also be correspondingly variable. For example, Lazarevic and colleagues [22] found that an intra-articular injection of 40 mg methylprednisolone acetate led consistently to decreased cortisol levels at 24 h but, by contrast, the plasma cortisol levels were erratic at 72 h: decreased in some patients, with little or no suppression in other patients at this time.

Corticosteroid esters are largely hydrolysed in the synovial fluid before diffusion into plasma

Methylprednisolone acetate is hydrolysed in plasma with a half-life of about 20 min [23]. Plasma proteins enter the inflamed joint readily and the ester corticosteroids, such as methylprednisolone acetate and triamcinolone hexacetonide (see Fig. 12.1) should be hydrolysed rapidly in synovial fluid.

Corticosteroids in solution diffuse readily out of synovial fluid

Corticosteroids have low but appreciable aqueous solubilities. There has been no direct measurement of the rate of diffusion of corticosteroids in solution out of synovial fluid but it is predicted that they should readily diffuse out. The endothelial cell layer is the only membranous barrier to drugs entering or leaving the synovial compartment. The synovial capillaries are moderately fenestrated [24] and should provide little barrier to the efflux of corticosteroids in solution.

The kinetics of the non-steroidal anti-inflammatory drugs have been studied in considerable detail and some predictions about corticosteroids can be made from this work. Methylprednisolone, for example, is moderately strongly protein bound at 78% but the transfer in the protein-bound form is probably a minor part of its transfer into and out of synovial fluid. This prediction is derived largely from data on the uptake and loss of non-steroidal anti-inflammatory drugs in synovial fluid. For example, diclofenac is more than 99% bound to plasma proteins but less than 50% of its transfer out of synovial fluid is in the bound form [25]. The lower protein binding of the corticosteroids means that their diffusion in the unbound form should be favoured but they have larger molecular masses than the non-steroidal anti-inflammatory agents, thus decreasing the diffusion of the unbound forms. The high proportion in the unbound form should, however, more than compensate and the efflux from the synovial compartment should largely be in the unbound form. Nevertheless, there should be high concentrations of corticosteroids in lymphatics draining injected joints. This is demonstrated in occasional patients by the development of a hypopigmented pattern around the knee in some patients [13].

It is anticipated that the synovial pharmacokinetics of corticosteroids alter as a result of the powerful anti-inflammatory properties of these drugs. Consistent with this view, the rate of loss of protein from the rabbit knee is slowed by the intra-articular injection of triamcinolone hexacetonide [26]. Synovial fluid volume and pressure, which are affected by the position and movements of the joint, have a profound effect on the oxygenation of the synovium [27] and the kinetics of corticosteroids should be altered by these factors although no formal studies have been conducted.

Interactions between the intra-articular corticosteroids and other drugs are short-lived

There has been no study of the influence of inhibitors of drug metabolism on the systemic effects of the intra-articular corticosteroids. It is, however, known that the metabolism of methylprednisolone is inhibited substantially by ketoconazole and the macrolide antibiotics, such as erythromycin [28,29]. The systemic effects of intra-articular methylprednisolone should therefore be increased substantially by the administration of these drugs. The intra-articular dose should not be altered although more intense short-term systemic effects, such as inhibition of cortisol secretion, may be produced.

There are relatively few proven effects of corticosteroids on the metabolism of other drugs. One is the increased clearance of salicylate by corticosteroids. Intra-articular injections of corticosteroids decrease the plasma concentrations of salicylate but the effect is short-lived with the plasma concentrations returning to previous levels mostly within 60 h [30]. Intra-articular corticoids also appear to increase the clearance of a sulphadimidine in some slow acetylators [31]. Sulphadimidine has been used as test drug for acetylator phenotype and this increased clearance in some slow acetylators may occur with other drugs which are acetylated.

Efficacy

The clinical experience and small trials which shaped the early and current use of intra-articular corticosteroids has been extensively reviewed by Gray and colleagues [13]. Comparatively little work has been published subsequently to enable the comparisons of the efficacy and safety of the various intra-articular steroid preparations. Few studies have compared intra-articular steroids with other agents and no published studies have compared local vs. systemic corticosteroids. The latter probably reflects the very different indications for these two approaches to corticosteroid therapy at present. Chronic oral dosage with corticosteroids is indicated to help control widespread synovitis whereas intra-articular steroids are generally reserved for the treatment of problematic individual joints on an 'as needed' basis.

One trial involved the comparison of intra-articular triamcinolone acetonide 20 mg with joint washout alone and a combination of joint washout and triamcinolone in the treatment of patients with RA and symptomatic knee effusions [32]. All three groups showed some symptomatic improvement at 3 months but the groups receiving triamcinolone acetonide also showed decreased joint size and increased range of movement. There was no statistical difference between the two groups receiving triamcinolone acetonide. This trial demonstrated prolonged, clinically important improvement with intra-articular corticosteroids compared with an intervention which would be expected to produce an equivalent placebo response. Corticosteroid injections into the shoulder similarly show superior results to manipulation [33].

Blyth and colleagues [34] compared hydrocortisone succinate with triamcinolone acetonide and hexacetonide in the intra-articular treatment of RA of the knee. Their study looked at efficacy in terms of pain relief in patients selected because of symptoms or requests for injections. This single blind comparative study between triamcinolone preparations and hydrocortisone succinate was stopped after only 60 patients had been randomized because of lack of efficacy of hydrocortisone succinate. How-ever, patients treated with hydrocortisone had larger volumes of aspirated joint fluid suggesting that this group had more severe disease. Although reported as a single study, patients were subsequently randomized to either of the two triamcinolone preparations. The hexacetonide showed superior efficacy with significantly more patients pain-free at 4 weeks, a difference which was sustained throughout the 12-week period of follow-up. At 12 weeks 18% of patients treated with triamcinolone hexacetonide were pain-free compared with 9% treated with the acetonide. Although this study was only single blind and methods of randomization were described incompletely, it does suggest that triamcinolone hexacetonide may be the more effective agent at the doses used.

Overall, intra-articular corticosteroids produce many changes in-dicative of decreased inflammation. Pain, swelling, blood flow, histological evidence of synovitis, volume of synovium and synovial fluid are all decreased. The composition of synovial fluid is altered, with decreased pro-tein and numbers of neutrophils [9] and, from animal studies, increased hyaluronate [35]. Gene expression, particularly that of collagenase and tissue inhibitor of metalloproteinases, is decreased [36]. The strength of extensor muscles of injected knees is increased [37].

Intra-articular corticosteroids have been used in a variety of conditions including RA, psoriatic arthritis, gout, pseudogout, and OA. Gray and col-leagues [13] considered that the intra-articular steroids were of little value in the treatment of OA, although, in a recent review, Towheed and Hochberg [38] concluded that intra-articular corticosteroids were of benefit. Inflam-mation of joints may occur in OA and the intra-articular corticosteroids may be useful in the treatment of acutely inflamed joints in this disease. Recent studies indicate that these preparations may be useful in the treat-ment of spondyloarthropathies [39], haemophiliac arthropathy [40] and polymyalgia rheumatica [41], although their usefulness in these syndromes is based on very limited studies. In the treatment of polymyalgia rheumatica, intra-articular corticosteroids control the symptoms although the synovitis may continue for a longer time in some patients [41]. Corticosteroid injec-tions have also been used in juvenile chronic arthritis, with triamcinolone hexacetonide appearing to be more useful than methylprednisolone acetate [42]. Favourable long-term efficacy in children was greater if the patients were young, had a short duration of disease and higher doses (within the range 20–40 mg) of triamcinolone hexacetonide had been given into the knees of the children [17]. Methylprednisolone acetate is, however, pre-ferred if the intra-articular route cannot be guaranteed because of a higher chance of adverse events such as subcutaneous atrophy with triamcinolone hexacetonide [42,43].

Newer methods of studying the anti-inflammatory effects of intra-articular steroids

More recently studies have looked at the efficacy of intra-articular steroids using new imaging techniques. Østergaard and colleagues [44] evaluated the effects of intra-articular steroids using quantitative magnetic resonance imaging to measure volumes of synovia and effusions and to look at cartilage and bone erosions. The technique is particularly useful after dosage with the gadolinium contrast agent, gadopentate dimeglumine. In a small sample of 18 patients treated with intra-articular methylprednisolone acetate 80 mg, rapid decreases in the volumes of both synovial tissues and effusions were noted [44]. Clinical relapse was associated with an increase to pretreatment levels of synovial tissue but not effusion volumes. Higher pretreatment synovial volumes were associated with a shorter duration of clinical remission. Magnetic resonance imaging has also been used to evaluate the decrease in inflammation of sacroiliac joints after the intra-articular injection, the injections being placed in the joints by the use of computed tomography [39]. Magnetic resonance imaging appears to be a very useful agent for further investigations of intra-articular steroids, in comparing different agents and also in determining the groups of patients likely to respond to this group of agents. The detection of early changes and a lack of observer bias may also be useful aspects of this technique [45,46].

Another new imaging technique which has been used to determine the extent of inflammation and the effect of intra-articular corticosteroids is positron emission tomography (PET) [47]. This involves the injection of a ^{11}C-labelled tracer, D-deprenyl, and location of the marker by the detection of the emitted positrons. High uptake of ^{11}C-labelled D-deprenyl in inflamed joints was reduced by ≈ 50% after the corticosteroid injection but the low resolution of PET does not allow the distinction between the uptake into synovial tissue or synovial fluid. Furthermore, the pathophysiological basis of the uptake of the D-deprenyl remains to be elucidated. Other labelled compounds may also be useful. PET is not a routine procedure but is a useful research tool.

Rest and efficacy of intra-articular corticosteroids

Bed rest or joint splinting for prolonged periods has commonly accompanied intra-articular corticosteroids [48]. As bed rest or splinting of joints is thought to have beneficial effects on inflamed joints, this becomes a potential confounder in the assessment of intra-articular corticosteroids. Rest may also alter efficacy of the intra-articular steroids by altering their pharmacokinetics. One possibility is that rest may change the areas of deposition of the steroid on the synovium.

Chakravarty and colleagues [49] examined this issue with a randomized controlled study comparing post-injection rest (24 h of in-patient bed rest) with out-patient injection and presumably normal activities in a group of patients receiving intra-articular triamcinolone hexacetonide for inflammatory arthritis. The clinical response was significantly better in the rest group at 12 and 24 weeks. The prolonged duration of improvement in the rest group was the most striking feature of this trial. Given the equivalent early response and short duration of bed rest, this difference is likely to be due to alterations in the pharmacology of the intra-articular steroid rather than any effect of the bed rest *per se* but the nature of the pharmacological alterations remains to be elucidated. However, another study conducted entirely in an in-patient setting [50] failed to detect a difference between patients rested after the injection and those who did not.

Safety

The risks associated with intra-articular corticosteroid injections have been reviewed recently by Cooper and Kirwan [51]. Compared with systemic corticosteroid use, they appear relatively free of toxicity. This is the common view of rheumatologists and orthopaedic surgeons, but the injections do have the potential for some specific adverse effects related to their intra-articular delivery.

Septic arthritis can occur with penetration of the joint for intra-articular delivery, either through direct inoculation or through predisposing to haematogenous spread of organisms from distant sites. Despite the widespread use of intra-articular steroids, with varying degree of attention to antisepsis or asepsis, infection is an uncommon event. Hollander [52] reported an incidence of less than one infection per 7000 injections and Gray and colleagues [13] an incidence of approximately one infection per 50 000 injections. Infections may, of course, be initially difficult to detect because of the anti-inflammatory effect of the corticosteroids.

Concern has arisen that a destructive arthropathy similar to Charcot's arthropathy may occur in joints receiving repeated intra-articular injections of corticosteroid. This concern has developed from a series of case reports [51,53] and from sub-primate animal studies [54] showing acceleration of joint damage. Osteonecrosis of joints repeatedly injected has also been reported [52].

Intra-articular corticosteroids do have catabolic effects on bone and cartilage including decreased proteoglycan synthesis and collagen production. Conversely, in inflamed joints, corticosteroids decrease the production of metalloproteinases and may protect against joint damage by this anti-catabolic effect. Joint damage is also postulated to arise as a result of the analgesic effects of intra-articular steroids allowing increased activity and therefore more damage to vulnerable joints. The inflammatory arthropathies for which intra-articular corticosteroids have been used are known to be associated with joint destruction and osteonecrosis so attributing causation of these events to intra-articular corticosteroids in the cases reported is problematic.

Roberts and colleagues [55] identified a group of patients who had received multiple (defined as greater than four in a year) injections of corticosteroids into a single joint without receiving multiple injections in the corresponding contralateral joint. These patients were then followed prospectively for 5 years. No significant relationship emerged between 'frequent' intra-articular steroid injections and subsequent arthroplasty. There was even a trend for the frequently injected joints to be less likely to require arthroplasty than joints with less frequent injections. Therefore, this study indicates a possible chondroprotective effect of intra-articular corticosteroids in inflammatory arthropathy. However, the study is small, of limited statistical power and is non-randomized and observational rather than experimental. Growth of children also does not appear to be affected [56].

A single intra-articular corticosteroid injection reduces serum osteocalcin, a marker of bone formation but had no effect on urinary pyridinoline, a breakdown product of collagen [57]. The effects on osteocalcin are transient (less than 2 weeks) and again, likely to be of far less clinical significance than the effects on bone metabolism of continued oral corticosteroid therapy. In horses, three intra-articular corticosteroids over 2 weeks greatly increased the concentrations of proteoglycan, indicating cartilage degradation [35].

Overall, it is concluded that intra-articular corticosteroids may, theoretically, be associated with catabolic effects which could cause a 'steroid arthropathy'. Conversely, it is possible that aspects of their anti-inflammatory effect could protect inflamed joints.

Conclusion

Several questions and controversies remain about the benefits and safety of intra-articular corticosteroids. These questions will remain until (if ever) they are answered by properly designed randomized controlled trials. The risk of any possible 'steroid arthropathy' does appear low and provided some caution is entertained about overfrequent intra-articular injections their evident symptomatic benefit should justify their continued use.

Future directions

Intra-articular injection techniques have the potential to localize drug action in the synovium limiting systemic adverse reactions. Rapid systemic absorption has limited this benefit from being realized completely although with corticosteroids the development of relatively insoluble esters has been partially successful. Other methods are being developed with the potential to deliver corticosteroids and other agents into the joint while limiting or substantially slowing systemic absorption. For example, liposomes have been used in animal models to deliver both intra-articular triamcinolone and methotrexate and showed advantages over free drug in the suppression of arthritis. This method of delivery results in efficient retention within the articular cavity and would appear to be a promising method for the delivery of both corticosteroids and other therapies such as anticytokine agents for which oral equivalents are not available currently or which are associated with systemic side-effects.

References

1 Haslock I, MacFarlane D, Speed C. Intra-articular and soft-tissue injections: a survey of current practice. *Br J Rheumatol* 1995; 34: 449–52.

2 Centeno LM, Moore ME. Preferred intraarticular corticosteroids and associated practice: a survey of members of the American College of Rheumatology. *Arthritis Care Res* 1994; 7: 151–5.

3 Kirwan JR. The effect of glucocorticoids on joint destruction in rheumatoid arthritis. *N Engl J Med* 1995; 333: 142–6.

4 Perretti M, Croxtall JD, Wheller SK *et al.* Mobilizing lipocortin 1 in adherent human leukocytes down-regulates their transmigration. *Nature Med* 1996; 2: 1259–62.

5 Flower RJ, Rothwell NJ. Lipocortin 1: cellular mechanisms and clinical relevance. *Trends Pharmacol Sci* 1994; 15: 71–6.

6 Cato ACB, Wade E. Molecular mechanisms of anti-inflammatory action of glucorticoids. *Bioessays* 1996; 18: 371–8.

7 Hollander JL, Brown EM Jr, Jessar RA, Brown CY. Hydrocortisone and cortisone injected into arthritic joints. Comparative effects of and use of hydrocortisone as a local antiarthritic agent. *JAMA* 1951; 147: 1629–35.

8 Dixon AStJ, Bywaters EGL. The effect of intra-articular injection of cortisone acetate and hydrocortisone acetate in rheumatoid arthritis. *Clin Sci* 1953; 12: 15–31.

9 Murdoch WR, Will G. Methyl-prednisolone acetate in intra-articular therapy. Clinical, biochemical and chro-matographic studies. *Br Med J* 1962; 1: 604–6.

10 Möllmann H, Rohdewald P, Schmidt EW, Salomon V, Derendorf H. Pharmacokinetics of triamcinolone acetonide and its phosphate ester. *Eur J Clin Pharmacol* 1985; 29: 85–9.

11 Zacco M, Richardson EM, Crittenden JO, Hollander JL, Dohan FC. Disposition of intraarticularly injected hydrocortisone acetate, hydrocortisone and cortisone acetate in arthritis. I. Concentration in synovial fluid and cells. *J Clin Endocrinol* 1954; 14: 711–18.

12 Wilson H, Glyn J, Scull E, Ziff M. Rate of disappearance and metabolism of hydrocortisone and cortisone in the synovial cavity in rheumatoid arthritis. *Proc Soc Exp Biol Med* 1953; 83: 648–54.

13 Gray RG, Tenenbaum J, Gottlieb NL. Local corticosteroid injection treatment in rheumatic disorders. *Semin Arthritis Rheum* 1981; 10: 231–54.

14 Derendorf H, Möllman H, Grüner A, Haack D, Gyselby G. Pharmacokinetics and pharmacodynamics of gluco-corticoid suspensions after intra-articular injection. *Clin Pharmacol Ther* 1986; 39: 313–17.

15 Bird HA, Ring EFJ, Bacon PAA. Thermographic and clinical comparison of three intra-articular steroid preparations in rheumatoid arthritis. *Ann Rheum Dis* 1979; 38: 36–9.

16 Toutain PL, Alvinerie M, Fayolle P, Ruckebusch Y. Bovine plasma and synovial fluid kinetics of methylprednisolone and methylprednisolone acetate after intra-articular administration of methylprednisolone acetate. *J Pharmacol Exp Ther* 1986, 236: 794–802.

17 Allen RC, Gross KR, Laxer RM *et al.* Intraarticular triamcinolone hexacetonide in the management of chronic arthritis in children. *Arthritis Rheum* 1986; 29: 997–1001.

18 Armstrong RD, English J, Gibson T, Chakraborty J, Marks V. Serum methylprednisolone level following intra-articular injection of methyl-prednisolone acetate. *Ann Rheum Dis* 1981; 40: 571–4.

19 Bertouch JV, Sallustio BC, Meffin PJ, Brooks PMA. Comparison of plasma methylprednisolone concentrations following intra-articular injection in patients with rheumatoid arthritis and osteoarthritis. *Aust NZ J Med* 1983; 13: 583–6.

20 Albert KS, Brown SW, DeSante KA *et al.* Double Latin square to determine variability and relative bioavailability of methylprednisolone. *J Pharm Sci* 1980; 39: 22–4.

21 Taylor HG, Fowler PD, David MJ, Dawes PT. Intra-articular steroids: confounder of clinical trials. *Clin Rheumatol* 1991; 10: 38–42.

22 Lazarevic MB, Skosey JL, Djordjevic-Denic G *et al.* Reduction of cortisol levels after single intra-articular and intramuscular steroid injection. *Am J Med* 1995; 99: 370–3.

23 Garg DC, Ng P, Weidler DJ, Sakmar E, Wagner JG. Preliminary *in vitro* and *in vivo* investigations on methylprednisolone and its acetate. *Res Commun Chem Pathol Pharmacol* 1978; 22: 37–48.

24 Hadler NM. The biology of the extracellular space. *Clin Rheum Dis* 1981; 7: 71–97.

25 Owen SG, Francis HW, Roberts MS. Disappearance kinetics of solutes from synovial fluid after intra-articular injection. *Br J Clin Pharmacol* 1994; 38: 349–55.

26 Jakobsen J, Christensen KS, Stockel M. The effect of a corticosteroid on the absorption of ^{131}I-albumin from rabbit knee joint. *Z Rheum* 1986; 45: 152–4.

27 Mapp PI, Grootveld MC, Blake DR. Hypoxia, oxidative stress and rheumatoid arthritis. *Br Med Bull* 1995; 51: 419–36.

28 Glynn AM, Slaughter RL, Brass C, D'Amrosio R, Jusko WJ. Effects of ketoconazole on methylprednisolone pharmacokinetics and cortisol secretion. *Clin Pharmacol Ther* 1986; 39: 654–9.

29 La Force CF, Szefler SJ, Miller MF, Ebling W, Brenner M. Inhibition of methylprednisolone elimination in the presence of erythromycin therapy. *J Allergy Clin Immunol* 1983; 72: 34–9.

30 Baer PA, Shore A, Ikeman RL. Transient fall in serum salicylate levels following intraarticular injection of steroid in patients with rheumatoid arthritis. *Arthritis Rheum* 1987; 30: 345–7.

31 Reeves PT, Hanrahan P, Edelman J, Ilett KF. Effect of intra-articular glucocorticoids on the disposition of sulphadimidine in chronic osteoarthritis patients. *Br J Clin Pharmacol* 1988; 26: 563–8.

32 Srinivasan A, Amos M, Webley M. The effects of joint washout and steroid injection compared with either joint washout or steroid injection alone in rheumatoid knee effusion. *Br J Rheumatol* 1995; 34: 771–3.

33 Winters JC, Sobel JS, Groenier KH, Arendzen HJ, Meyboom de Jong B. Comparison of physiotherapy, manipulation, and corticosteroid injection for treating shoulder complaints in general practice:

randomised, single blind study. *Br Med J* 1997; 314: 1320–5.

34 Blyth T, Hunter JA, Stirling A. Pain relief in the rheumatoid knee after steroid injection. A single-blind comparison of hydrocortisone succinate, and triamcinolone acetonide or hexacetonide. *Br J Rheumatol* 1994; 33: 461–3.

35 Roneus B, Lindblad A, Lindholm A, Jones B. Effects of intraarticular corticosteroid and sodium hyaluronate injections on synovial fluid production and synovial fluid content content of sodium hyaluronate and proteoglycans in normal equine joints. *Zentralbl Veterinarmed A* 1993; 40: 10–16.

36 Firestein GS, Paine MM, Littman BH. Gene expression (collagenase, tissue inhibitor of metalloproteinases, complement and HLA-DR) in rheumatoid arthritis and osteoarthritic synovium. Quantitative analysis and effect of intraarticular corticosteroids. *Arthritis Rheum* 1991; 34: 1094–105.

37 Geborek P, Mansson B, Wollheim FA, Moritz U. Intraarticular corticosteroid injection into rheumatoid arthritis knees improves extensor muscles strength. *Rheumatol Int* 1990; 9: 265–70.

38 Towheed TE, Hochberg MCA. A systemic review of randomized controlled trials of pharmacological therapy in osteoarthritis of the knee, with an emphasis on trial methodology. *Semin Arthritis Rheum* 1997; 26: 755–70.

39 Mutze S, Seyrekbasan F, Wolf KJ, Hamm BCT. Guided intraarticular corticosteroid injection into the sacroiliac joints in patients with spondyloarthropathy. Indication and follow-up with contrast-enhanced MRI. *J Comput Assist Tomogr* 1996; 20: 512–21.

40 Shupak R, Teitel J, Garvey MB, Freedman J. Intraarticular methyl-prednisolone therapy in hemophilic arthropathy. *Am J Hematol* 1988; 27: 26–9.

41 Meliconi R, Pulsatelli L, Uguccioni M *et al.* Leukocyte infiltration in synovial tissue from the shoulder of patients with polymyalgia rheumatica. Quantitative analysis and influence of corticosteroid treatment. *Arthritis Rheum* 1996; 39: 1199–207.

42 Honkanen VE, Rautonen JK, Pelkonen PM. Intra-articular glucocorticoids in early juvenile chronic arthritis. *Acta Paediatr* 1993; 82: 1072–4.

43 Job-Deslandre C, Menkes CJ. Complications of intra-articular injections of triamcinolone hexacetonide in chronic arthritis in children. *Clin Exp Rheumatol* 1990; 8: 413–16.

44 Østergaard M, Stoltenberg M, Gideon P *et al.* Changes in synovial membrane and joint effusion volumes after intraarticular methylprednisolone. Quantitative assessment of inflammatory and destructive changes in arthritis by MRI. *J Rheumatol* 1996; 23: 1151–61.

45 Østergaard M, Stoltenberg M, Henriksen O, Lorenzen I. Quantitative assessment of synovial inflammation by dynamic gadolinium-enhanced magnetic resonance imaging. A study of the effect of intra-articular methylprednisolone on the rate of early synovial enhancement. *Br J Rheumatol* 1996; 35: 50–9.

46 Creamer P, Keen M, Zananiri F *et al.* Quantitative magnetic imaging of the knee: a method of measuring response to intra-articular treatments. *Ann Rheum Dis* 1997; 56: 378–81.

47 Danfors T, Bergström M, Feltelius N *et al.* Positron emission tomography with ^{11}C-D-deprenyl in patients with rheumatoid arthritis. *Scand J Rheumatol* 1997; 26: 43–8.

48 McCarty DJ, Harman JG, Grassanovich JL, Qian C. Treatment of rheumatoid joint inflammation with intrasynovial triamcinolone hexacetonide. *J Rheumatol* 1995; 22: 1631–5.

49 Chakravarty K, Pharoah PD, Scott DGA. Randomised controlled study of post-injection rest following intra-articular steroid therapy for knee synovitis. *Br J Rheumatol* 1994; 33: 464–8.

50 Chatham W, Williams G, Mooreland L *et al.* Intraarticular corticosteroid injections: should we rest the joints? *Arthritis Care Res* 1989; 2: 70–4.

51 Cooper C, Kirwan JR. The risks of local and systemic corticosteroid administration. *Baillière's Clin Rheumatol* 1990; 4(2): 305–8.

52 Hollander JL, Jessar RA, Brown RR. Intrasynovial corticosteroid therapy: a decade of use. *Bull Rheum Dis* 1969; 11: 239–40.

53 Owen DS Jr. Aspiration and injection of joints and soft tissues. In: Kelley WN, Harris ED, Ruddy S, Sledge CB, eds. *Textbook of Rheumatology*, 5th edn. Philadelphia: WB Saunders, 1997; 591–608.

54 Behrens F, Shepard N, Mitchell N. Alteration of rabbit articular cartilage by intra-articular injections of glucocorticoids. *J Bone Joint Surg* 1975; 57A: 70–6.

55 Roberts WN, Babcock EA, Breitbach SA, Owen DS, Irby WR. Corticosteroid injection in rheumatoid arthritis does not increase rate of total joint arthroplasty. *J Rheumatol* 1996; 23: 1001–4.

56 Huppertz H-I, Tschammler A, Horwitz AE, Schwab KO. Intraarticular corticosteroids for chronic arthritis in children: efficacy and effects on cartilage and growth. *J Pediatr* 1995; 127: 317–21.

57 Emkey RD, Lindsay R, Lyssy J *et al.* The systemic effect of intraarticular administration of corticosteroid on markers of bone formation and bone resorption in patients with rheumatoid arthritis. *Arthritis Rheum* 1996; 39: 277–82.

13: Should disease-modifying drugs be used alone or in combination?

P.M. Brooks

Introduction

It is now recognized that rheumatoid arthritis (RA) causes significant morbidity and mortality [1–3]. Yelin and colleagues have demonstrated that 50% of RA patients have a significant impairment of work capacity 10 years after diagnosis and it is also clear from early arthritis clinics that, once the disease has been established with persisting synovitis of over 3 months' duration, it is unusual for remission to occur spontaneously or with drug therapy [4,5]. Extensive research on the aetiopathogenesis of joint destruction in RA has defined to a very large extent the multiplicity of interacting cells and mediators that result in joint destruction (Fig. 13.1) and with these interacting pathways it is unlikely that one single agent, unless directed specifically at the triggering mechanism for the disease, will significantly dampen down the pathological process.

It is now clear that cartilage destruction and subsequent bony erosion occur extremely early in the course of RA, with recent magnetic resonance imaging (MRI) data suggesting the development of cartilage damage even before clinical synovitis is apparent [6]. This has given rise to the concept that the management of RA should be approached as an acute medical emergency and that aggressive therapy needs to be commenced at the earliest possible stage [7]. The prescribing practices of rheumatologists vary considerably but over the last few years there has been a significant shift to early use of disease-modifying anti-rheumatic drugs (DMARDs) [8] although the majority of rheumatologists would commence with single agents rather than using these drugs in combination [9].

Over the last decade the strategy for management of rheumatoid arthritis has also changed with suggestions of the step-down approach [10] where more potent drugs are used initially to dampen down inflammation and synovitis and then withdrawn, or the so-called sawtooth approach suggested by Fries, where the patient is reviewed at frequent

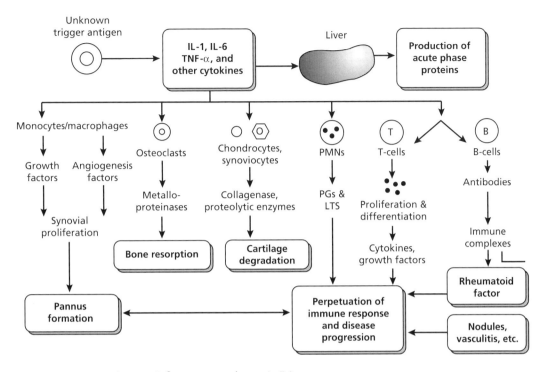

Fig. 13.1 Inflammatory pathways in RA.

intervals with goals set *a priori* in terms of inflammation control and the patient reviewed at frequent intervals from the perspective of achieving those goals [11].

Drugs available

An increasing number of DMARDs have now been shown to retard the progression of erosions in RA and can reduce progression of disability [12]. These drugs and their proposed mechanisms of action are shown in Table 13.1. The rationale for using combinations of DMARDs is that, by using drugs which have a different mechanism of action and, in particular, a different side-effect profile, it might be possible to have synergistic effects on efficacy without additive adverse events. One of the difficulties with this thesis has been that the differences between DMARDs, in their ability to slow erosions, may not be very great and trials of combination therapy have usually been either poorly designed or underpowered [13,14].

Table 13.1 Mechanism of action of disease-modifying anti-rheumatic drugs.

Drug	Mechanism of action
Antimalarials	Inhibition of lysosomal enzymes Inhibits PMNs and lymphocytes (*in vitro*) Inhibits IL-1 release (*in vivo*) ? Cartilage protection (*in vitro*)
Sulphasalazine	Inhibits PMN migration Reduces lymphocyte responses Inhibits angiogenesis
Gold	Inhibits PMN function Inhibition of T- and B-cell activity Inhibits macrophage activation (*in vitro*)
d-penicillamine	Inhibits neovascularization (*in vitro*) Inhibits PMN myeloperoxidase Scavenges free radicals Inhibits T-cell function Impairs antigen presentation
Corticosteroids	Increases lipocortin levels leading to inhibition of phosphilipase A_2 Reduced cytokine production Inhibits Fc receptor expression Suppresses lymphocyte function Redistributes circulating leucocytes
Methotrexate	Decreases thymidilate synthetase activity and subsequent DNA synthesis Diminishes PMN chemotaxis
Azathioprine	Interferes with DNA synthesis Inhibits lymphocyte proliferation
Cyclophosphamide	Cross-links DNA leading to cell death Decreases circulating T and B cells
Chlorambucil	Similar to cyclophosphamide
Cyclosporin	Blocks synthesis/release of IL-1 and IL-2

PMN, polymorphonuclear leucocyte; IL, interleukin.

Trial design issue

Trial design issues in the use of combination therapy in RA have been summarized by Johnson [15] and include the problems of:
• choice of controls, trial design and sufficient patients to ensure a fair comparison between therapies;
• the issue of safety assessment as well as efficacy;
• the problems of maintaining some blinding over a significant period of time.

Although the issues of outcome assessment in RA have now been addressed to a large extent with the development of the Outcome Measures in Rheumatoid Arthritis Clinical Trial (OMERACT) core set [16], careful definition of erosions at an early stage remains either elusive, or expensive to carry out in large-scale trials. The duration of the study is also important since small differences in the slowing of erosion rates may only be detectable over a 1- or 2-year period. Cost-effective issues need to be considered since use of combination therapy may be associated with an increase in the frequency or type of monitoring that is required to be carried out from a safety perspective and these cost issues need to be considered particularly if only small gains are seen with the combination treatment over single agents.

Pharmacokinetics

Potential pharmacokinetic interactions between DMARD combinations are usually not considered. If formal combination therapy is to be used, then an investigation of pharmacokinetic interactions should be carried out at an early stage to make sure that the concentration of one of the drugs in the combination is not being significantly increased. If that is so, then this needs to be incorporated into the design in that it would be more appropriate to test two dose levels of a single drug against the combination. This is particularly so for drugs within a combination that might act on renal function and therefore decrease excretion of a drug such as cyclosporin. Cyclosporin and methotrexate combinations are now widely suggested as a treatment of choice in RA although the benefits seem to be relatively small and the cost of increased monitoring, potential for adverse drug reactions, particularly with hypertension and renal dysfunction, may be significant [17,18]. The rationale for combinations in terms of mechanism, pharmacokinetics and toxicity has recently been summarized by Furst and is shown in Table 13.2 [19].

Table 13.2 Kinetics of disease-modifying anti-rheumatic drugs. (Adapted from [19] with permission.)

	AZA	CSA	DPA	GST	HCQ/CQ	MTX	SSZ
Bioavailability (%)		20–50	50–70	> 95	74	70	25–33
Tissue binding*				3+*	4+	3+	
Serum protein binding (%)	70	90		> 90	40–60	50	
Renal clearance (%)		6	47	30–60	20	30–80	60–95
Biliary clearance (%)		94	35			3–23	5
Hepatic clearance*	2+*		3+		4+	3+(H)	4+(H,A)

AZA, azathioprine; CSA, cyclosporin A; DPA, d-penicillamine; GST, gold sodium thiomalate; HCQ/CQ, hydroxychloroquine; MTX, methotrexate; SSZ, sulphasalazine; H, hydroxylation; A, acetylation.
* On a qualitative scale of 0–4+, where '0' = none, 4+ is 'major effect'.

In vitro data

A number of *in vitro* systems have been used to study the effect of drug combinations. Danis and colleagues [20] examined the effects of a variety of DMARD combinations on the production of interleukin 1 (IL-1) and tumour necrosis factor alpha (TNF-α) by purified human monocytes stimulated with the cytokines granulocyte–macrophage colony-stimulating factor (GM-CSF) and interferon gamma (IFN-γ). In this system the inhibition of IL-1 and TNF-α production by monocytes was seen with many DMARDs although there were individual differences. Interestingly, combinations of gold sodium thiomalate plus auranofin, and hydroxychloroquine plus sulphasalazine were extremely effective at suppressing cytokine production although other combinations were not so effective. In a further study by this group [21], chloroquine was shown to decrease the inhibition of pokeweed mitogen-stimulated blast formation of monocytes that was induced by d-penicillamine—suggesting that this particular combination would not be useful. In a recent study of IFN-γ production by CD4+ and CD8+ T-cell clones the combination of chloroquine and cyclosporin were found to synergistically inhibit production [22]. These data would suggest that certain combinations of DMARDs might be particularly useful in inhibiting the inflammatory responses in RA but further work needs to be done to establish whether *in vitro* assays can predict subsequent clinical response.

Another reason for using combination therapy is that it might slow the development of so-called drug resistance. It is clear from long-term drug studies that a significant number of patients with RA, who are initially controlled on a DMARD or combination of DMARDs, will then have a flare of their disease despite initial control [23]. Studies from the cancer literature have clearly demonstrated the development of drug resistance to anticancer agents as being associated with the generation of P-glycoproteins [24] and it has been hypothesized that this might operate for DMARDs as well [25]. The P-glycoprotein mediates a cell membrane pump which rapidly transports anticancer drugs out of tumour cells, thus reducing their effect. There are some data to suggest that anti-arthritic effects of antimalarials, cyclosporin and possibly corticosteroids are at least in part attributable to the inhibition of the P-glycoprotein function which blocks TNF-α release by macrophages, TNF-α activation of natural killer (NK) cells and NK-cell secretion of cytokines within the rheumatoid joint [25,26]. Whether 'drug resistance' in RA is associated with an increase in P-glycoprotein is not known but a number of DMARDs including cyclosporin A and chloroquine have been shown to competitively inhibit the efflux function of P-glycoproteins [26]. Glucocorticoids have also been shown to induce increased P-glycoprotein expression in cell line [27] suggesting that glucocorticoid resistance maybe explained by P-glycoprotein efflux function. Salmon and Dalton hypothesize that the use of a DMARD which has an effect on the P-glycoprotein function (such as cyclosporin and antimalarials) together with drugs that are not subject to P-glycoprotein efflux such as methotrexate might provide added benefit in RA [25] and this seems to be reflected in clinical trials [17,28].

Animal models

Despite the fact that animal models of inflammation have significantly influenced the development of DMARDs for use in humans, few studies have been carried out using combinations of DMARDs [29]. The combinations of anti-rheumatic and other drugs used in animal models are shown in Table 13.3. In the collagen-induced arthritis rat model low doses of cyclosporin A do not significantly affect the disease process although when combined with low doses of methotrexate significant reduction in inflammation and joint damage is seen [30]. A combination of cyclosporin A and calcitriol has again been shown to be suppressive of inflammation in the adjuvant arthritis model when both drugs used singly have little effect (and in fact may promote inflammation) [31]. Studies with a potent angiogenesis inhibitor AGM-1470 either alone or in combination with an anti-CD5 pan-T-cell monoclonal antibody [32,33] or taxol have also demonstrated that combinations are better than single agents in a collagen-induced arthritis model [34]. Although it is often difficult to extrapolate the results of treatment of animal models to humans, they may provide a useful screening milieu in which single drugs and combinations can be tested to see whether drug synergy is obtained.

Table 13.3 Drug combinations in animal models. (From [32].)

		Efficacy	
Drug or combination	Animal model	Single agent	Combination
Cyclosporin			
+ Methotrexate	CIA	–	++
+ Calcitriol	AA	–	+
+ AGM-1470	CIA	+	++
AGM-1470			
+ Anti-CD5 Mono	CIA	–	++
+ Taxol	CIA	–	++

AA, adjuvant arthritis; CIA, collagen-induced arthritis.

Clinical trials of DMARD combination in RA

Rheumatologists have been using combinations of DMARDs for a long period of time. Corticosteroids have often been added to a regimen of non-steroidal anti-inflammatory drugs (NSAIDs) or DMARDs. This has usually been on the premise that if one drug works a little, then two drugs or three will work better. Formal clinical trials of combinations of DMARDs are relatively recent and are summarized in Table 13.4. Some of these trials are relatively underpowered and the trials can often be criticized in terms of the patients that are entered into the studies, the duration of the study and the size of the benefit. Pharmacokinetic issues are very rarely taken into account and the trial design should consider these factors.

The major pitfalls with published trials of combination therapy have been well summarized by a number of authors [35–38]. In a study carried out by Scott and colleagues [39] gold therapy (Myocrisin) was compared with a combination of gold plus hydroxychloroquine. Patients with an average disease duration of 2 years were randomized to receive hydroxychloroquine or placebo in addition to their gold treatment. Hydroxychloroquine dosage was 400 mg daily for 6 months followed by 200 mg for the following 6 months as well as background NSAIDs and analgesics. Significantly more patients in the combined group developed side-effects (particularly rash) but more patients withdrew from gold therapy than from the combination therapy because of lack of benefit. There were statistically significant benefits in overall disease activity and c-reactive protein levels in those patients completing the 12 months of combination therapy.

Bunch and colleagues [40] reported a 2-year, randomized, double-blind comparison of hydroxychloroquine, d-penicillamine and a combination in patients with an average duration of disease of over 6 years. The d-penicillamine-only group felt better, while toxic events were less frequent in the combination group than in the d-penicillamine-only group. This study only had 56 patients and therefore is grossly underpowered.

A study by McKenna [41] reported only in abstract form showed that patients treated with a combination of gold and d-penicillamine showed an earlier response than to gold or d-penicillamine alone. Again this study is underpowered.

Taggart and colleagues [42] assessed in a double-blind fashion a combination of d-penicillamine with sulphasalazine in patients who had either failed or showed a partial response to a year's treatment with d-penicillamine alone. Their data suggest a small benefit of combination treatment over sulphasalazine alone.

Faarvang and colleagues [43] conducted a 6-month, randomized, double-blind study comparing hydroxychloroquine and sulphasalazine alone and

Table 13.4 Combination therapy in rheumatoid arthritis (RA).

Reference		Combination	No. of patients	Results
Double-blind randomized				
Scott *et al.* (1989)	[39]	Gold and hydroxyloroquine	101	Combination more effective than gold or placebo
Bunch *et al.* (1984)	[40]	d-penicillamine and hydroxychloroquine	56	Combination not as effective as d-penicillamine
McKenna *et al.* (1985)	[41]	Gold and d-penicillamine	45	Combination showed earlier response compared with gold or d-penicillamine alone
Faarvang *et al.* (1993)	[43]	Hydroxychloroquine and sulphasalazine	91	No advantage of combination
Williams *et al.* (1992)	[44]	Methotrexate and auranofin	335	No advantage. More withdrawals with combination due to side-effects
Willkens *et al.* (1992)	[45]	Methotrexate and azathioprine	209	Combination and methotrexate alone superior to azathioprine alone
Clegg *et al.* (1997)	[46]	Hydroxychloroquine and methotrexate	141	Combination more effective, using flare of RA as the outcome measure
O'Dell *et al.* (1995)	[48]	Methotrexate, hydroxychloroquine and sulphasalazine	100	Triple combination more effective than sulphasalazine plus hydroxychloroquine or methotrexate alone
Tugwell *et al.* (1995)	[47]	Cyclosporin-A and methotrexate	148	Combination more effective than methotrexate alone
Ferraz *et al.* (1994)	[28]	Methotrexate and chloroquine		
Non-blinded				
Bitter (1984)	[50]	Gold and d-penicillamine, levamisole or chlorambucil	71	d-penicillamine plus gold effective, other combinations not effective
Tiliakos (1986)	[51]	Methotrexate, cyclophosphamide and hydroxychloroquine	12	Combination effective. Recortication of erosions
Taggart *et al.* (1987)	[41]	d-penicillamine and sulphasalazine	30	Combination more effective than sulphasalazine alone
Haasgsma *et al.* (1994)	[52]	Methotrexate and sulphasalazine	40	Combination more effective than methotrexate alone
Bensen *et al.* (1994)	[58]	Cyclosporin and methotrexate Cyclosporin and gold	20 in each arm	Non-randomized, non-blinded combination better
Boers *et al.* (1997)	[49]	Methotrexate, prednisolone, sulphasalazine		Combination better

in combination. The patients treated with the combination responded more rapidly and to a greater extent than those treated with hydroxychloroquine alone although the difference did not reach statistical significance. With only 91 patients, this trial is significantly underpowered.

Drug treatment of RA over the last few years has been strongly focused on combinations with methotrexate and/or cyclosporin. Methotrexate has been studied in combination with azathioprine, hydroxychloroquine, sulphasalazine and cyclosporin while cyclosporin has been in trials in combination with gold.

The effect of combining auranofin and methotrexate was investigated in a well-conducted, double-blind, randomized study comparing 6 mg/day auranofin, 7.5 mg/week methotrexate and a third group given the combination [43]. There were no statistical differences in response between the groups although withdrawals because of lack of efficacy were less frequent in the combination group who on the other hand had more terminations due to adverse events [44]. Willkens and colleagues [45] compared azathioprine, methotrexate and a lower-dose combination of each. Combination therapy and methotrexate alone were slightly better than azathioprine alone although the differences were not large.

Clegg [46] reported an interesting study where 121 patients who had responded to a combination of methotrexate and hydroxychloroquine were randomized to one of three treatments. Forty patients continued on hydroxychloroquine with pulse methotrexate for a flare (Group 1), 41 patients continued on hydroxychloroquine with placebo pulse for a flare (Group 2) and 40 patients were randomized to placebo with pulse methotrexate for a flare (Group 3). Half of the patients in Groups 1 and 3 flared within 8 weeks of randomization. Of those not flaring in the first 8 weeks, 61% of Group 1, 72% of Group 2 but only 21% of Group 3 remained 'flare-free' for the duration of the study (36 weeks). 'Flares' seen in Group 2 were also much longer lasting than those seen in Groups 1 and 3. In summary, patients improved on a combination of methotrexate and hydroxychloroquine while maintenance of hydroxychloroquine delayed the onset and seemed to shorten the duration of flares when methotrexate was discontinued.

Tugwell and colleagues [47] conducted a 6-month randomized trial of cyclosporin (2.5–5 mg/kg body weight/day) and methotrexate to maximal tolerated dose in patients who had had a partial response to methotrexate. Patients were randomized to receive cyclosporin or placebo and continue their methotrexate. At the end of the 6-month period the combination group had a net improvement in tender joint count of 25% and three times the number of patients (36) on the combined regimen fulfilled 20% American College of Rheumatology (ACR) improvement criteria than on placebo (12 patients). On the negative side, serum creatinine concentrations increased significantly in those patients on cyclosporin.

In a 2-year, double-blind, randomized study O'Dell and colleagues [48] compared methotrexate alone (7.5–17.5 mg/week), sulphasalazine (1 g/day) plus hydroxychoroquine (400 mg/day) or all three drugs. The primary endpoints of the study were 50% improvement in composite symptoms of

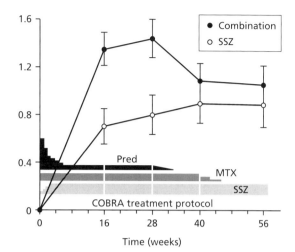

Fig. 13.2 Drug regimen and clinical outcome of methotrexate (MTX), sulphasalazine (SSZ) and prednisolone (Pred) combination. (With permission from [49].)

arthritis and no evidence of drug toxicity. Fifty of 102 patients had a 50% improvement at 9 months and maintained at least that degree of improvement for the 2-year period. Of these 'responders', 24 of 31 were treated with the three-drug combination, 12 of 36 treated with methotrexate alone and 14 of 35 were treated with sulphasalazine and hydroxychloroquine. A slightly higher number of patients (7) in the methotrexate group discontinued treatment because of drug toxicity.

Boers and colleagues [49] have recently conducted an interesting study of an initial high-dose prednisolone combination regimen in early RA. This double-blind, randomized controlled trial (RCT) compared a combination of sulphasalazine (2 g/day), methotrexate (7.5 mg/week) and prednisolone reducing from an initial dose of 60 mg/day to 7.5 mg/day after 6 weeks, with sulphasalazine alone. The interesting feature with this study was that it enrolled patients with early RA (median duration 4 months). The drug regimen is shown in Fig. 13.2 along with the clinical outcomes. At week 28 the mean pooled index in the combined treatment group was significantly higher than in the sulphasalazine group with 72% of the combined group improving according to ACR criteria in contrast to 49% in the sulphasalazine group. The differences between the groups was only maintained while prednisolone was given. At 28 weeks the radiographic damage score had increased by a median of one in the combined therapy group and four in the sulphasalazine group—again this was a statistically significant difference. These differences in radiographic scores remained throughout the duration of the trial (80 weeks).

Over the years a number of open studies have been carried out to suggest that high doses of gold plus d-penicillamine, gold plus chlorambucil and gold plus levamisole were effective in suppressing in RA. These studies unfortunately were of poor design and with few patients [50]. Tiliakos [51] reported a 50–90% improvement in a small group of patients treated with hydroxychloroquine, cyclophosphamide and methotrexate and noted recortication of erosions in seven of 12 patients. Haagsma and colleagues [52] studied the addition of methotrexate (7.5–15 mg/week) to patients not responding to 3 g of sulphasalazine. In a 24-week, unblinded study patients continued on 2 g daily of sulphasalazine alone or in combination with 7.5–15 mg weekly of methotrexate. At the end of the study the combination appeared superior to methotrexate in terms of efficacy and had comparable toxicity.

Farr and colleagues [53] demonstrated that d-penicillamine in a dose of 125–1000 mg/day or aurothiomalate produced a favourable response in over 70% of patients when added to sulphasalazine treatment (1.5–3.0 g daily). A third of patients discontinued gold and d-penicillamine because of side-effects and the number of patients in the study were small.

Porter and colleagues [54] studied the combination of hydroxychloroquine and intramuscular gold in 142 patients who had a suboptimal response to 6 months of intramuscular gold therapy. Patients continued with gold and were randomized to receive either hydroxychloroquine 400 mg daily or placebo, and followed for a 6-month period. No significant differences between treatments were seen in terms of either efficacy or toxicity and these authors felt there was no justification for using combination of intramuscular gold and hydroxychloroquine in patients with RA not responding to gold treatment.

In a further open study, Gibson and colleagues [55] compared chloroquine, 200 mg daily, d-penicillamine, 250–750 mg daily, and a combination in a randomized, non-blinded study of 1 year's duration. At the end of 12 months no significant differences were seen between the patient groups in terms of efficacy although adverse events and withdrawals due to side-effects were significantly more frequent in the combination therapy group.

In a retrospective review of 32 patients treated with a combination of methotrexate and salazopyrin, Nisar and colleagues [56] showed that the combination of methotrexate and salazopyrin was well tolerated in comparison to methotrexate alone.

Van Gestel and colleagues [57] have pointed out the importance of using combinations of DMARDs early in rheumatoid arthritis and review the new sulphasalazine/methotrexate combinations demonstrating good response to methotrexate, sulphasalazine or the combination with most efficacy endpoints favouring the combination although not reaching statistical significance.

A number of other studies of various combinations have been published, but many of these are of small number and are open and unblinded as in the studies reported on the combination of cyclosporin and methotrexate and cyclosporin and gold [58].

Table 13.5 Numbers required in trials to detect differences in efficacy between anti-rheumatic drugs used to treat rheumatoid arthritis. (From [61].)

	Actual differences in efficacy (standardized effect units)				
	0.1	0.2	0.3	0.4	0.5
Two-drug comparison					
No. per drug	1500	400	170	96	62
No. per trial	3000	800	340	192	124
Three-drug comparison					
No. per drug	1300	325	143	80	52
No. per trial	3900	975	429	240	156

Power = 80%; α = 0.05 (2 tailer).

Conclusion

McCarty and Carrera were among the first to report treatment of rheumatoid arthritis patients with multiple therapies [59]. Recent follow-up of these patients demonstrated an impressive response with complete remission being achieved in 43% of patients and a low incidence of side-effects [60]. This open study does provide powerful evidence that combination therapy is beneficial in RA but of course it is uncontrolled. Subsequent randomized studies have failed to produce the impressive evidence seen in uncontrolled studies and the continuing publication of underpowered, non-randomized and unblinded studies has only confused the database. Felson and colleagues [61] have reported the patient numbers required to detect differences in efficacy between DMARDs used to treat RA (Table 13.5). Obviously the trial size in excess of 3000 patients needed to achieve the appropriate statistical power to detect a clinically important difference between single drugs and combination therapy is impractical [62]. Careful attention to trial design, however, could improve the database on these combinations considerably.

Editors of medical journals should adopt clear principles for the publication of all clinical trials but particularly those on combination therapy in RA. These should include:

- adequate numbers;
- appropriate design including randomization;
- an indication of consideration of pharmacokinetic interactions;
- an indication of cost benefit of the combined therapy.

Pharmacokinetic interactions are very rarely considered in these studies although the study of Haagsma and colleagues [52] comparing a combination of methotrexate and sulphasalazine with methotrexate alone did address this issue and demonstrated no change in methotrexate kinetics in a small subset of patients. On the other hand, Seideman and colleagues [63] demonstrated a reduced bioavailability of methotrexate in patients with RA which might explain the observation that patients on this combination have a lower incidence of liver function abnormalities [64]. These data are very important and really should be available for combinations such as methotrexate and cyclosporin where, because of the effect of cyclosporin on renal function, it might be expected that interactions would occur. In combination studies it is also important to look at the size of the effect and weigh that up against the potential cost. This is particularly so with expensive combinations such as cyclosporin where there is the added risk of increase in blood pressure and decrease in renal function. Given the known increase in cardiovascular mortality in RA [65,66], these factors may well be contributory.

Cost implications are also important although with drugs such as cyclosporin, dosing requirements may be decreased by use of such things as grapefruit juice [67].

Combinations of DMARDs will continue to be used and already there is some experience combining drugs like methotrexate with anti-CD4 monoclonals or anti-CD5 immunocongates [68]. These combinations would also have to be evaluated extremely carefully [69]. It is now time to review combination therapy and to encourage appropriately designed studies to answer critical questions, such as:

• Should all patients with RA receive combination therapy?
• Are there ways of predicting who will respond?
• When should combinations be commenced?
• Which combinations are best?
• Is there a variability amongst patients?
• After an excellent response, should drugs be tapered or discontinued?
• What is the role of biologicals and how will they perform as combination therapy [70]?

It would seem that some combination of DMARDs do provide added efficacy although few if any studies have been appropriately designed to address the issue of dose of drug. Pharmacokinetic interactions have rarely been explored and the added cost is often significant both in economic and health terms.

It is now time for rheumatologists to take a leaf from our cardiological and oncological colleagues and establish large multicentre trials with appropriate numbers of patients to clearly demonstrate one way or the other the benefits of combination therapies.

References

1 Wolfe F, Mitchell DM, Sibley JT *et al*. The mortality of rheumatoid arthritis. *Arthritis Rheum* 1994; 37: 481–94.

2 Yelin E, Henke C, Epstein WV. The work dynamics of the person with rheumatoid arthritis. *Arthritis Rheum* 1987; 30: 507–12.

3 Yelin E, Callahan L. The economic cost and social and psychological impact of musculoskeletal conditions. *Arthritis Rheum* 1995; 38: 1351–62.

4 Eberhardt KB, Rydgen LC, Petterson H, Wollheim FA. Early rheumatoid arthritis: onset, course and outcome over two years. *Rheumatol Intern* 1990; 10: 135–42.

5 Mottonen T, Paimela L, Ahonen J *et al*. Outcome in patients with early rheumatoid arthritis treated according to the 'sawtooth' strategy. *Arthritis Rheum* 1996; 39: 996–1006.

6 McConagle D, Gibbon W, Green M, Proudman NS, O'Conner P, Emery P. A longitudinal MR study of bone changes of the MCP joints in early rheumatoid arthritis. *Arthritis Rheum* 1997; 40: S246.

7 Emery P. The optimal management of early rheumatoid disease: the key to preventing disability. *Br J Rheumatol* 1994; 33: 765–8.

8 Conaghan PG, Crotty M, Oh E-S, Day RO, Brooks PM. Antirheumatic drug prescribing behaviour of Australasian Rheumatologists 1984–94. *Br J Rheumatol* 1997; 36: 487–90.

9 Galindo-Rodriquez G, Avina-Zubieta JA, Fitzgerald A *et al*. Variations and trends in the prescription of initial second-line therapy for patients with rheumatoid arthritis. *J Rheumatol* 1997; 24: 633–8.

10 Wilske KR, Healey LA. Challenging the therapeutic pyramid: a new look at treatment strategies for rheumatoid arthritis. *J Rheumatol* 1990; 17 (Suppl. 25): 4–7.

11 Fries JF. Evaluating the therapeutic approach to rheumatoid arthritis: The 'sawtooth' strategy. *J Rheumatol* 1990; 22 (Suppl.): 12–15.

12 Fries JF, Williams CA, Morefeld D, Singh G, Sibley J. Reduction in long-term disability in patients with rheumatoid arthritis by disease modifying antirheumatic drug-based treatment strategies. *Arthritis Rheum* 1996; 36: 616–22.

13 Bombardier C, Tugwell P. Controversies in the analysis of long term clinical trials of slow acting drugs. *J Rheumatol* 1998; 12: 403–5.

14 Felson D, Anderson J, Meenan R. The efficacy and toxicity of combination therapy in rheumatoid arthritis: a meta-analysis. *Arthritis Rheum* 1994; 37: 1487–91.

15 Johnson K. Efficacy assessment in trials of combination therapy for rheumatoid arthritis. *J Rheumatol* 1996; 23 (Suppl. 44): 107–9.

16 Tugwell P, Boers M, OMERACT Committee. Developing consensus and preliminary core efficacy endpoints for rheumatoid arthritis clinical trials. *J Rheumatol* 1993; 20: 555–61.

17 Tugwell P, Pincus T, Yocum D *et al*. Combination therapy with cyclosporin A and methotrexate in severe rheumatoid arthritis. *N Engl J Med* 1995; 333: 137–41.

18 Chaudhuri K, Torley H, Madhok R. Cyclosporin. *Br J Rheumatol* 1997; 36: 1016–21.

19 Furst DE. Clinical pharmacology of combination DMARD therapy in rheumatoid arthritis. *J Rheumatol* 1996; 23 (Suppl. 44): 86–90.

20 Danis VA, Franic GM, Brooks PM. The effect of slow acting antirheumatic drugs (SAARDs) and combinations of SAARDs on monokine production *In Vitro Drugs Exptl Clin Res* 1991; 17: 549–54.

21 Danis VA, Kulesz AJ, Nelson DS. Cytokine regulation of human monocyte interleukin-1 production *in vitro*. Enhancement of IL-1 production by interferon-γ, tumour necrosis factor-α, IL-2 and IL-1 and inhibition by interferon. *Clin Exp Immunol* 1990; 8: 435–43.

22 Landewe R, Miltenberg A, Breedfeld F, Daha M, Kijkmans B. Cyclosporin and chloroquine synergistically inhibit the interferon-gamma production by CD4 positive and CD 8 positive synovial T cell clones derived from a patient with

rheumatoid arthritis. *J Rheumatol* 1993; 19: 1353–7.

23 Wolfe F. The epidemiology of drug treatment failure in rheumatoid arthritis. *Baillière's Clin Rheumatol* 1995; 9: 619–32.

24 Shulstik C, Dalton W, Gros P. P-glycoprotein-mediated multidrug resistance in tumour cells: Biochemistry, clinical relevance and modulation. *Mol Aspects Med* 1995; 16: 1–78.

25 Salmon SE, Dalton WS. Relevance of multidrug resistance to rheumatoid arthritis: Development of a new therapeutic hypothesis. *J Rheumatol* 1996; 23 (Suppl. 44): 97–101.

26 Klimecki WT, Taylor CW, Dalton WS. Inhibition of cell-mediated cytolysis and P-glycoprotein function in natural killer cells by verapamil isomers and cyclosporin A analogs. *J Clin Immunol* 1995; 15: 152–8.

27 Bourgeoi S, Gruol DJ, Newby BRF, Rajah FM. Expression of an MDR gene is associated with a new form of resistance to dexamethasone-induced apoptosis. *Mol Endocrinol* 1993; 7: 840–51.

28 Ferraz MB, Pinheiro GRC, Helfenstein M *et al.* Combination therapy with methotrexate and chloroquine in rheumatoid arthritis: a multicentre randomised placebo controlled trial. *Scand J Rheumatol* 1994; 23: 231–6.

29 Oliver SJ, Brahn E. Combination therapy in rheumatoid arthritis. The animal model perspective. *J Rheumatol* 1996; 23 (Suppl. 44): 56–60.

30 Brahn E, Peacock DJ, Banquerigo ML. Suppression of collagen-induced arthritis by combination cyclosporin A and methotrexate. *Arthritis Rheum* 1991; 34: 1282–8.

31 Boissier MC, Chioccha G, Fournier C. Combination of cyclosporin A and calcitriol in the treatment of adjuvant arthritis. *J Rheumatol* 1992; 19: 754–7.

32 Oliver SJ, Cheng TP, Banquerigo ML, Brahn E. Suppression of collagen-induced arthritis by an angiogenesis inhibitor, AGM-1470, in combination with cyclosporin reduction of vascular endothelial growth factor (VEGF). *Cell Immunol* 1995; 166: 196–206.

33 Peacock DJ, Banquerigo ML, Brahn E. An angiogenesis inhibitor in combination with anti-CD5 Mab suppresses established collagen-induced arthritis significantly more than single agent therapy. *Arthritis Rheum* 1992; 35: S140 (Abstract).

34 Oliver SJ, Banquerigo ML, Brahn E. Suppression of collagen-induced arthritis using an angiogenesis inhibitor AGM 1470, and a microtubule stabilizer, Taxol. *Cell Immunol* 1994; 157: 291–9.

35 Brooks PM, Schwartzer AC. Combination chemotherapy in rheumatoid arthritis. *Ann Rheum Dis* 1991; 50: 507–9.

36 Boers M, Ramsden M. Long acting drug combinations in rheumatoid arthritis: a formal review. *J Rheumatol* 1991; 18: 316–24.

37 Tugwell P, Boers M. Long acting drug combination in rheumatoid arthritis: an updated overview. In: Wolf F, Pincus T, eds. *Rheumatoid Arthritis Pathogenesis, Assessment, Outcome and Treatment.* New York: Marcel Dekker, 1994: 357–71.

38 Borgini M, Paulus HE. Combination therapy. *Baillière's Clin Rheumatol* 1995; 9: 689–710.

39 Scott DL, Dawes PT, Tunn E *et al.* Combination therapy with gold and hydroxychloroquine in rheumatoid arthritis: a prospective, randomised, placebo-controlled study. *Br J Rheumatol* 1989; 28: 128–33.

40 Bunch TW, O'Duffy JD, Tompkins RB *et al.* Controlled trial of hydroxychloroquine and d-penicillamine singly or in combination in the treatment of rheumatoid arthritis. *Arthritis Rheum* 1984; 27: 267–76.

41 McKenna F, Hopkins R, Hinchcliffe KD *et al.* Gold and d-penicillamine, alone and in combination, in active rheumatoid arthritis. *16th International Conference of Rheumatology*, Sydney, Australia, 1986 (Abstract).

42 Taggart AJ, Hill J, Ashbury C *et al.* Sulphasalazine alone or in combination with d-penicillamine in rheumatoid arthritis. *Br J Rheumatol* 1987; 26: 32–6.

43 Faarvang KL, Egmose C, Krgar P *et al.* Hydroxychloroquine and sulphasalazine alone and in combination in rheumatoid arthritis: a randomised double blind trial. *Ann Rheum Dis* 1993; 52: 711–15.

44 Williams HJ, Ward JR, Reading JC
    et al. Comparison of auranofin,
    methotrexate and the combination of
    both in the treatment of rheumatoid
    arthritis: a controlled trial. *Arthritis
    Rheum* 1992; 35: 259–69.

45 Willkens RF, Urowitz MB, Stablein DM
    et al. Comparison of azathioprine,
    methotrexate, and a combination of
    both in the treatment of rheumatoid
    arthritis: a controlled clinical trial.
    Arthritis Rheum 1992; 35: 849–56.

46 Clegg DO, Dietz F, Duffy J *et al.* Safety
    and efficacy of hydroxychloroquine as
    maintenance therapy for rheumatoid
    arthritis after combination therapy with
    methotrexate and hydroxychloroquine.
    J Rheumatol 1997; 24: 1896–902.

47 Tugwell P, Pincus T, Yocum D *et al.*
    Combination and cyclosporin and
    methotrexate in severe rheumatoid
    arthritis. *N Engl J Med* 1995;
    333: 137–41.

48 O'Dell JR, Haire CE, Erikson N *et al.*
    Treatment of rheumatoid arthritis with
    methotrexate alone, sulphasalazine and
    hydroxychloroquine, or a combination
    of all three medication. *N Engl J Med*
    1996; 334: 1287–91.

49 Boers M, Verhoeven AC, Markusse
    HM *et al.* Randomised comparison
    of combined step-down prednisolone,
    methotrexate and sulphasalazine
    with sulphasalazine alone in early
    rheumatoid arthritis. *Lancet* 1997;
    350: 309–18.

50 Bitter T. Combined disease modifying
    chemotherapy for intractable
    rheumatoid arthritis. *Rheumatic Dis
    Clin North Am* 1984; 10: 417–28.

51 Tiliakos HA. Low dose cytotoxic drug
    combination therapy in intractable
    rheumatoid arthritis: Two years later.
    Arthritis Rheum 1986; 29: S79
    (Abstract).

52 Haagsma CJ, Van Reil PLCM, van
    de Putte LBA. Continuation of
    methotrexate and sulphasalazine vs.
    methotrexate alone: a randomised
    clinical trial in rheumatoid arthritis
    patients resistant to sulphasalazine
    therapy. *Br J Rheumatol* 1994;
    33: 1049–55.

53 Farr M, Kitas G, Bacon PA.
    Sulphasalazine in rheumatoid
    arthritis, combination therapy
    with d-penicillamine or sodium
    aurothiomalate. *Clin Rheumatol*
    1988; 7: 242–8.

54 Porter D, Capell H, Hunter J.
    Combination therapy in rheumatoid
    arthritis: no benefit of addition of
    hydroxychloroquine to patients with a
    sub-optimal response to intra-muscular
    gold therapy. *J Rheumatol* 1993;
    20: 645–9.

55 Gibson T, Emery P, Armstrong RD
    et al. Combined d-penicillamine and
    chloroquine treatment of rheumatoid
    arthritis: a comparative study. *Br J
    Rheumatol* 1987; 26: 279–84.

56 Nisar M, Carlisle L, Amos RS.
    Methotrexate and sulphasalazine in
    combination therapy in rheumatoid
    arthritis. *Br J Rheumatol* 1994;
    33: 651–4.

57 Van Gestel AM, Haagsma CJ, Furst
    DE, Van Riel PLCM. Treatment of
    early rheumatoid arthritis patients
    with slow acting anti-rheumatic drugs
    (SAARDS). *Baillière's Clin Rheumatol*
    1997; 11: 65–82.

58 Bensen W, Tugwell P, Roberts R *et al.*
    Combination therapy of cyclosporin
    with methotrexate and gold in
    rheumatoid arthritis (2 pilot studies).
    J Rheumatol 1994; 21: 2034–8.

59 McCarty DJ, Carrera GF. Treatment
    of intractable rheumatoid arthritis
    with combined cyclophosphamide,
    azathioprine and hydroxychloroquine.
    JAMA 1982; 248: 1718–23.

60 McCarty DJ, Harman JG, Grassanovich
    JL, Qian C, Klein JP. Combination drug
    therapy of seropositive rheumatoid
    arthritis. *J Rheumatol* 1995; 22:
    1636–45.

61 Felson DT, Anderson JJ, Meenan RF.
    The comparative efficacy and toxicity
    of second-line drugs in rheumatoid
    arthritis: Results of two meta-analyses.
    Arthritis Rheum 1990; 30: 1449–61.

62 Tugwell P. Combination therapy in
    rheumatoid arthritis: Meta-analysis. *J
    Rheumatol* 1996; 23 (Suppl. 44): 43–6.

63 Seideman P, Albertoni F, Beck O *et al.*
    Chloroquine reduces the bioavailability
    of methotrexate in patients with
    rheumatoid arthritis. *Arthritis Rheum*
    1994; 37: 880–3.

64 Fries JF, Singh G, Lenert L *et al.*
    Aspirin, hydroxychloroquine and

hepatic abnormalities with methotrexate in rheumatoid arthritis. *Arthritis Rheum* 1990; 33: 1611–19.

65 Wålleberg-Johnson S, Öhman M-L, Dahlquest SR. Cardiovascular morbidity and mortality in patients with seropositive rheumatoid arthritis in Northern Sweden. *J Rheumatol* 1997; 24: 445–51.

66 Raynauld J-P. Cardiovascular mortality in rheumatoid arthritis: How harmful are corticosteroids? *J Rheumatol* 1997; 24: 415–16.

67 Ioannides-Demos LL, Christophides N, Ryan P *et al.* Dosing implications of a clinical interaction between grapefruit juice and cyclosporin E and metabolite concentrations in patients with autoimmune disease. *J Rheumatol* 1997; 24: 49–54.

68 Moreland LW. Initial experience combining methotrexate with biologic agents for treating rheumatoid arthritis. *J Rheumatol* 1996; 23 (Suppl. 44): 78–83.

69 Strand V. The future use of biologic therapies in combination for the treatment of rheumatoid arthritis. *J Rheumatol* 1996; 23 (Suppl. 44): 91–6.

70 O'Dell JR. Combination DMARD therapy for rheumatoid arthritis: a step closer to the goal. *Ann Rheum Dis* 1996; 55: 781–3.

14: Does immunotherapy have a role?

J.D. Isaacs

Introduction

In the context of autoimmune disease, immunotherapy refers to treatments which specifically target the diseased immune system, with the aim of arresting tissue damage and destruction, and restoring immune homeostasis. In particular, the 'holy grail' of immunotherapy is the restoration of self-tolerance and therefore the achievement of long-term disease remission from relatively short-term therapy. Two major factors have contributed to the increased popularity of immunotherapy during the past 10 years. The first has been a substantially improved understanding of the mechanisms underlying the induction and regulation of immunological self-tolerance, which has provided a theoretical framework for novel treatments; the second has been the development of necessary technologies, enabling the design and production of novel therapeutics such as humanized monoclonal antibodies (mAbs) and immunoadhesins [1,2].

During the 1980s and 1990s, immunotherapies have been applied extensively and successfully to animal models of autoimmune disease and transplant rejection. For example, anti-T cell or anticlass II mAbs have been used to prevent, and treat, induced animal diseases such as experimental allergic encephalomyelitis (EAE) [3], and collagen-induced arthritis (CIA) [4], and also spontaneous diseases such as systemic lupus erythematosus (SLE) [5] and diabetes [6]. Furthermore, when the inciting autoantigen and/or pathogenic T-cell clone(s) are known, treatment can be suitably focused. Thus, EAE has been treated by vaccination with peptides derived from target proteins [7], or even by inducing immune responses against the pathogenic T cells themselves [8,9].

The history of immunotherapy in rheumatoid arthritis (RA) is shorter: it is less than 10 years since the first open clinical trials were published [10,11], and just a few years for controlled studies. In general, the data have been less impressive than those derived from animal models but important lessons have been learned, and the aim of this chapter is to review the field, and form an opinion concerning the future of such treatments for RA.

The development of immunotherapy

To illustrate the potential power of immunotherapy it is necessary to start by highlighting some important milestones in its history. A central tenet of the field is that T cells are central to, and coordinate, all immune responses both beneficial and pathological. Therefore if pathogenic T cells could in some way be controlled and rendered non-aggressive, immunopathological responses might be reversible. Early studies in animals highlighted the useful, immunosuppressive properties of mAbs but it was not until the mid-1980s that mAbs were shown to be tolerogenic. Thus, animals could be rendered tolerant of foreign proteins by administering them concomitantly with depleting T cell (usually anti-CD4) mAbs [12,13]. At that time, self-tolerance was believed to be predominantly a central (thymic) process involving deletion of autoreactive cells. Depleting mAbs were assumed to act by eradicating the recipient's immune system, with subsequent regeneration and thymic deletion of lymphocytes reactive with the introduced foreign antigen. Appropriate regimens could be used to induce tolerance not only to foreign proteins but also to entire foreign tissues, including bone marrow. In that situation, the resultant haemopoietic chimerism permitted tolerance to develop to a variety of tissues from the marrow donor [14].

Despite the power of such strategies, and although experimental animals remained healthy, there was some concern surrounding the potential dangers of clinical lymphocyte depletion. Consequently, attention was switched to the use of non-depleting agents, initially chemically modified fragments of mAbs [15] and, subsequently, mAb isotypes that could not harness conventional effector functions [16]. Such agents were found to be as potent as and, in some instances, more effective than conventional depleting mAbs. A significant milestone was reached when it was demonstrated that non-depleting mAbs could reverse ongoing skin graft rejection, simultaneously inducing tolerance to the graft antigens such that subsequent identical grafts were tolerated [17]. In other words, non-depleting mAbs could be used to induce tolerance to antigen even in the context of an ongoing agressive immune response against that antigen. The mechanisms underlying such effects were uncertain, but the then recently described phenomenon of immune 'anergy' could be demonstrated in at least some experimental systems [14]. *In vitro*, anergy induction could be achieved by blockade of signals through CD28 which had recently been described as a T-cell co-receptor responsible for receiving the 'second signal' necessary for activation of naive T cells. Predictably, once agents were available for blocking CD28 *in vivo*, these proved to be particularly potent, non-depleting tolerogens. Thus, CTLA4-Ig, an immunoadhesin which blocked the interaction between CD28 and its ligands, facilitated islet transplantation between MHC mismatched rat strains [18], and was also an extremely effective treatment for murine SLE [19].

The definition of immune tolerance suggested that short-term mAb treatments might provide long-term therapeutic sequelae, and the demonstration of 'infectious tolerance' provided a basis for such robust effects. Those experiments demonstrated definitively that mAb-induced immune tolerance could be associated with the appearance of regulatory cells which subsequently maintained the tolerant state [20]. These were shown to be CD4+ T cells [21] although their relationship to the regulatory cells recently described under different circumstances remains to be defined [22,23]. 'Immune deviation' (a switch in the cytokine secretion profile of organ-infiltrating or circulating T cells) could also be achieved using mAbs and was demonstrable *in vivo* [24,25], although the interrelationships between anergy, regulation and deviation also awaits clarification.

It should be evident from the foregoing that the potential power of appropriately targeted immunotherapy in human autoimmune disease is great. Although some of the above work focused on models of transplantation rather than autoimmunity, the pathogenic mechanisms are similar, and equivalent regimens are effective in both systems. Furthermore, as knowledge of normal immune homeostasis increases, an expanding spectrum of novel methods for artificially inducing tolerance are being applied successfully to animal models. Strategies not referred to in this section include

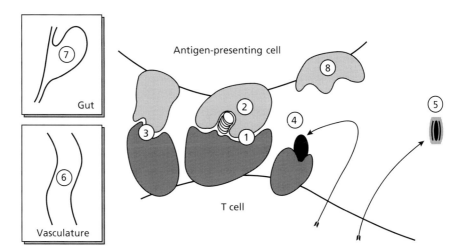

Fig. 14.1 Potential sites of action of immunotherapeutic agents. The figure illustrates some of the membrane interactions between T cells and antigen-presenting cells, and the activation-dependent release of autocrine growth factors and other cytokines by the T cell. Insets show the vascular endothelium and gut epithelium. Numbers denote sites targeted by various immunotherapeutic strategies as shown in Table 14.1. All of these strategies have been applied in animal models.

1 T-cell receptor/class II MHC interaction:	**Table 14.1** Sites targeted by various immunotherapeutic strategies.

1 T-cell receptor/class II MHC interaction:
   Anti-CD4 mAbs*
   Anti-CD3 mAbs
   Anti-TCR mAbs
   Anti-class-II mAbs
   TCR/TCR peptide vaccination*
2 MHC/peptide interaction:
   Altered peptide ligands
   MHC-blocking peptides
3 Co-stimulatory molecules:
   Anti-CD28 mAbs
   Anti-B7 mAbs
   CTLA4-Ig
   Anti-CD40
   Anti-CD40L
4 Growth factor/receptor interactions:
   Anti-CD25 mAbs
   IL-2-toxin fusion proteins*
5a Anticytokine reagents:
   Anti-TNF-α mAbs*
   TNF-α receptor immunoadhesins*
   IL-1 receptor antagonist protein*
   IL-1 receptor immunoadhesins*
5b Cytokine therapy:
   IL-4, IL-10*
6 Lymphocyte/endothelium interaction:
   Anti-selectins
   Anti-integrins (CD18, VLA-4)
   Anti-CD44
   Anti-ICAM-1
   Anti-VCAM-1
   Chemokine antagonists
7 Gastrointestinal tract:
   Oral tolerance strategies*
8 T-cell surface molecules used as targets for
lymphocytotoxic mAbs:
   Anti-CD5*
   Anti-CD52*

* Refer to clinical strategies discussed in the context of RA.

tolerance induction via peptide administration, direct manipulation of the cytokine milieu, and mucosal tolerance (Fig. 14.1). Each of these is theoretically applicable in the clinic although it is critical that this occurs rationally and in a controlled manner.

Is RA an autoimmune disease?

Whilst it is generally accepted that T cells control the generation of immune responses, their role in RA remains controversial [26,27]. Chapter 4 reviews the evidence for lymphocyte involvement in RA and I shall merely summarize the strongest arguments. CD4+ T cells are certainly abundant in early RA synovium although attempts to identify T-cell products such as interferon gamma (IFN-γ) and interleukin 4 (IL-4) have met with limited success [28]. Synovial T cells may influence their neighbours via direct membrane interactions, however [29], and recent evidence also demonstrates their active suppression, arguably for the purposes of damage limitation [30,31]. Additionally lymphapheresis, thoracic duct drainage, total lymphoid irradiation and lymphocytotoxic mAb therapy each provided transient symptomatic relief of RA in open studies [32–35], and the presence of rheumatoid factor and its link with severe disease also implicates immune-mediated damage. The strong linkage of RA to specific haplotypes of the HLA-DRB1 locus provides circumstantial evidence of a role for T cells and, whilst there are alternative explanations for this finding [36], RA is inherited in family studies alongside undisputed autoimmune diseases such as type I diabetes and autoimmune thyroid disease. Lastly the numerous animal models of RA, although imperfect, practically all implicate immune mechanisms in their pathogenesis [37].

A more relevant question is whether T cells can account for all of the damage in RA, and here the answer is almost certainly no. The fibroblastic and monocytic synovial lining layer cells (synoviocytes) proliferate in RA, in a quasi-autonomous fashion [38]. They secrete cytokines and enzymes which attack bone and cartilage and are undoubtedly responsible for much of the destruction and damage that occurs. Similar changes are seen in other rheumatological diseases, however, and it seems likely that synoviocytes have a limited repertoire of responses to injury. In RA therefore synoviocytes may become dysregulated secondary to an autoimmune attack on the joint and a unifying theory is that T cells are critical for initiation but that, in established RA, additional factors contribute to the poor outcome. It is unknown, however, whether adequate control of the immune response will enable the synoviocytes to subsequently return to their resting state.

Perhaps the clearest evidence that T cells play a role in RA comes from studies of modern immunosuppressive drugs such as cyclosporin A, FK506 and rapamycin. These drugs specifically target T cells and have only recently been introduced as therapeutics for autoimmunity. Controlled studies demonstrate considerable benefit, however, including some evidence for a reduction in joint damage [39,40] which provides support for the above contention that damage-inducing synoviocytes are controlled by pathogenic T cells.

What are the aims of immunotherapy in RA?

The advantages of an immunotherapeutic approach to RA are clear. It is a disease with significant associated morbidity and mortality [41], but there is no currently available therapy that predictably slows the progression to joint damage and destruction. Restoration of self-tolerance, on the other hand, should switch off the disease process. If this could be achieved with short courses of immunomodulatory reagents, their therapeutic ratio would be extremely high, particularly in comparison with our standard, relatively ineffective and moderately toxic, yet chronically administered, drug treatments.

How should we judge individual immunotherapies when responses fall short of self-tolerance, however? It took many years to devise regimens for tolerance induction in animal models and, in general, such regimens comprised improved applications of existing agents rather than the discovery of new agents. Potential outcome in RA is also dependent upon the stage at which the disease is treated: the application of successful immunotherapy at disease onset might result in a 'cure' with complete normalization of joint function. Investigations of early RA, however, continue to suggest that there is a significant preclinical phase and that irreversible joint damage already exists at presentation, at least in some patients [42]. Furthermore, aggressive, conventional treatment fails to control disease in a significant proportion of patients at that time [43,44]. Additionally, even if we successfully treat the autoimmune element of the disease, this may not prevent progressive joint destruction mediated by synoviocytes, which in turn could rekindle autoreactivity.

Our aim, then, should be to look for immunotherapeutic regimens which adequately control the immuno-inflammatory element of RA, removing or at least reducing the requirement for other anti-inflammatory medications. Ideally, short-term treatments should be followed by prolonged therapeutic benefit although, as with animal models, this is likely to require an iterative approach [45]. Given the high level of expectation induced in physician and patient by new therapies, particularly when parenterally administered, only randomized, double-blind, placebo-controlled studies can provide useful efficacy information. This does not, however, preclude a role for small, open studies when analysing the biological properties of novel reagents [46].

Immunotherapy trials in RA

T-cell-specific reagents

Most studies performed in RA since 1987 have been open and uncontrolled and the majority have been reviewed previously [47,48]. Although occasional long-term remissions of symptoms were seen, these studies were inadequate for formal assessment of therapeutic efficacy. Some provided useful information regarding the biological properties of mAbs, however,

16: Will there be a role for gene therapy?

C.H. Evans and P.D. Robbins

Introduction

So long as it remains incurable and resists effective treatment, rheumatoid arthritis (RA) will continue to attract novel therapeutic ideas. Gene therapy represents the latest of those strategies which attempt to use the resources provided by biology in this regard [1,2]. Whether gene therapy will find a use in the treatment of RA, and what that use may be depends on several factors. These can be stated in the form of the following questions.

- Will gene therapy provide a clinically useful outcome?
- If so, will it be clinically superior to those provided by competing treatments?
- Will gene therapy be cost effective?
- Will the application of gene therapy be hindered by insurmountable ethical problems?

Before considering each of these questions, readers who are not familiar with the field of gene therapy may appreciate the following orientation.

Gene therapy for arthritis

Gene therapy, as its name suggests, involves the transfer of genes to patients for therapeutic purposes. Its potential is most obvious in the treatment of monogenic diseases, such as haemophilia, where the successful transfer and prolonged expression of a functional gene will provide a cure. However, in most human trials gene therapy is used in the context of acquired diseases. Here the aim is not necessarily to compensate for a genetic defect, but to deliver therapeutic gene products. This is the strategy for treating RA with genes.

Two circumstances led to the suggestion of using gene therapy for RA. The first was the continuing failure of traditional therapeutic approaches to provide adequate control over the disease. The second was the great strides that were being made in understanding the biology of RA [1]. In particular, a number of proteins with anti-rheumatic properties had been identified, but their clinically usefulness was limited by problems in delivering them to patients for extended periods of time. Intra-articular delivery was a particularly difficult problem. Because proteins are the products of genes, and because of major advances being made in gene transfer technology, it became possible to contemplate the transfer to patients of genes encoding anti-rheumatic products, be these proteins or therapeutic types of RNA, such as anti-sense RNA, ribozymes or decoy RNA. These genes could be delivered to individual rheumatoid joints (local delivery), or to extra-articular locations where the gene products, if secreted, could enter the systemic circulation (systemic delivery). Later extensions of these concepts included the possibility of using DNA to vaccinate against arthritogenic T lymphocytes or to express arthritogenic antigens at sites or in a manner where they provoke immune tolerance.

To implement a successful gene therapy for RA it is necessary to identify anti-arthritic genes and to have a way of delivering the genes to the targeted anatomical sites. Once delivered, the gene will need to be expressed for as long as is necessary to cure or treat the patient. As the chances of a cure are far fewer than those of a treatment, it will probably be necessary to achieve prolonged gene expression unless ways can be found to make repeated gene delivery facile. Once prolonged gene expression has been accomplished, it may be advantageous to regulate the level of gene expression in accordance with the level of disease activity.

At present, a number of very promising anti-arthritic genes have been identified. Several of these have shown efficacy in animal models of RA (Table 16.1). A variety of viral and non-viral vectors have been used in these studies, including those derived from retroviruses and adenoviruses, liposomes and naked, plasmid DNA. Each of these vectors has its own advantages and disadvantages. In general, viral vectors are far more efficient than non-viral vectors, but raise greater safety concerns because of the pathogenic properties of the wild-type viruses from which they were derived. The safety of gene therapy is discussed later in this chapter.

Two human trials of gene therapy for RA have been initiated, one at the University of Pittsburgh in the USA and one at the University of Düsseldorf in Germany. Both use a retrovirus to transfer a human interleukin 1Ra (IL-1Ra) complementary DNA (cDNA) to the metacarpophalangeal (MCP) joints of postmenopausal or ovariectomized women with RA (Fig. 16.1). These are *ex vivo* procedures in which autologous synovium is removed as part of an earlier joint surgery and then used as a source of fibroblastic cells. These cells are expanded in culture and half the population is then retrovirally transduced with the IL-1Ra cDNA. After detailed safety testing, MCP joints 2–5 are injected with either transduced or

Table 16.1 Successful gene therapy of animal models of rheumatoid arthritis. (From [2] with permission.)

Animal model	Gene product	Vector	Ex vivo (E) or in vivo (I)	Transduced cells (E) or application route (I)
Local delivery				
a.i.a.	IL-1Ra	Retrovirus	E	Synovial fibroblasts
s.c.w.	IL-1Ra	Retrovirus	E	Synovial fibroblasts
z.i.a., c.i.a.	IL-1Ra	Retrovirus	E	3T3 cells
a.i.a.	vIL-10, sIL-1R sTNFR	Adenovirus	I	i.a.
c.i.a.	vIL-10	Adenovirus	I	i.a.
c.i.a.	Fas L	Adenovirus	I	i.a.
s.c.w.	None*	Liposome	I	i.a.
c.i.a.	IL-10	Plasmid	I	i.a., i.d.
Systemic delivery				
c.i.a.	sTNFR, TGF-β	Retrovirus	E	Splenocytes
c.i.a.	vIL-10	Adenovirus	I	i.v.
s.c.w.	TGF-β$_1$	Plasmid	I	i.m.
c.i.a.	IL-4, -IL-13	Plasmid	E	CHO cells†

a.i.a., antigen-induced arthritis; c.i.a., collagen-induced arthritis; s.c.w., streptococcal cell-wall-induced arthritis; z.i.a., zymosan-induced arthritis; IL, interleukin; sTNFR, Soluble tumour necrosis factor receptor; TGF, transforming growth factor.
* Oligonucleotides containing the NFkB recognition sequence were used.
† CHO, Chinese hamster ovary cells. These cells were transfected, selected and used subcutaneously as xenografts.
References to the studies summarized in this table are to be found in [2].

non-transduced cells 1 week before total joint replacement surgery in the American trial, or 1 month before synovectomy in the German one. The retrieved tissues are then analysed for evidence of successful gene transfer and gene expression. Patients are closely monitored for safety. Details of these protocols are to be found in [3]. The early data from these trials suggest that the procedure is safe, successful and well accepted by the patients. Because of the advanced stage of the disease and the short dwell time of the gene, no clinical improvement is expected.

More detailed information on the application of gene therapy to arthritis can be found in a number of recent review articles [2,4–6].

Will gene therapy provide a clinically useful outcome?

Progress towards the gene therapy of RA is occurring with remarkable speed. The idea to use gene therapy in this way arose in 1989, the first paper was published in 1992 [7], the first detailed animal data were published in 1993 [8] and the first efficacy data were published in 1996 [9,10], the year

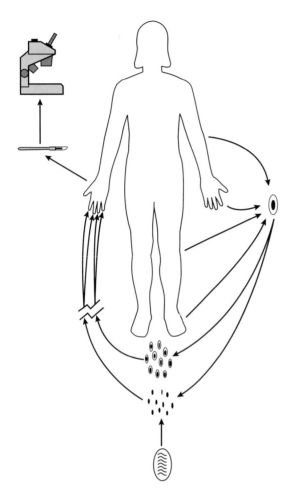

Fig. 16.1 Gene therapy for rheumatoid arthritis. This is an *ex vivo* procedure in which human IL-1Ra cDNA is retrovirally transferred to the metacarpophalangeal joints of patients with rheumatoid arthritis. For details see text. (From [6] with permission.)

in which the first human trial began. At the time of writing, there are 14 published studies related to the efficacy of gene therapy in animal models of RA (Table 16.1), and two human protocols are in progress. Increasing numbers of scientists at various centres are becoming involved in this field of research, partly because the National Institutes of Health in the USA have issued several 'Requests for Applications' in this and related areas. In addition, a number of biotechnology companies are interesting themselves in the gene therapy of RA. Thus, there is every reason to predict a successful outcome from these endeavours: the underlying concept is robust and reasonable, we are approaching a critical mass of accomplished investigators, funding is available and there is already an impressive track record of accomplishment.

Before a useful clinical product results from this activity, however, there are still a number of scientific and technical matters to be addressed. Although we have a good idea of which genes to use and which methods to use to introduce them into various sites in the body, long-term gene expression is rare. We have been able to express potentially anti-arthritic genes for life in mice by transduction of haematopoietic stem cells [11,12], but this is unlikely to be of general use in humans so long as the procedure involves ablation of the recipient's bone marrow. Transfer of genes to synovium, a favoured site in the present context, fails to give expression beyond 6 weeks [8].

Although transient gene expression thus remains a present limitation, it is a problem susceptible to resolution. As discussed elsewhere [2,6] there are various possible strategies for prolonging gene expression, including improvements in vector design, the use of different promoters and the judicious choice of target cells. Little effort has yet been put into achieving regulated gene expression for treating RA, but advances in other areas of gene therapy promise to provide such capabilities in the future.

As an alternative to accomplishing prolonged gene expression, there is the prospect of simplifying gene delivery so that genes may be administered easily on a regular basis. This is presently not possible but, again, is an achievable aim.

The evidence thus justifies a cautious optimism about the ability of gene therapy eventually to provide a clinically useful treatment for RA. Whether and to what degree it becomes used in clinical practice depends upon the answers to the following three questions.

Will gene therapy be clinically superior to competing treatments?

As stated in the previous section, it was the inadequate pharmacological control over RA that encouraged the concept of using gene therapy. The development of a simple cure for RA would render gene therapy unnecessary. Predicting the answer to the above question thus becomes a matter of judging how likely it is that the non-genetic treatment of RA will improve to the point where gene-based therapies are not needed.

If we take history as our guide, we may be forgiven for predicting that there is little to be gained by continuing to try to improve the treatment of RA by the traditional pharmacological approach. With the possible exception of sulphasalazine, no commonly used pharmaceutical was specifically designed to treat arthritis. In many cases their use in arthritis was based upon false assumptions about disease mechanisms. Gold drugs, for instance, were being used to treat tuberculosis and entered rheumatology in the belief that RA was caused by a bacillus. Methotrexate was designed as an anticancer drug and its anti-arthritic properties were only discovered by accident. Non-steroidal anti-inflammatory drugs (NSAIDs) are probably the only pharmaceutical agents designed around a specific mechanism, but the ability to inhibit cyclooxygenase also explains the actions of acetyl-salicylate, a drug that has existed for over 100 years. Selective COX-2 inhibitors are likely to reduce side-effects and thus permit higher dosing but it is not clear whether their anti-arthritic properties will be enhanced. The accelerating trend towards early intervention with existing drugs may improve the results obtained with them [13], but this remains to be demonstrated [14].

Considerations such as these suggest that the traditional pharmacological approach of synthesizing small, diffusable orally active molecules will not lead to any major improvements in RA therapy. The power of combinatorial chemistry and high throughput screening may prove us wrong, but at present, it seems that the strongest challenge to any gene treatment will come from other areas of biological therapy [1].

At the time of writing, impressive results are being described for the treatment of RA with proteins that block the actions of tumour necrosis factor (TNF) or IL-1. These results are important because they confound the predictions of those who argued that it would not be possible to treat this disease by blocking only one cytokine. The findings also suggest that, in many cases, patients are willing to endure the inconvenience and unpleasantness of injecting themselves several times a week with the protein. Other cohorts of patients are willing to report to clinics every few weeks for intravenous infusions.

Systemic gene therapy may provide a more attractive method for achieving these same ends, especially if improvements in the longevity of gene expression mean that the genes need be administered only once. For proteins with a long biological half-life this would represent only an improvement of convenience rather than a major qualitative leap forward. Patients would presumably prefer an infrequent and facile gene treatment to the frequent, invasive delivery of protein.

For proteins with a short biological half-life, such as IL-1Ra, it may not be possible to inject enough protein often enough to maintain therapeutic levels within the patients' tissues. In this case, continuous endogenous production of the protein as a result of gene transfer would be a major advantage and would avoid the peaks and troughs in serum concentration that follow protein delivery.

Safety becomes a possible factor because such treatments involve the systemic production of sustained, high levels of immunosuppressive proteins. This issue has already become manifest in the trials of TNF blockade where several patients have had infections and another has lost an eye through infection. There are also concerns about malignancies and the appearance of lupus symptoms. Chronic antagonism of IL-1 might not have such drastic consequences, but hard data are lacking. However, it is likely that any anti-rheumatic protein given in this manner will run the risk of increasing the incidence of infections and malignancies, if given for long periods. As anti-TNF therapy seems to be a treatment, rather than a cure, patients are likely to be on such regimens for decades. Systemic gene therapy is only slightly better equipped to deal with these complications than systemic protein therapy. Although we will in the future be able to switch off gene expression if risk of infection or malignancy is suspected, this would only be of the equivalent of suspending injection of the protein.

Where gene therapy does, however, have a distinct advantage is in local delivery to joints. The advantages of introducing anti-arthritic genes into individual diseased joints are several. It is a strategy which ensures maximum local therapeutic effect with minimum side-effects. In the context of the foregoing discussion, it should be noted that local delivery might ameliorate disease in joints without causing generalized immunosuppression. Another advantage of local, intra-articular, gene therapy is that, unlike systemic gene therapy, it can achieve what competing methods of delivery cannot—the sustained, high concentration of gene products selectively within the joint.

Critics of local, intra-articular delivery point out that the genetic treatment of individual joints in a polyarticular disorder is likely to be extremely tedious and, as one commentator put it, 'turn patients into pin cushions'. In response, we may observe that this does so to no greater a degree than when intra-articular steroids are administered, and it is certainly less invasive than total joint replacement. Furthermore, our most recent data suggest that local delivery of anti-arthritic genes to one joint of an arthritic animal suppresses disease in not only the injected joint, but also non-injected joints on the same animal [15,16]. This indicates that patients may require injection of only one or a few joints to suppress disease in all joints.

A second criticism of local delivery is that RA is a systemic disease which cannot be adequately treated by addressing only the joints. Be this as it may, most patients with RA suffer joint dysfunction as their overriding symptomatic concern. Only a minority have serious extra-articular manifestations of disease, and all would be helped dramatically if the joints could be protected. In addition, our studies lead us to wonder whether pathophysiological processes within the joint, particularly within the synovium, contribute to systemic aspects of the disease to a far greater degree than is generally realized [2].

When comparing local gene delivery to systemic protein delivery, there is also the matter of chondroprotection. Although the inflammatory component of RA is more symptomatic, it is loss of the articular cartilage that leads to the failure of joints as organs of locomotion. The view that loss of cartilage is solely a direct consequence of inflammation is no longer tenable; instead, erosion of cartilage needs to be studied as a separate pathophysiological entity. No existing drugs are convincingly chondroprotective, and it is too early to tell whether systemic blockade of TNF or IL-1 is anti-erosive. By delivering anti-erosive molecules in close proximity to the articular cartilage, local gene therapy has a distinct advantage as an anti-erosive strategy. The principle of protecting the articular cartilage by genetic means has been demonstrated [17–19].

Oral tolerance is another competing biological strategy. If it can be achieved it will probably put all other therapies out of business. There is also the possibility of tolerizing through genetic means by, for instance, introducing appropriate antigens to areas, such as the intestinal mucosa, where tolerance is to be expected, or by altering the behaviour of T lymphocytes. It is too early to predict the outcome of these efforts. If, as some maintain, immune mechanisms are not the primary pathophysiological driving force in established RA, there may be only a narrow therapeutic window during early disease when tolerization strategies might work.

Will gene therapy be cost effective?

Although most progress has been made with laborious and expensive *ex vivo* protocols, these are mainly being used to establish proof of principle. We will continue with them as long as we have to, but the aim is to develop an *in vivo* gene therapy that needs infrequent administration—ideally only once. Such a treatment need not be prohibitively expensive, especially if the vector is non-viral.

The unit price of a genetic treatment is unlikely ever to rival that of a NSAID pill, but if the genes only need to be administered once or infrequently, the cumulative price could well be competitive. It has, for example, been estimated that the average patient with RA spends over $2000 (£1500) a year on drugs. There is an additional burden of $20 000 (£15 000) p.a. from loss of working days and disability payments. For those who progress to total joint replacement, the costs become huge. When cashed out over the life of the patient, gene therapy has the potential to provide greater therapeutic benefit for lower cumulative cost.

An effective, *in vivo* gene therapy that needs to be given at rare intervals may prove much cheaper than biological therapy with recombinant proteins or antibodies. Clinical grade proteins are expensive to prepare and need to be given at frequent intervals in large amounts. Clinical grade genes and vectors may be no less expensive to produce, but their use may be cheaper in the long term because they are given infrequently in much smaller amounts;

a single gene can, after all, direct the synthesis of millions of molecules of the protein for which it codes.

Oral tolerance again emerges as the dark horse. Unless some strange and expensive manipulation is required for clinical success, an effective tolerizing pill would be impossible to beat in terms of price.

Will the application of gene therapy be hindered by insurmountable ethical questions?

The term 'gene therapy' triggers a conditioned negative reflex in the minds of those concerned about future brave new worlds. Within such groups lies a hard core of individuals who will never yield to the possibility of using gene therapy beneficently. This possibility is, nevertheless, a real one.

It is important that, for the purposes of treating arthritis, we are proposing to employ *somatic* gene therapy. This means that the genes do not enter the germ line and are not passed on to subsequent generations. Under these conditions, it is possible to argue that the issues surrounding somatic gene therapy are qualitatively no different from those accompanying the evaluation of any new drug [2]. That is to say, the key issues are safety and risk/benefit ratios.

Many of the safety issues in using gene therapy stem from the appropriation of infectious agents as the gene delivery vehicles. For use as gene therapy vectors, the viruses are genetically disabled to minimize pathogenicity. Nevertheless, concerns remain.

One potential problem is the formation of viruses that have regained their ability to replicate through recombination events. Recombinant, replicating virus might produce the same diseases in the patient as those produced by the original wild-type virus (Table 16.2). In addition, there may be infection of other individuals with consequential unintentional lateral transfer of the transgene.

Advances in methods used to generate viral vectors continue to reduce the theoretic frequency of such recombinants to ever smaller levels. As a result of such manipulations, replicating recombinant viruses have been

Table 16.2 Diseases caused by wild-type viruses from which viral vectors are derived.

Virus	Disease
Retrovirus (MMLV-based)	Murine cancer
Adenovirus	'Colds', fluish symptoms
Adeno-associated virus	None
Herpes simplex virus I	Cold sores and other skin lesions

MMLV, Moloney murine leukaemia virus.

virtually eliminated as an issue that impedes the development of human gene therapy.

Preparations of viral vectors can be screened thoroughly for the presence of recombinants. Nevertheless, once viruses have been introduced into the patient by *in vivo* delivery no further control is possible. An advantage of *ex vivo* gene therapy is that it permits screening of the transduced cells for recombinant virus prior to re-implantation.

An additional safety concern surrounds the use of retroviral vectors. Although replication-competent retroviruses can be eliminated in the manner described above, the viral genome integrates into the genomic DNA of the host cell. Unlike wild-type adeno-associated virus, retroviruses lack a specific site of integration. Random integration raises the theoretical possibility of insertional mutagenesis. In its worst case, this could generate malignant cell transformation or some other fatal condition.

Future manipulation of the retroviral genome may provide site-specific integration. Until this occurs, the matter can be dealt with in several ways. *Ex vivo* gene therapy permits the transduced cells to be assayed for malignant transformants prior to reimplantation. Given the delay in generating a transformed phenotype, such screening may be imperfect. A more secure approach is to introduce into the viral genome a conditionally lethal gene which permits any problematic cells to be eradicated as necessary. The herpes thymidine kinase gene is one example of such a gene. Its product is only toxic to the cell when the drug ganciclovir is administered. Herpes thymidine kinase may be antigenic, but a variety of improved 'silent' systems are becoming available. It may also be possible to place the thymidine kinase gene under the control of an inducible promoter.

Insertional mutagenesis in response to transduction by retroviral vectors is a theoretical possibility that has so far remained theoretical. The most commonly used of these vectors is derived form the Moloney murine leukaemia virus. The wild-type virus causes cancer in mice, but preparation of replication-defective vectors derived from this virus has not been observed to do so in any animal in the absence of contaminating replication competent retrovirus. Over 2000 human patients have undergone retrovirally mediated gene transfer, without incident. As the first of these was only treated in 1989, there has been insufficient time for late effects to have shown themselves; nevertheless, the safety record of retroviral vectors to date is impressive.

The first gene therapy human trial in progress for RA is an *ex vivo* protocol utilizing retroviruses. Because this was the first human trial proposed for a disease that is not normally considered lethal, the study design pays particular attention to safety (Table 16.3).

To carry out this trial it was necessary to get permission from two

Table 16.3 Safety measures incorporated into the first two human rheumatoid arthritis gene therapy protocols.

1 Patients are unable to bear children—no germline transmission
2 All vector production and human cell manipulation is performed in GMP facilities according to strict governmental requirements
3 All vectors and cells are extensively screened for replication-competent retrovirus and various other adventitious agents
4 Use of an *ex vivo* strategy ensures that vectors are not introduced directly into the body. This method permits screening of cells prior to reimplanation
5 Cells are surgically removed from the patients shortly after injection
6 Patients undergo life-long follow-up including annual testing for evidence of replication-competent retrovirus

GMP, good manufacturing practice.

Table 16.4 Gene therapy for arthritis—progress to the clinic.

Event	Year
Concept	1989
Approval from local IRB and IBC	1994
Provisional RAC approval	1994
Final RAC approval	1995
Approval by Director of NIH	1995
FDA approval	1996
First patient treated	1996

IRB, Institutional Review Board; IBC, Institutional Biohazard Safety Committee; RAC, Recombinant DNA Advisory Committee; NIH, National Institutes of Health; FDA, Food and Drug Administration.

local institutional committees before applying to the Recombinant DNA Advisory Committee (RAC) of the National Institutes of Health (NIH), and the federal Food and Drug Administration (FDA). Progress through these various committees took several years (Table 16.4), during which time the protocol was scrutinized from various points of view including science, ethics, feasibility, study design and risk/benefit ratio. The NIH, as a condition of funding this trial, required additional oversight in the form of an external monitoring board. This board is independent and contains a rheumatologist, an orthopaedic surgeon, a molecular biologist and an ethicist. This committee had to give permission for us to treat the first patient, and continues to monitor the trial as it progresses.

A similar trial started last year at the University of Düsseldorf, as discussed earlier in this chapter. The German trial contains the features of the American trial and, in addition, had to be approved by the local ethics committee in accordance with German law.

The response to these trials has been almost uniformly favourable. Indeed, some of our colleagues would have supported a more ambitious protocol in which the genes were introduced into early disease and not removed. Safety considerations restrained us from doing so.

At the other end of the spectrum, there have been isolated expressions of anger. A prominent German rheumatologist is quoted [20] as saying, '... one is operating on the edge between legality and illegality ... because the treatment is totally untested, safety is not sufficiently documented and thus the experiment ethically questionable'. Such extremist outbursts have been rare, and no sign of official resistance has emerged. Indeed, as described earlier in this chapter, the field of arthritis gene therapy is growing rapidly.

Overall, the authorities are taking a more relaxed attitude towards gene therapy. In the USA, the RAC is no longer required to approve every protocol, and investigators may apply directly to the FDA. The RAC now deals only with new and unusual protocols, such as the recent request to introduce adenoviral vectors into normal individuals, and examines the larger issues. For example, it recently held a conference on genetic enhancement.

The increasing societal acceptance of gene therapy and the overwhelmingly favourable response to the first human arthritis trial auger well for the future acceptance of this treatment modality.

Conclusion

We are optimistic gene therapy will provide a clinically useful treatment for RA at an acceptable price. There should be no ethical, regulatory or safety barriers to its implementation. Whether gene therapy finds widespread clinical practice will depend upon the success of competing approaches to treatment, especially other biological therapies.

References

1 Moreland LW, Heck LW, Koopman WJ. Biologic agents for treating rheumatoid arthritis. Concepts Progress. *Arthritis Rheum* 1997; 40: 397–409.

2 Evans CH, Ghivizzani SC, Kang R *et al*. Gene therapy for rheumatic diseases. *Arthritis Rheum*, 43: 1–16, 1999.

3 Evans CH, Robbins PD, Ghivizzani SC *et al*. Clinical trial to assess the safety, feasibility, and efficacy of transferring a potentially anti-arthritic cytokine gene to human joints with rheumatoid arthritis. *Hum Gene Ther* 1996; 7: 1261–80.

4 Evans CH, Robbins PD. Pathways to gene therapy in rheumatoid arthritis.

Curr Opin Rheumatol 1996; 8: 230–4.

5 Evans CH, Whalen JD, Ghivizzani SC, Robbins PD. Gene therapy in auto-immune diseases. *Ann Rheum Dis* 1998; 57: 125–7.

6 Evans CH, Ghivizzani SC, Robbins PD. Blocking cytokines with genes. *J Leuk Biol* 1998; 64: 55–61.

7 Bandara G, Robbins PD, Georgescu HI *et al*. Gene transfer to synoviocytes: prospects for gene treatment for arthritis. *DNA Cell Biol* 1992; 11: 227–31.

8 Bandara G, Mueller GM, Galea-Lauri J *et al*. Intraarticular expression of

biologically active interleukin-1 receptor antagonist protein by *ex vivo* gene transfer. *Proc Natl Acad Sci USA* 1993; 90: 10764–8.

9 Otani K, Nita I, Macaulay W, Georgescu HI, Robbins PD, Evans CH. Suppression of antigen-induced arthritis by gene therapy. *J Immunol* 1996; 156: 3558–62.

10 Makarov SS, Olsen JC, Johnston WN *et al*. Suppression of experimental arthritis by gene transfer of interleukin-1 receptor antagonist cDNA. *Proc Natl Acad Sci USA* 1996; 93: 402–6.

11 Boggs SS, Patrene KD, Mueller GM *et al*. Prolonged systemic expression of human IL-1 receptor antagonist protein in sera of lethally irradiated mice reconstituted with hematopoietic stem cells transduced with a retrovirus containing the IL-1ra gene. *Gene Ther* 1995; 2: 632–8.

12 Doughty LA, Patrene KD, Evans CH, Boggs SS, Robbins PD. Constitutive expression of IL-1Ra or soluble TNF receptor by genetically modified hematopoietic cells suppresses LPS induction of IL-6 and IL-10. *Gene Ther* 1997; 4: 252–7.

13 Emery P, Salmon M. Early rheumatoid arthritis: time to aim for remission. *Ann Rheum Dis* 1995; 54: 944–7.

14 Emery P. Rheumatoid arthritis: not yet curable with early intensive therapy. *Lancet* 1997; 350: 304–5.

15 Ghivizzani SC, Lechman ER, Kang R *et al*. Direct adenoviral-mediated gene transfer of IL-1 and TNF-α soluble receptors to rabbit knees with experimental arthritis has local and distal antiarthritic effects. *Proc Natl Acad Sci USA* 1998; 95: 4613–18.

16 Whalen JD, Lechman ER, Carlos CA *et al*. Adenoviral transfer of viral IL-10 gene periarticularly to mouse paws suppresses development of collagen-induced arthritis in both injected and uninjected paws. *J Immunol*, in press.

17 Müller-Ladner U, Roberts CR, Franklin BN *et al*. Human IL-1Ra gene transfer into human synovial fibroblasts is chondroprotective. *J Immunol* 1997; 158: 3492–8.

18 Müller-Ladner U, Evans CH, Gay S *et al*. Gene transfer to cytokine inhibitors into human synovial fibroblasts in the SCID mouse model. *Arthritis Rheum*, in press.

19 Pelletier JP, Caron JP, Evans CH *et al*. *In vivo* suppression of early experimental osteoarthritis by IL-1Ra using gene therapy. *Arthritis Rheum* 1997; 40: 1012–19.

20 Translated from the *Süddeutsche Zeitung*, July 3, 1997.

17: Do prostheses last longer? Should joints be replaced earlier?

I. Stockley

Over the last 30 years, the management of patients with joint disabilities has been revolutionized. The development of total hip replacement in the 1960s by Sir John Charnley represents a milestone in orthopaedic surgery. Hip replacement is a highly successful operation in terms of improvement in quality of life and cost effectiveness [1–5]. Of all the treatments studied to date, Williams [6] found that hip replacement produced the greatest improvement in quality of life for its cost. Quality of life is recognized as an important outcome measure in arthroplasty surgery. It focuses on health as perceived by the patient, rather than on the status of the prosthesis or other technical concerns which may not be directly related [7].

The indications for total hip replacement have evolved since the procedure was first introduced. Persistent pain and disability despite appropriate conservative treatment is the main indication for surgery. Although one would now consider all patients with chronic pain and functional impairment for surgery irrespective of age, this was not always the case. Charnley in 1979 [8] stated, 'When total hip replacement becomes a true science, as the author believes some day it will, there ought to be no need for a chapter on how to select patients, because then perhaps all hip disorders will be treated by total replacement. This happy situation in fact has already been achieved for patients over 65 years of age. Below 45 years of age we are still only at the beginning of our experience.'

In the past two decades, a number of innovations and technological advances have been introduced. Many of these have had an important effect and have resulted in significant improvements with drastic reductions in failure rates. On the other hand, many innovations in technology have failed to live up to their promise. It is important for the surgeon and the patient to be aware of the shortcomings of the procedure. Hip arthroplasty cannot be successfully used in the young and active individual without a change in activity levels leading to a more sedentary lifestyle. Continuing to indulge in heavy manual labour or sport such as running and competitive racquet games will lead to premature failure of the implant.

Currently about 40 000 hip replacements are performed annually in the UK [9]. The revision rates vary between series but 10% at 10 years is an average figure [10–12]. Unfortunately some designs have impressive results at 5 years but by 10 years high failure rates present [12,13]. Revision procedures cost more both in financial terms and in respect of morbidity and mortality. It has been generally stated that the results following revision surgery are not as good as the primary surgery [14,15] but early to mid-term results with modern bone grafting techniques are very encouraging [16]. Despite advances in primary hip arthroplasty surgery, the number of revisions performed annually is increasing. It is therefore essential that implants are formally evaluated and only those with a proven track record are used.

Fixation of the prosthesis was initially thought to be the major problem with arthroplasty surgery and the most likely reason for failure. Aseptic loosening was attributed to the use of bone cement and hence the term 'cement disease'. This led to developments in cementless fixation, but again hips still failed. Finally, it was realized that the long-term problem affecting survivorship of the implant is wear and the resultant biological response to the wear debris. This is obviously a major problem in the young patient as there is a time factor to consider, in addition to the potential level of activity.

Aseptic loosening represents the most common indication for revision surgery. Malchau and colleagues [12] reporting from the Swedish Hip Registry found that between the years 1979 and 1990, 79% of all revisions performed were for aseptic loosening. Many of these failures may be the result of prosthetic design principles that were introduced as improvements but subsequently resulted in disastrous consequences. The original Exeter hip femoral component was manufactured with a polished surface from EN58J stainless steel. There was no particular reason for this at the time, except that it was the fashion for many femoral components of that era to have a polished finish. No particular significance was attached to the type of surface finish in 1969. Unfortunately, the rather weak and ductile EN58J produced a number of stem and neck fractures and so the stem design was changed to be slightly wider in the anteroposterior plane and the metal changed to 316L stainless steel. The surface finish was changed from polished to matt, representing an increase in surface roughness of two orders of magnitude. Again there was no special reason for this change, other than it had by 1976 become the fashion for femoral components to be manufactured with a matt finish. No particular significance was attached to this change, and no adverse effects were anticipated as its sequel. In fact, the consequences were serious. Introduction of the 316L stem almost entirely stopped femoral component fractures but it produced an increased incidence of aseptic loosening and endosteal bone lysis in comparison with the original polished stems. It gradually became clear that the difference between the behaviour of the polished and matt stems was profound. Ten per cent of the matt stems inserted in 1980 had been revised by 10 years. This was a loosening rate requiring revision almost four times higher than that shown by the original polished stems over 20 years. The conclusion was reached that the difference could be explained on the basis that the polished stem was functioning as a taper [17], and at the same time producing minimal debris as a consequence of fretting at the stem–cement junction. By acting as a taper there is a reduction in shear forces at the stem–cement junction but an increase in radial compressive forces.

Reduction in cement stresses is the desired effect when contemplating stem geometry. Sharp corners should be eliminated and proximal cross-sections should be trapezoidal. Straight or curved, collared or collarless are all debatable points as equally good results have been reported using each of these variables. The most critical factor in all clinical series appears to be the quality of the cement mantle. Incomplete mantles can lead to premature failure by allowing a communication for wear debris to enter the joint cavity. Wear particles from any interface, polyethylene from the joint articular surface, corrosion products generated at a Morse taper cone junction of the femoral head and from abraded cement or metal debris, have all been linked to a granulomatous reaction leading to membrane formation, osteolysis and eventual implant loosening. Although mechanical factors play a part, e.g. the repetitive nature of external loads generating stresses at the prosthesis and interfaces, in practice a mixture of biological and mechanical factors operate.

Fixation is best discussed under two separate headings: cement and cementless. Early reported results of cemented stems reported failure rates of up to 20–24% at 5 years which increased to 30–40% at 10 years [18]. Although similar results have been reported by others, Schulte and colleagues [19] reported excellent results in a minimum 20 years follow-up. Of the 98 hips in patients surviving at least 20 years, 85% had retained their original prosthesis. With improved cementing techniques, the long-term results of femoral component fixation have uniformly improved dramatically. Mulroy and colleagues [20] reviewing 102 hips at an average of 15 years found that two hips had been revised and a further seven were loose on radiographic criteria alone. Modern cementing techniques with initial preparation of the bone bed by pulsed lavage, cement application by retrograde filling with a gun, distal plugging and pressurization with a proximal seal are all measures which have been shown to improve femoral component longevity. Individually each of these steps reduces the risk for revision $\approx 25\%$ when compared with conventional finger packing [21].

Another factor to be considered is the choice of cement. Studies from the Swedish and Norwegian registries [21,22] have reported much inferior survivorship: 25% increase in the risk for revision if low viscosity cement had been used. Although there has been a documented improved survival for the femoral component, the same cannot be said for the acetabulum. Loosening rates of 7–40% at 10 years have been reported even with the use of modern cement techniques [23,24]. This is in part due to the shape of the respective bones. It is very difficult to make the acetabulum a closed contained system for extreme pressurization which one can achieve in the femoral canal. There may also be biological differences between the femoral and acetabular trabecular bone, but because of acetabular failure, cementless sockets have become more popular.

The evolution of cementless acetabular components is divided between those devices that were designed to achieve mechanical fixation in the pelvis and the more current designs that were intended to achieve biological fixation via bone ingrowth into a porous surface. In clinical practice all but the hemispherical designs have proven to have unacceptably high failure rates. Threaded ring designs appeared in the short term to be satisfactory but longer-term follow-up revealed high migration rates. Much less surface area of the cup comes into contact with the bone in the case of a threaded cup compared with a porous coated hemispherical cup. Cementless porous coated acetabular components have been used in clinical practice for over 10 years. In general, the clinical and radiographic results of these types of implants have been excellent. After a mean follow-up of 12.3 years, only one cup out of a series of 52 was loose radiologically but clinically all functioned well [25].

Although there are advantages to a two-piece acetabular component, e.g. the ability to exchange a worn or damaged polyethylene liner, there are disadvantages. These include the possibility of increased polyethylene wear, both from the articulating surface and the back side surface, problems with conformity of the polyethylene within the metal backing of the acetabular shell, and problems with the mechanism by which the modular liner was attached to the metal acetabular shell. However, for the vast majority of patients the performance of cementless sockets has been at least equivalent to that of cemented sockets. In those under the age of 50 years, cementless sockets appear to provide fixation superior to that which can be achieved with cemented sockets. The addition of screws adds very little to the fixation if a good press has been obtained, indeed they themselves may cause further problems by fretting. Although improvements have been made with polyethylene and the locking mechanism to the metal shell, the plastic portion of the socket continues to be the weak link in the system.

Despite the generally accepted concept of a cementless socket, cement-less stems are not as uniformly acknowledged. So-called first-generation stems were designed and implanted with little knowledge of the factors governing biological fixation. Manufacturing techniques were crude and porous coatings debonded. Second-generation stems were an improvement. Better fill of the bone and biological fixation became more predictable. Third-generation stems have much more improved modifications. Split distal stems to decrease the incidence of thigh pain and circumferential porous coating along with improved bearing surfaces to reduce osteolysis have been introduced. Despite the wide variety of different femoral components available, most stems fall into one of two main categories. The first is the anatomic type of stem that is proximally porous coated and designed for metaphyseal fixation with an anterior bow. The second is the straight stem which can be proximally or extensively coated. Although early to mid-term results are comparable to a cemented series, there has been no evidence to suggest that cementless joint replacements perform better in the long term than cemented [5]. Retrieval of non-cemented, porous coated hip and knee prostheses have revealed that many components are fixed to bone only by fibrous tissue, although some authors have reported greater amounts of bone ingrowth [26]. For these reasons there has been substantial research into methods of enhancing bone ingrowth into cementless prosthetic surfaces. Particular interest has been focused on hydroxyapetite which can be successfully coated on to metal surfaces by plasma spraying techniques. One of the effects of hydroxyapetite is its ability to enhance bone growth across a gap around an implant. A concern, however, is its degradability in the biological environment. This a potential complication, particularly with respect to third body wear. There is increasing clinical experience with hydroxyapetite coating; several studies have shown promising clinical and radiological results [27,28]. It is not yet clear whether the superior fixation of hydroxyapatite-coated prosthetic components will last longer than that of uncoated or cemented prostheses and so longer follow-up and randomized controlled trials are awaited.

One of the drawbacks to cementless femoral components is the problem of thigh pain. A number of patients continue to experience thigh pain despite apparently well fixed components and it is for this reason that the cementless stem tends not to be as popular as the cemented, particularly in the UK. North America and other parts of Europe tend to have a different philosophy and favour the cementless approach. However, this may change depending on the longer-term results of hydroxyapatite implants.

Irrespective of the combination of cementless and cemented components, the long-term problem affecting survivorship of the implant is wear and the resultant biological response to the wear debris. Furthermore, it is the young patient that is at risk, both because of the time factor involved and their potential level of activity. Osteolysis is common in loose cemented components. It can also be seen in stable cemented implants where a deficiency in the cement mantle and a communication between the joint and the focal lesion has been recognized. Cementless implants both fixed and loose have been associated with endostealysis. The histology of the lytic lesion is characterized by granuloma formation with foci of intense histiocytic infiltration and foreign body giant cells in association with dense fibrous tissue [29]. Fine, opaque, black granules can be seen within the histiocytes and under polarized light, minute strongly birefringent particles (characteristic of polyethylene) can be seen within the cytoplasm of the histiocytes. If the implant was cemented then large numbers of methylmethacrylate particles can also be seen. Seventy to eighty per cent of the particles retrieved from the lytic areas are ultra-high-molecular-weight polyethylene, the remainder being corrosion products, titanium alloy, unalloyed titanium, cobalt chrome, stainless steel and silicates. These wear particles migrate into the joint cavity and periprosthetic spaces and stimulate macrophages and phagocytosis. Cytokines are then produced which in turn set about osteoclastic bone resorption. Although the majority of the particles are polyethylene derived, fretting and corrosion from modular junctions are important potential sources of particulate debris. Modularity was introduced into hip systems as an important advance in prosthetic design for the surgeon as it brings more versatility to the surgical procedure. However, it has a disadvantage as a source of debris.

Although all wear particles are biologically active, it is polyethylene, particularly the fine micron and submicron particles, which are the most aggressive [30]. It therefore follows that if one can decrease the severity of polyethylene wear, implants may well last longer. Important factors to decrease wear are the avoidance of third body and surgical damage to the femoral heads, the use of damage-resistant ceramic and smaller heads (22–28 mm). The recent introduction of alternative or improved methods of sterilization for polyethylene, which avoid the use of gamma irradiation in the presence of oxygen, will also help to reduce polyethylene wear and delay osteolytic changes [31].

The use of alternative bearing systems such as metal on metal or ceramic on ceramic is currently under evaluation both experimentally and clinically. The advantage of these articulations is that the linear wear rates are less when compared with metal on polyethylene.

Although good long-term results can be achieved with a standard cemented hip arthroplasty most series relate to the elderly population. However, recent studies looking at young patients have been encouraging. Callaghan and colleagues [32] report on 20–25 years follow-up of patients undergoing primary hip arthroplasty under the age of 50 years. Twenty-nine per cent required revision, the majority being socket revision only. In another long-term follow-up study of young patients undergoing hip arthroplasty surgery, Emery and colleagues [33] found the overall survivorship was 90% at 10 years and 68% at 15 years. Despite these good results caution is rightly expressed when the young arthritic patient presents. However, the aim of surgery is to improve quality of life and so age must not be a definite contraindication to arthroplasty surgery. Conservative hip replacement with resurfacing of the femoral head and acetabulum has many attractions in the younger patient. Non-violation of the upper femur, retention of upper femoral bone stock and the absence of proximal stress protection are unique advantages of hip resurfacing. It is important to keep the bone stock, as success of any revision procedure depends upon the available bone. Therefore perhaps in the young the first operation is a resurfacing, the first revision a standard hip arthroplasty followed by, if necessary, a revision with bone grafting.

In the young patient, who should be doing the surgery? Should any orthopaedic surgeon or should it be the specialist hip surgeon? I think the latter, as longevity of the prosthesis may well be surgeon dependent. It has been reported that known improved techniques for cemented arthroplasty surgery are frequently not used [34] and so the need for revision surgery may well be reduced if a greater proportion of primary hip arthroplasties and particularly those in the young were performed in specialist centres or by surgeons with a specific interest in this field. To confirm this and to see how good or bad we are, a national register of hip replacements and revisions should be set up. This would allow the identification of implants that are doing badly and would allow individual units to compare their performance with national figures. In addition, appropriate outcome measures are needed for assessing new implants that are more sensitive to failure than revision. The Swedish hip registry has led to improved efficiency and clinical practice and will allow optimizing of resources. Total hip arthroplasty can advance only if the orthopaedic community takes joint responsibility for patient and prosthesis selection and improvement of surgical technique.

To answer the question 'Do prostheses last longer?', the answer is probably yes, but it depends upon the implant and who put it in. To the second question, 'Should joints be replaced earlier?', again, the answer is probably yes, but choose your surgeon and check what implant he or she uses.

References

1 Charnley J. The long term results of low friction arthroplasty of the hip performed as a primary intervention. *J Bone Joint Surg Br* 1972; 54B: 61–76.

2 Wilcock GK. Benefits of total hip replacement to older patients and the community. *Br Med J* 1978; 2: 37–9.

3 O'Boyle CA, McGee H, Hickey A, O'Malley K, Joyce CR. Individual quality of lie in patients undergoing hip replacement. *Lancet* 1992; 339: 1088–91.

4 Laupacis A, Bourne R, Rorabeck C *et al*. The effect of elective total hip replacement on health related quality of life. *J Bone Joint Surg Am* 1993; 75A: 1619–26.

5 Rorabeck CH, Bourne RB, Laupacis A *et al*. A double blind study of 250 cases comparing cemented with cementless total hip arthroplasty: cost effectiveness and its impact on health related quality of life. *Clin Orthop* 1994; 298: 156–64

6 Williams A. Economics of coronary artery bypass grafting. *Br Med J* 1985; 291: 326–9.

7 Gartland JJ. Orthopaedic clinical research: deficiencies in experimental design and determinations of outcome. *J Bone Joint Surg Am* 1988; 70A: 1357–64.

8 Charnley J. *Low Friction Arthroplasty of the Hip. Theory and Practice.* Berlin: Springer-Verlag, 1979.

9 Williams M, Frankel S, Nanchahal K, Coast J, Donovan J. Epidemiologically based needs assessment. Total hip replacement. *DHA Project: Research Programme Commissioned by the NHS Management Executive.* Crown Publisher, 1992: 287.

10 Alsema R, Deutman R, Mulder TJ. Stanmore total hip replacement: a 15–16 year clinical and radiographic follow up. *J Bone Joint Surg Br* 1993; 74B: 240–4.

11 Schulte KR, Callaghan JJ, Kelly SS, Johnston RC. The outcome of Charnley total hip arthroplasty with cement after a minimum twenty year follow up: the results of one surgeon. *J Bone Joint Surg Am* 1993; 75A: 961–75.

12 Malchau H, Herberts P, Ahnfelt L. Prognosis of total hip replacement in Sweden: follow up of 92675 operations performed 1978–90. *Acta Orthop Scand* 1993; 64: 697–506.

13 Owen TD, Moran CG, Smith SR, Pinder IM. Results of uncemented porous coated anatomic total hip replacement. *J Bone Joint Surg Br* 1994; 76B: 258–62.

14 Kershaw CJ, Atkins RM, Dodd CAF, Bulstrode CJK. Revision total hip arthroplasty for aseptic failure: a review of 276 cases. *J Bone Joint Surg Br* 1991; 71B: 564–8.

15 Pellicci PM, Wilson PD, Sledge CB *et al*. Long term results of revision total hip replacement. *J Bone Joint Surg Am* 1985; 67A: 513–16.

16 Gie GA, Linder L, Ling RSM *et al*. Femoral reconstruction: cement with graft. In: Galante JO, Rosenberg AG, Callaghan JJ, eds. *Total Hip Revision Surgery.* New York: Raven Press, 1995: 367–73

17 Timperley AJ, Gie GA, Lee AJC, Ling RSM. The femoral component as a taper in cemented total hip arthroplasty. *J Bone Joint Surg Br* 1993; 75B (Suppl. 1): 33.

18 Stauffer RN. A ten year follow up study of total hip replacements with particular reference to roentgenographic loosening of the components. *J Bone Joint Surg Am* 1982; 64A: 983–90.

19 Schulte KR, Callaghan JJ, Kelley SS, Johnston RC. The outcome of Charnley total hip arthroplasty with cement after a minimum of twenty year follow up. *J Bone Joint Surg Am* 1993; 75A: 961–75.

20 Mulroy WF, Estok DM, Harris WH. Total hip arthroplasty with use of so called second generation cementing techniques. *J Bone Joint Surg Am* 1995; 77A: 1845–52.

21 Herberts P, Malchau H. How outcome studies have changed total hip arthroplasty practices in Sweden. *Clin Orthop* 1997; 344: 44–60.

22 Haverlin LI, Espehaug B, Vollset SE, Engesaeter LB. The effect of the type of cement on early revision of Charnley total hip prostheses. *J Bone Joint Surg Am* 1995; 77A: 1543–50.

23 Hodgkinson JP, Maskell AP, Paul A, Wroblewski BM. Flanged acetabular

components in cemented Charnley hip arthroplasty. Ten year follow up of 350 patients. *J Bone Joint Surg Br* 1993; 75B: 464–7.

24 Ranawat CS, Deshmukh RG, Peters LE, Umlas ME. Prediction of long term durability of all-polyethylene cemented sockets. *Clin Orth* 1985; 317: 89–105.

25 Smith SE, Harris WH. Total hip arthroplasty performed with insertion of the femoral component with cement and the acetabular component without cement. *J Bone Joint Surg Am* 1997; 79A: 1827–33.

26 Engh CA, Hooten JP Jr, Zettl-Schaffer KF *et al*. Evaluation of bone ingrowth in proximally and extensively porous coated anatomic medullary locking prostheses retrieved at autopsy. *J Bone Joint Surg Am* 1995; 77A: 903–10.

27 Geesink RGT, Hoefnagels NHM. Six year results of hydroxyapetite coated total hip replacement. *J Bone Joint Surg Br* 1995; 77B: 534–47.

28 Onsten I, Calsson AS, Sanzen L, Besjakov J. Migration and wear of a hydroxyapetite coated hip prosthesis: a controlled roentgen stereophoto-grammetric study. *J Bone Joint Surg Br* 1996; 78B: 85–91.

29 Anthony PP, Gie GA, Howie CR, Ling RSM. Localised endosteal bone lysis in relation to the femoral components of cemented total hip arthroplasties. *J Bone Joint Surg Br* 1990; 72B: 971–9.

30 Amstutz HC, Campbell P, Kossovsky N, Clarke IC. Mechanism and clinical significance of wear debris induced osteolysis. *Clin Orthop* 1992; 276: 7–18.

31 Fisher J. Wear of polyethylene in artificial hip joints: superolateral wear of the acetabulum. *J Bone Joint Surg Br* 1998; 80B: 190–1.

32 Callaghan JJ, Forest EE, Olejniczak JP, Goetz DD *et al*. Charnley total hip arthroplasty in patients less than fifty years old. *J Bone Joint Surg Am* 1998; 80A: 704–14.

33 Emery DFG, Clarke HJ, Grover ML. Stanmore total hip replacement in younger patients. *J Bone Joint Surg Br* 1997; 79B: 240–6.

34 Timperley AJ, Jones PR, Roosen R, Porter ML. Their hip in your hands—what is the contemporary total hip? *J Bone Joint Surg Br* 1991; 73B: 71–2.

18: Are occupational therapy and physiotherapy cost effective?

A.K. Clarke

Introduction

In many respects rheumatological services are fairly cheap. Our drugs are inexpensive, we are not high users of expensive investigation and we are well used to collaborative care with primary physicians which can significantly reduce cost. Admittedly there are a lot of patients, which does represent considerable cost to the healthcare system but when seen as cost per case then we are seemingly good value for money. However, no self-respecting rheumatologist would be happy to offer a service without physiotherapy (PT) or occupational therapy (OT) support. Preferably the therapists would have special experience and be dedicated to the rheumatology service. This adds to the cost of the service in a number of ways, mostly from the manpower aspect and therefore raises the important question of cost effectiveness.

At this point it is worth reminding ourselves that the cheapest service is not necessarily the best or even adequate. In any patient-related activity the totality of the intervention must be considered and proper outcome measures, if they exist, should be used. Looking beyond rheumatoid arthritis (RA) we know that two very expensive treatments used in locomotor disease, pain management for back pain and intensive in-patient programmes for ankylosing spondylitis make little difference, respectively, to long-term pain levels or spinal movements, but do considerably improve quality of life [1,2]. We must therefore resist the temptation to dismiss PT and OT if we find insufficient evidence for cost effectiveness at the present time. Rather we should be planning ways of identifying what it is we require from our colleagues and testing if they can then deliver. Those of us who work in large multidisciplinary teams have no doubt of their value and neither do our patients. Having said that the published evidence is inconclusive. Vliet Vlieland and Hazes undertook a meta-analysis of multidisciplinary team care programmes [3]. Thirty-five clinical trials were identified.

Of these only 15 were of a controlled design, of which nine were randomized. Twelve studies compared such multidisciplinary programmes with standard out-patient follow-up: six in-patient and six out-patient. The in-patient programmes were demonstrated to have a positive outcome, lasting up to a year, on disease activity. The results of the out-patient programmes were much less impressive, with only one [4] showing an advantage in terms of functional outcome. Three trials compared in-patient with out-patient multidisciplinary programmes [5–7]. Only one showed that the in-patient programme was better than that offered to out-patients, the other two showing the two approaches to be equally effective. The authors conclude that there is good evidence in favour of short-term in-patient programmes when compared with standard out-patient follow-up, but that the evidence in favour of out-patient programmes was scanty. They further state, however, that the results comparing in-patient with out-patient team care remains inconclusive. This is, of course, paradoxical and underlines the difficulties of undertaking such studies because of the need to compare like with like. In general terms, until proven otherwise, it seems that the team approach in clinical terms is likely to be useful, even if we do not know which elements are important.

This analysis did not address the question directly of cost effectiveness. There is some evidence that rheumatology services are generally of value in societal terms. Lee and colleagues looked at the overall cost benefit of an in-patient programme and were able to show a definite benefit [8]. Anderson and colleagues did address the comparison in cost of an in-patient programme with standard care [9]. They compared the healthcare cost of 16 patients with active RA who accepted admission in the early stages of the disease with 10 patients who refused to come in. The study showed not only a clinical advantage for the admitted patients but also that after the initial higher cost due to the admission ($5065) the follow-up care costs were significantly lower in this group ($99 less per year—all costs at 1985 prices). The clinical advantage was achieved in 2 weeks as opposed to the same effect taking nearly 2 years in the out-patient group. It is important to underline that this was not a randomized study. The two groups were self-selected and there could well be other factors, not least compliance, which led to this result, but the speed of recovery might well have had significant effects on quality of life, including economic activity. When translated to a large population of people with RA the savings to society could be considerable.

We do have a difficulty that the number of studies looking at the costs of PT and OT overall are few in number and very sparse in terms of RA. The rest of this chapter is divided into two sections, firstly dealing with the range of activities therapists undertake in the management of RA and the second looking at cost comparisons with alternative methods of treatment.

In the first section where studies do exist I have highlighted them. It would seem safe to assume that if a treatment or modality has been shown not to work, then it cannot be cost effective. This is on the basis that therapists, especially those with specific training in rheumatology, are in short supply and are relatively expensive. In the second section I have looked at a number of treatments that are either of proven efficacy or are likely to be so if adequately tested and tried to do a simple cost comparison with other interventions.

What do therapists offer?

At this point we should look at what therapists at present offer. This gives the opportunity to look at the published evidence on cost effectiveness and clinical efficacy as mentioned above.

Physiotherapy

Some data are available to help us with our quest. However, it is surprisingly thin on the ground as far as RA is concerned.

Assessment

Before any physiotherapist starts treatment he or she will do a thorough assessment. This complements that undertaken by the physician and will concentrate on those areas likely to be treated. Such assessments will frequently include measurements that are likely to be more reliable and reproducible, at least as far as intraobserver error is concerned, than those undertaken by the average physician. Moreover, the recording of the data obtained is likely to be of high quality.

The obvious way of harnessing the assessment skills is to look to doctor substitution, especially in drug-monitoring clinics and in clinical trials. I will return to whether this is truly cost effective later.

Exercise

There is evidence in favour of exercise as a useful modality in the treatment of all forms of arthritis, including RA. A number of studies have now shown that for the majority of patients with RA exercise will have improved outcome as judged by reduction in pain and increased function. Lyngberg and colleagues showed that a physical training programme undertaken with patients with moderately active RA led not only to an improvement in the number of swollen joints but also a rise in the level of haemoglobin in the blood [10]. Brighton and colleagues showed highly significant improvements in hand function in patients on a 4-year hand exercise programme, when compared with a control group who received no exercises [11].

It is generally agreed that very inflamed joints, however, should be rested. Traditionally bed rest has been used to treat an acute flare of RA and this is effective in selected patients [12] but the use of steroid pulsing has by and large superseded bed rest, as it is a much more cost effective form of treatment. It must also be remembered that bed rest will rapidly lead to loss of muscle bulk and tone and that this loss has to be reversed once the patient is mobilized.

Apart from formal exercises it does appear that general fitness exercises are of value and have the added benefit of helping cardiovascular health. Swimming is particularly suitable for many patients. Patients also benefit from undertaking simple limbering-up exercises on rising in the mornings. It is worth remembering that by exercising the patient is taking control of his or her own treatment and this is in itself likely to be of benefit. Work by such authors as Skevington [13] shows that if the locus of control passes to the patient, then the outcome will be improved.

Other modalities

Hydrotherapy is a direct descendant of the old spa therapies and as such is held in high regard as a treatment modality in RA. I am unaware of any cost-effectiveness data, and early clinical trials suggested that very similar results could be obtained on dry land, at least as far as muscle strengthening is concerned [14]. Later work has shown a more positive result. Thus, Hall and colleagues undertook a randomized controlled study of hydrotherapy, seated immersion, land exercises, and progressive relaxation over a 4-week period. Physical and psychological measures were made before and after the intervention and at a 3-month follow-up [15]. They were able to demonstrate that all four groups of patients improved but that hydrotherapy gave the best improvement, which was maintained at 3 months. Stenstrom and colleagues looked at the effects of undertaking dynamic training in water in patients with RA, comparing with a control group, over a 4-year period [16]. They were able to show that the training group had a significantly better grip strength and higher activity levels.

There is little evidence that any of the electromagnetic wave forms are of value in RA. Indeed a number of studies have shown that such interventions are at best no better than placebo. Examples include laser in the rheumatoid hand and short-wave diathermy for knee pain [17–19]. Ultrasound has been shown to be helpful in encouraging healing of skin ulcers [20], although this work has been challenged [21]. However, ultrasound may be of use in the treatment of vasculitic lesions. Therefore from the clinical effectiveness point of view there may be a very limited place for the use of most 'machines' in the treatment of RA.

Education

Because physiotherapists spend considerable time with patients and are more 'user-friendly' than physicians, they are in an excellent position to act as educators, especially as they are seen as being well informed by their patients. Unlike OT there are, however, no good controlled studies looking at PT as an educational tool.

Occupational therapy

Information about the effectiveness of OT in RA is as hard to come by as it is in PT. There is a variety of studies looking at some components of the process and also in the context of the wider rehabilitation team.

Assessment

As with PT, there is a strong tradition of assessment in OT. It tends to be more functionally based and the recording of data has, until fairly recently in rheumatology at least, been qualitative rather than quantitative. More recently a number of measures have been developed which are more applicable to the rheumatic patient, as opposed to the neurologically disabled individual. Of the general disability measures the best is probably the functional independence measure (FIM) [22]. Although many of the items in the scale are still more applicable to neurological disability, such as those referring to incontinence, it is reasonably sensitive to changes in locomotor function. It is certainly a measure that cannot be ignored, as many purchasers of health care, especially in North America, are using changes in the scores to judge the effectiveness of treatment programmes.

However, it is important to remember that global scores may not be appropriate in certain circumstances. An example might be the assessment of hand function when a specific measure, almost certainly an observational test looking at a variety of grips and other actions, would be much more useful.

A specific OT score, AMPS, has been introduced [23]. Like the FIM, it requires specific training, and licensing agreements are also in place. Also like the FIM, it is relatively time consuming to administer. In the rheumatological setting it needs to be compared with an assessment approach that might include the use of the Health Assessment Questionnaire (HAQ), which is self-administered by the patient [24], and a problem-orientated clinical enquiry.

Splinting

The OT frequently uses upper limb splinting. Few controlled studies exist showing that such splinting is of value. Rennie, in 1996, described a study in which a metacarpophalangeal ulnar deviation (MUD) orthosis was tested against no splint [25]. The study showed that anatomical alignment improved in all fingers except in the index finger. Pinch was also improved but significantly there was no change in the hand function score, pain score or gross grip strength. This is not very good evidence for the effectiveness of the MUD splint but only small numbers of patients were involved (26) and it could be that methodological problems in the study, including the crudeness of the outcome measures, did not give a fair picture of the usefulness. It is of some interest that 25 of the patients continued to the splint. Ansell's group reported a comparative study of two wrist splints in juvenile chronic arthritis [26], and my group recently provided a comparison of a number of ready-made wrist splints in RA [27], but neither study addressed the issue directly as to whether the splints were actually influencing outcome. Certainly such splints ease pain but it is far from certain that they prevent anatomical or pathological change.

Joint protection

Intuitively it seems reasonable to expect that if inflamed joints are used properly and protected from unnecessary stress then the outcome will be better. Considerable effort is put into joint protection but there is little evidence that this is indeed useful. Furst and colleagues were able to show that a programme for energy conservation and joint protection, using a workbook, resulted in a change of behaviour in those subjects undertaking the programme as opposed to a control group [28]. Crucially, however, they did not demonstrate that the outcome in clinical or personal terms was better in the treatment group as opposed to the controls. It is worth pointing out that if followed such programmes do give considerable control back to the patient and this may in itself be a benefit but that too needs to be proven.

Activities of daily living

For the rheumatic patient, the OT is usually seen as the prime source of advice about activities of daily living (ADL). This is very specific advice about the use of strategies and of technical equipment to assist people maintain independence, usually in the home but also at work and at leisure. It requires an adequate and appropriate assessment of the patient's needs and then the choice of what help would be best. Much of this work, although seen as essential and of great value, is arrived at empirically. Joint protection is mentioned below. I would like to quote two examples of frequently given advice, one of equipment, the other of environmental change, which we have shown are not based on any sound assessment of usefulness.

Perhaps the simplest of all OT aids is the tap turner, frequently given to people with RA who have trouble with domestic taps. We undertook a comparative study of the tap turners available on the British market, as part of the Department of Health's Disability Equipment Assessment Programme [29]. We did not find any previous studies described in the world literature. Much to our surprise we found that the tap turners were difficult to use and that patients preferred to either get other members of the family to turn the taps on for them, or left the taps just lightly turned off. A number of the tap turners actually required more physical strength and dexterity than the unadapted tap. A subsequent study showed that replacing the normal tap head with a lever tap was the proper strategy to adopt [30].

We compared, in another study for the Department of Health, portable ramps, used to enable wheelchair users to overcome steps when entering or leaving buildings [31]. To enable the ramps to be portable the slope on the overwhelming majority of them was greater then the 1 in 12 or 1 in 14 usually recommended. Despite this the majority of our wheelchair users were able to cope with the slopes. This did not matter if the wheelchair was being self-propelled, pushed by an attendant, or was motorized. Indeed a number of users commented to us that they found long, shallow ramps harder to negotiate than short, steep ramps. We therefore went again to the literature to see where the 1 in 12 and 1 in 14 figures came from. We could find no comparative data looking at the ideal rake of a ramp and recommended that, for the majority of people, a 1 in 8 ramp, and as steep as a 1 in 6 ramp for a power chair, was to be preferred.

These two examples do not, of course, invalidate the majority of the ADL activities undertaken by the OT. What it does remind us is that equipment needs to be properly evaluated and particular care taken to carefully evaluate the patient, preferably in their own home, before supplying or recommending an item. This item should be able to be demonstrated to achieve an improvement in the quality of life of the recipient.

Education

Apart from joint protection, the OT frequently undertakes other forms of education and instruction. There is some support for the effectiveness of this role as far as improving compliance. Thus, Feinberg [32] examined the effects of the approach of the therapist on the use of resting hand splints by patients with RA. The study, involving 40 patients, demonstrated that what is described as a compliance-enhancement approach improved significantly the number of days that the splint was worn, and more experimental patients wore their splints daily as opposed to the control group (nine as opposed to four). However, there was no difference in the levels of pain in the two groups and of course this study does not address the central issue of whether splints made any difference in the long term. Certainly the therapists are making a modest improvement in compliance with treatment but is this effort worthwhile? Until we can be sure that splints do improve the outcome, especially when compared with alternative strategies, such as injection and better disease control, it is far from clear as to whether the amount of professional time spent on patient education, in this area at least, is well spent.

Costs of therapy vs. other forms of treatment

It is at this point that we need to address the relative costs of OT and PT in comparison with other management methods. In the health service approximately 70% of costs relate to personnel. However, it must be remembered that does not just mean clinical staff. Each patient contact includes in its cost a proportion of the administrative salaries, for instance. Heat, light and power, postage, telephone and local taxation are all part of the calculation that has to be made in defining the cost of a service.

Hydrotherapy

Because this is such an expensive form of treatment it seems sensible to start here. We will assume that capital costs are not an issue at this stage. We need to consider running costs, which includes water supply, heating of the water, chlorination, heating and air conditioning of the pool room, council tax, pool attendants, the therapists, laundry and any number of sundry items. Maintenance is an important issue. General maintenance includes replacement of plant components, filters and redecoration. Health and safety maintenance includes microbiological testing, cleaning materials and attention to hoists. Typically this amounts to £18 000 per annum (see Table 18.1). Staff costs include the PTs and pool assistants. To get 48 h of hands-on treatment per week will require 2.3 whole time equivalents of both grades, which with on-costs comes to approximately £72 000 per annum. Those 48 h will provide approximately 100 one-to-one treatments.

Table 18.1 The cost of operating a typical hydrotherapy pool (with thanks to Miss Helen Whitelock).

Non-therapy staff costs	
Maintenance—general	£4500.00
Maintenance—health and safety	£7100.00
Equipment replacement	£1500.00
Running costs	£3000–£5000.00
Total	£18 100.00
Daily cost, i.e.,	£18 100 ÷ 365 = £49.59
Hourly cost	£49.59 ÷ 24 = £2.066
Therapy staff costs	
Senior 1 Physiotherapist to provide 48 hours per week actual 'hands on' treatment for a full year will require 2.3 whole time equivalent (WTE)	
Salary (approx)	£44 102.50
On costs (approx)—National Insurance	£4851.00
—NHS Pension contribution	£2646.00
Physiotherapy assistant 2.3 WTE	
Salary (approx)	£20 700.00
On costs (approx)	£3519.00
Total	£75 818.50

Assuming the pool works for 50 weeks in the year, this gives an approximate cost per treatment of £18. This compares with approximately £48 000 for 48 h weekly for dry land treatment. In the same period 150 treatments would be given, making £6.50 per treatment the main department.

Although there is a significant difference in cost, it really becomes startling when we do consider capital costs. It is impossible to give a typical cost because of such considerations as land purchase, the cost of new building as opposed to conversion of an existing building, the size of pool to be constructed, ancillary buildings and plant and the quality of materials used. An entirely new pool will be more expensive, as a rule, than one constructed as part of larger project. Costs are likely to be in excess of £100 000, and may be much more. This puts it in the same cost bracket as a computed tomography scanner. Few organizations would be prepared to give priority to a pool over other items of new high-technology equipment that the hospital might require, especially if it was not likely to produced significantly better results in terms of patient outcome.

Electrical modalities

The various electromagnetic machines vary greatly in price. A standard ultrasound machine costs approximately £800, an interferential machine £1000, a pulsed short-wave machine £2300, and a simple laser for rheumatic diseases, with a variety of probes, £3000. There are maintenance costs, accessories, and the cost of the therapist to operate the equipment. We also need to add in the heat, light and power for the portion of the department occupied by the equipment, replacement costs and other less easily quantified costs, such as patient transport and time lost from work to come for treatment. Bearing in mind that there is little evidence of efficacy for any of these modalities in RA the continued use of such methods must surely be highly questionable.

Exercise

Exercise is effective and has the advantage that once taught can be continued by the patient at home, or in their local gymnasium or health club if they wish (and have the financial freedom to do so!). Chamberlain and colleagues examined the effectiveness of exercise in managing osteoarthritis of the knee [33]. They were able to show that if patients were taught how to do quadriceps exercises, using weights, it made no difference if the patient was treated in the physiotherapy department or was allowed to do the exercises at home. What did make a difference was ensuring that the patient was reviewed regularly, if infrequently. If a patient was aware that he or she was to be seen again, then it was much more likely that the exercises would be maintained. It is true that this study was undertaken in osteoarthritis, but it seems reasonable to extrapolate the results to inflammatory arthritis. Supervised home exercises represent good value for money, reduce patient travel costs and time away from work or home and free up therapists' time for those activities that they do best.

Patient education

As noted above, teaching exercises is likely to be cost effective. Similarly other focused educational activities may well be a good use of therapists' time. This is particularly true if groups can be used and if the therapist involved is sufficiently experienced and knowledgeable to be able to assist with areas beyond that strictly related to treatment. It is for this reason perhaps more than any other that a rheumatology department should have dedicated therapists who are full and active members of the clinical team. This means that they need to be actively involved in the educational programme of the department, an area traditionally the preserve of the medical staff. It is also important that they have access to good library facilities and have the opportunity to take appropriate study leave. This adds to cost as the amount of 'down time', when the therapist is not in contact with the patient, will be significantly increased.

Doctor substitution

This is an attractive idea superficially. Doctors, especially consultants, are expensive. It would seem sensible to get the cheaper PT or OT to see patients coming up for routine follow-up, including drug-monitoring clinics. There are, however, a number of factors to take into account before declaring this as an obvious value-for-money strategy. Firstly, the clinical salaries represent a part of the overall cost of an out-patient consultation. Other outgoings include such items as estate costs (including capital or replacement costs), pathology and radiological investigations, secretarial and administrative support, and transport. Therapists are likely to be reluctant to discharge patients back to their general practitioners and may miss unusual clinical events. Their advice might also be held not to be so authoritative as that given by the hospital doctor. Many general practitioners are now wishing to take on more of the day-to-day management of their own patients and may therefore resist 'routine' follow-up at the hospital clinic. This is especially true if it means long or difficult journeys for the patient.

Activities of daily living

This area is potentially a minefield. A simple approach would be to ask the patient what functional problems they have and then provide them with a range of simple items of equipment from a stock or catalogue. This is a cheap option, which almost certainly would not tackle many of the real-life problems that the patient faces. These can be addressed by doing an observational assessment in the OT department and this is likely to produce a much better result. However, there are two drawbacks to this approach. The first is that the OT kitchen or bathroom may bear no relationship to the dwelling back to which the patient will return. Although housing standards are improving, we still find elderly patients in particular who have outside lavatories or who are virtual kleptomaniacs, with every spare inch of their house or flat being covered with the collected artefacts of 60 years. Both of these circumstances will make the use of various items of equipment very difficult. The second problem is that of patient compliance. Above I have mentioned the problems related to inappropriate items being provided, i.e. tap turners and shallow ramps. Many specific aids designed for disabled people are in fact less functional than those produced for the population at large. There is mounting pressure to look at design and the built environment in such a way that it facilitates ease of use for all, rather than stigmatize by a separate approach for disadvantaged people [34]. It is always alarming to go to a patient's home and find all manner of items still in the wrappings in which they were delivered.

The best answer, of course, is the home visit. This can be a very expensive operation. It will mean that the OT will spend half a day undertaking the visit, longer if the hospital is a specialist unit at some distance from the patient's home. There will be transport costs, and time spent liaising with local services, especially as there are very few Social Service departments that will accept the assessment of the hospital OT. However, the OT is likely to get a much better view of the abilities of the patient and his or her requirements. I am unaware of any studies that have looked at the cost effectiveness of home visiting for ADL purposes, or indeed any that show a better outcome in clinical terms.

What does the future hold?

There are two major problems when we consider the question of value for money when it comes to PT and OT in RA. The first is that much of what is done at the moment is ineffective and therefore clearly not value for money. The second is that much of what is done has never been subjected to critical assessment, despite the fact that intuitively such interventions seem valuable. In more leisurely times this would really not have mattered but worldwide the health budget is getting out of hand and the demands increasing. The purchasers, especially institutional ones, such as governments and insurance companies, are demanding evidence that they are spending wisely. We do know a number of things from the available research. The positive ones are as follows.
- In-patient multidisciplinary teams appear to improve outcome.
- Exercise is effective in preserving function and improving outcome.
- OTs are good educators.

The negative areas include the following.
- There is little or no evidence to support the use of most electrical modalities in the treatment of RA.
- Hydrotherapy is expensive.
- There appears to be little evidence to support doctor substitution on cost grounds.

However, we are left with large areas that at the moment have not been put to the test and which need to be addressed. Further questions include such items as the following.
- Does joint protection improve outcome?
- Is home visiting cost effective?
- Does splinting improve outcome?
- Should we continue with hydrotherapy?
- What are the best outcome measures to use to show effectiveness of the various therapies?

- What is the best mix of skills in a multidisciplinary team?
- What is the ideal length of a treatment session?
- Would we do better to teach patients their exercises to do at home?

Few people would seriously challenge that all PT and OT is of little clinical value or even poor value for money. What many are doing is challenging the notion that the whole package is of value, especially when they see that treatments that have been proven not to work, such as laser, are still frequently being used. A particularly worrying trend is for purchasers to demand that a specific numerical outcome measure should be applied, such as FIMS or the Barthell Index, when judging outcome of rehabilitation. As long as we in rheumatology are not in a position to show the overall effectiveness of our packages or to provide evidence that the individual components of that package are sound, then we will face scepticism and hostility. There are undoubted difficulties in coming up with the answers but on the other hand there is scope for a wide range of exciting research projects which potentially may be far more beneficial to patient care than quite a lot of the cellular and immunological research at present being undertaken.

References

1 Rose MJ, Reilly JP, Pennie B et al. Chronic low back pain rehabilitation programs: a study of the optimum duration of treatment and a comparison of group and individual therapy. Spine 1997; 22: 2246–51.

2 Bakker C, Hidding A, van der Linden S, van Doorslaer E. Cost effectiveness of group physical therapy compared to individualized therapy for ankylosing spondylitis. A randomized controlled trial. J Rheumatol 1994; 21: 264–8.

3 Vliet Vlieland TP, Hazes JM. Efficacy of multidisciplinary team care programs in rheumatoid arthritis. Semin Arthritis Rheum 1997; 27: 110–22.

4 Spiegel JS, Spiegel TM, Ward NB et al. Rehabilitation for rheumatoid arthritis patients: a controlled trial. Arthritis Rheum 1986; 29: 628–37.

5 Helewa A, Bombardier C, Goldsmith CH, Menchions B, Smythe HA. Cost-effectiveness of inpatient and intensive outpatient treatment of rheumatoid arthritis. A randomized, controlled trial. Arthritis Rheum 1989; 32: 1505–14.

6 Lambert CM, Hurst NP, Lochhead AJ et al. A pilot study of the economic cost and clinical outcome of day patients vs inpatient management of active rheumatoid arthritis. Br J Rheumatol 1994; 33: 383–8.

7 Nordstrom DC, Konttinen YT, Solovieva S, Friman C, Santavirta S. In- and out-patient rehabilitation in rheumatoid arthritis. A controlled, open, longitudinal, cost-effectiveness study. Scand J Rheumatol 1996; 25: 200–6.

8 Lee P, Kennedy AC, Anderson J, Buchanan WW. Benefits of hospital admission in rheumatoid arthritis. Q J Med 1974; 43: 205–14.

9 Anderson RB, Needleman RD, Gatter RA, Andrews RP, Scarola JA. Patient outcome following inpatient vs outpatient treatment of rheumatoid arthritis. J Rheumatol 1988; 15: 556–60.

10 Lyngberg K, Danneskiold-Samsoe B, Halskov O. The effect of physical training on patients with rheumatoid arthritis: changes in disease activity, muscle strength and aerobic capacity.

A clinically controlled minimized cross-over study. *Clin Exp Rheumatol* 1988; 6: 253–60.

11 Brighton SW, Lubbe JE, van der Merwe CA. The effect of a long-term exercise programme on the rheumatoid hand. *Br J Rheumatol* 1993; 32: 392–5.

12 Alexander GJ, Hortas C, Bacon PA. Bed rest activity and the inflammation of rheumatoid arthritis. *Br J Rheumatol* 1983; 22: 134–40.

13 Skevington SM. Psychological aspects of pain in rheumatoid arthritis: a review. *Soc Sci Med* 1986; 23: 567–75.

14 Harrison RA, Allard LL. An attempt to quantify the resistances produced using the Bad Ragaz ring method. *Physiotherapy* 1982; 68: 330–1.

15 Hall J, Skevington SM, Maddison PJ, Chapman K. A randomized and controlled trial of hydrotherapy in rheumatoid arthritis. *Arthritis Care Res* 1996; 9: 206–15.

16 Stenstrom CH, Lindell B, Swanberg E *et al.* Intensive dynamic training in water for rheumatoid arthritis functional class II—a long-term study of effects. *Scand J Rheumatol* 1991; 20: 358–65.

17 Heussler JK, Hinchey G, Margiotta E *et al.* A double blind randomized trial of low power laser treatment in rheumatoid arthritis. *Ann Rheum Dis* 1993; 52: 703–6.

18 Hall J, Clarke AK, Elvins DM, Ring EF. Low level laser therapy is ineffective in the management of rheumatoid arthritic finger joints. *Br J Rheumatol* 1994; 33: 142–7.

19 Hamilton DE, Bywaters EGL, Please NW. A controlled trial of various forms of physiotherapy in arthritis. *Br Med J* 1959; i: 542–4.

20 Dyson M, Franks C, Suckling J. Stimulation of healing of varicose ulcers by ultrasound. *Ultrasonics* 1976; 14: 232–6.

21 Lundeberg T, Nordstrom F, Brodda-Jansen G *et al.* Pulsed ultrasound does not improve healing of venous ulcers. *Scand J Rehabil Med* 1990; 22: 195–7.

22 Granger CV, Hamilton BB, Sherwin FS. *Guide to the Use of the Uniform Data Set for Medical Rehabilitation.* UDS for MR Project Office, Buffalo General Hospital, New York, 1986.

23 Fisher AG, Lui Y, Velozo CA, Pan AW. Cross-cultural assessment of process skills. *Am J Occup Ther* 1992; 46: 876–85.

24 Kirwan JR, Reeback JS. Stanford Health Assessment Questionnaire modified to assess disability in British patients with rheumatoid arthritis. *Br J Rheumatol* 1986; 25: 206–9.

25 Rennie HJ. Evaluation of the effectiveness of a metacarpophalangeal ulnar deviation orthosis. *J Hand Ther* 1996; 9: 371–7.

26 Eberhard BA, Sylvester KL, Ansell BM. A comparative study of orthoplast cock-up splints versus ready-made Droitwich work splints in juvenile chronic arthritis. *Disabil Rehabil* 1993; 15: 41–3.

27 Catchpole N, Clarke AK. *Wrist Splints for People with Rheumatological Disease—A Comparative Evaluation.* London: Medical Devices Agency, 1997.

28 Furst GP, Gerber LH, Smith CC, Fisher S, Shulman B. A program for improving energy conservation behaviors in adults with rheumatoid arthritis. *Am J Occup Ther* 1987; 41: 102–11.

29 Swinkels A, Clarke AK. 'What's on tap?'—An assessment of tapturners and taphead adapters. *Br J Occup Ther* 1993; 56: 173–6.

30 Sweeney GM, Catchpole N, Clarke AK. Choosing lever taps for people with rheumatoid arthritis. *Br J Occup Ther* 1994; 57: 263–5.

31 Sweeney GM, Clarke AK. Gradients of portable ramps. *Br Med J* 1991; 302: 1277.

32 Feinberg J. Effect of the arthritis health professional on compliance with use of resting hand splints by patients with rheumatoid arthritis. *Arthritis Care Res* 1992; 5: 17–23.

33 Chamberlain MA, Care G, Harefield B. Physiotherapy in osteoarthrosis of the knees: a controlled trial of hospital versus home exercises. *Int Rehab Med* 1982; 4: 101–6.

34 Goldsmith S. *Designing for the Disabled; The New Paradigm.* Oxford: The Architectural Press, 1997.

19: Is rheumatoid arthritis declining in incidence and severity? A critical appraisal

L.A. Mandl and M.H. Liang

Introduction

Twenty years ago Buchanan and Murdoch in a paper entitled 'That rheumatoid arthritis will disappear' [1] hypothesized; '. it is possible that we may now expect the current pandemic to disappear. Perhaps by the end of the next century [rheumatoid arthritis] will be mild and rare or even non-existent'. As the new millennium approaches we revisit this prophecy and critically review the literature suggesting the putative evolution of rheumatoid arthritis (RA) from a severe, relatively common disease to a more benign, less frequent disease. The original suggestion that RA might diminish in incidence and severity was based on the observation that RA has features consistent with an 'infectious' aetiology, and thus may be subject to cyclical changes in both incidence and virulence of the aetiological agent [2]. Although this hypothesis has been overshadowed by studies on the mechanisms of disease, a recent review concedes 'it remains possible that an infection of the synovial lining is the initiating event' in RA [3]. It is likely that the cause of RA is multifactorial, the result of a genetic predisposition, such as polymorphism of the DRβ locus [4], intersecting with environmental factors.

We review the indirect evidence from art, literature, medical writings, palaeopathology and epidemiological studies. Whether RA is becoming less frequent and/or milder and why is of more than academic interest since the answer may provide clues to its aetiology and would inform what we tell patients and their families.

Clues from ancient literature and historical medical writings

For a disease of such striking physiognomy, there is a lack of references to RA in both ancient literature and medical writings. In searching the ancient Greek and Roman medical literature for allusions to RA, Short [5] concludes that the earliest mention is by Scribonious Largus (AD 40), Julius

Caesar's chief medical officer. Largus describes a chronic polyarthritis occurring mostly in 'elderly' (by Roman standards), women, which would be compatible with RA. A reference is made by Aretaeus (AD 81–138?), who described a polyarthritis which 'is a general pain of all the joints— the disease lies concealed for a long time, when the pain and the disease are kindled up by any slight cause'. Soranus of Ephesus (AD 98–138) describes a deforming polyarthritis with pronounced morning stiffness [6]. Short points out that some of these may have been chronic tophaceous gout, as there are references to discharging tophi and the incidence of the disease was least common in women and most common in middle-aged men. There is also a reference in the *Caraka Samhita*, an ancient Indian text of the first century AD, to a deforming polyarthritis consistent with RA [7]. The Emperor Constantine IX Momomachus (980–1055) had a severe crippling polyarthritis, but it is difficult to know if this was RA or a reactive or gonococcal arthritis as his biographer, Michael Constantine Psellus, states the Emperor was 'naturally inclined to sexual indulgence' [8]. Thomas Sydenham (1624–1689) published his *Medical Observations Concerning the History and the Cure of Acute Diseases* in 1676 [9]. In it he describes some of the main disease attributes of RA, including its intermittent progressive course, the possibility of disability, as well as classic swan neck deformities [5].

The first unequivocal reference to RA in the medical literature is in 1800 by Landre-Beauvais, a French medical student [10]. His doctoral thesis, which quoted Sydenham on its title page, was entitled 'Should we Recognize a New Type of Gout, to be called Primary Aesthenic Gout?' Landre-Beauvais felt this 'new' syndrome differed from classical gout in that:
• patients were mostly women;
• those affected where aesthenic and poor rather than corpulent and wealthy;
• initially, multiple not single joints were affected;
• the time course of attacks were longer;
• the intensity of the pain less;
• residual deformity remained even after resolution of symptoms.
For a disease that has such an easily recognized phenotype, it is significant that in 1800 it was felt to be unique enough to be posited as a 'new' syndrome. The 19th century continued to see descriptions of what would be recognized today as typical RA by Jean Charcot, Sir Alfred Garrod and Sir Archibald Garrod [11–16]. Sir Alfred Garrod gave the syndrome its modern name of 'rheumatoid arthritis' in 1859.

Clues from the arts and literature

There are no references to RA in the Bible or in the works of Shakespeare

[17,18]. A number of paintings done prior to 1800 have been presented as evidence that RA existed in Europe prior to Landre-Beauvais' description. 'Praying Hands' by Albrecht Durer (1471–1528) is a possible example of RA [19]. 'The Temptation of St Antony', an early 16th century painting of the Flemish–Dutch school, shows a beggar who has ulnar deviation of the digits and flexion contractures of the extremities [20]. A portrait of Seibrandus Sixtius, a 17th century Dutch priest born in 1568, also shows typical hand deformities of RA [21,22]. However, diagnosing diseases from artistic representations is fraught with potential problems. At an international meeting on art history and the antiquity of rheumatic disease it was 'concluded that style and artistic license precluded attribution of diagnostic significance' to works of art examined in isolation [23], a conclusion also of others in the field [24].

Clues from palaeopathology

A precise method of identifying cases of RA in the past is by examining skeletal remains. While there is good palaeopathological evidence that osteoarthritis, spondyloarthritis and gout have existed for at least 4000 years [25–29], there are no European, Egyptian or Asian skeletons showing definitive changes of RA. Some 580 skeletons from archaeological sites in France, Iran, Israel, Egypt and Sudan have been examined, and none had signs of RA [25,30,31]. A symmetrical erosive arthritis has been found in Native American skeletons from the Archaic period in Pre-Columbian America, 3000–5000 years ago [32], and most experts believe that the findings are consistent with RA existing in North America at this time. The findings of RA in Pre-Columbian America were seen in eight distinct populations centring around the west branch of the Tennessee River. Clustering by place is sometimes a clue of a common environmental factor in disease aetiology. Sixty-three other geographical populations in nearby areas were examined, for a total of 6364 additional skeletons, none of which showed any evidence of RA. Interestingly, the areas in which evidence of RA has been found are some of the most historically isolated to 'Old World' influences, being the last areas in the north-east to be explored by the English, Dutch, French and Spanish explorers [31,33–35]. This might explain the 300 years 'lag time' in the export of RA to Europe.

The marked difference in skeletal evidence of RA between North America and 'the Old World' leads to an intriguing hypothesis, put forth by Rothschild and colleagues [31]. Christopher Columbus found the New World in 1492, and European penetration of areas of the north-east containing skeletal evidence of RA occurred only by the late 18th century [33–35]. The first clear account of RA in Europe appears in the medical literature in 1800, and is then followed by increasing numbers of descriptions until it is a well-established disease [36]. If the frequency of its mention in the literature is any reflection of increased incidence and recognition, then— and this is a major leap—the pattern is consistent with the hypothesis that RA has an infectious aetiology, perhaps a virus [37]. A disease which progresses rapidly to a 1% prevalence fits an 'epidemic' pattern. It would therefore not be surprising to see a decrease in the frequency and severity of the disease, as those with the least resistance to disease die off and herd immunity is acquired, leading to diminished incidence and severity, fitting with the cyclic pattern of infectious epidemics [38].

Clinical studies

An apparent temporal change has occurred in the pattern of RA [39]. Anecdotal observations appear to be buttressed by studies from Europe and North America, which support the prediction of a 'milder' RA. Although individual studies have limitations, almost every study published in the last 15 years has shown a decreasing trend in incidence and severity. Given the inherent problems in studying the epidemiology of RA in different populations, using different methods of assembling patients and using different criteria, the consistency of the findings are impressive.

The first modern study of secular trends in RA is by Linos and colleagues who reviewed medical records at the Mayo clinic [40]. She looked at the rates of RA in Rochester, Minnesota from 1950 to 1974 and found an average incidence of 28.1/100 000 for men and 65.7/100 000 for women using the 1958 American Rheumatism Association (ARA) criteria for RA [41]. When only cases of definite RA were included, the rates were 21.6/100 000 and 48.0/100 000 for men and women, respectively, one of the lowest rates yet recorded [42]. One of the striking findings was an increase in the incidence of RA, peaking in the early sixties and then falling dramatically over the next decade. This decrease was accounted for almost exclusively by a decrease in female incidence, as the male rate remained relatively stable. Incidence rates for women went from 68.0/100 000 in 1950–54 to 92.3/100 000 in 1960–64, to 39.7/100 000 in 1970–74, a decline of 41%. The investigators speculated that the differential decline among women was due to the burgeoning use of oral contraceptives and hormone replacement therapy, supporting the findings of an earlier study in England which reported a 50% lower rate of RA in users of oral contraceptives than non-users [43]. The study, despite its inherent limitations, was the first to suggest a declining incidence of RA in women but not men—in the late 60s to early 70s. Other studies from this period showed slightly higher or similar figures [44–46]. The Linos study missed patients who had not sought medical attention, and because the ARA criteria used require a minimum duration of signs and symptoms, led to the exclusion of 25% of qualifying patients. This led to lower rates than previous studies, which had used modified criteria [42]. The peak rate may have been influenced by increased awareness of RA due to the introduction in the early 1960s of the test for rheumatoid factor. This may have increased or strengthened the clinical impression in mild cases, allowing them to swell the early numbers and create the impression of a subsequent declining incidence. It should be noted, however, that a reclassification of the cases is ongoing because it is suspected that non-cases were included (S. Gabriel, personal communication, 1997) [47].

Other studies also show a declining trend [48,49]. Hochberg analysed data from a national morbidity and mortality study in England and Wales from 1970 to 1972 and 1981–82 and found a fall of 30% in the age-adjusted incidence of RA in women, from 3.7/1000 to 2.6/1000, with essentially no change in men [50]. Unfortunately, the diagnosis of RA was only based on a general practitioner's clinical diagnosis which was not externally validated or standardized. In addition, ankylosing spondylitis was coded within the same diagnostic category as RA, and therefore could not be separated out in the analysis. This makes impossible a valid comparison of these results with those from other studies. The incidence may have declined or there may have been a change in diagnostic practices with improved education regarding rheumatic diseases that led to appropriately fewer diagnosis of RA in the 1980s creating the appearance of decreased incidence. Silman found a decrease of 50% in both sexes over an 11-year period, from almost 160/100 000 to 80/100 000, although reanalysis suggested ascertainment bias may have influenced results [51]. Rates of rheumatoid factor seropositivity in four of five cohorts peaked in the early 1960s—the same time Linos and colleagues noted peak rates in Minnesota. Another British study drawing on the Royal College of General Practitioners' database found a 46% decrease in incidence among women who had never used hormonal contraception [52]. Dugowson and colleagues looked at the incidence rate of RA in Seattle, Washington from 1987 to 1989 [53]. This was a prospective case–control study looking at newly diagnosed RA in women, ages 18–64, based on the 1958 ARA criteria. The incidence rate for definite/classic RA was 23.9/100 000, 44.7% lower than the Rochester, Minnesota data from 1950 to 1974. Incidence rates in women also increased with age.

Two studies look at the incidence of RA prospectively. Symmons and colleagues studied all new cases of inflammatory arthritis in a regional health district, as defined by the 1987 ARA criteria [54] who presented for the first time in 1990 to the end of 1991. They found an age-adjusted incidence of 34.3/100 000 in women and 12.7/100 000 in men. These were lower rates than the previous UK rates but were similar to the data found in the USA [40,53]. Incidence in women increased up to age 45, stabilized after age 75, and then declined dramatically in the over-85 years group. In men incidence rose consistently with age. In a longitudinal epidemiological study, Jacobsson and colleagues looked at rates of RA in Pima Indians from 1965 to 1990 [55]. This is a particularly good population for epidemiological studies as Native Americans have a high rate of RA, but the findings are less generalizable to other populations [56,57]. The 1961 Rome Criteria were used, which are based on eight of 11 of the 1958 ARA criteria. They found a 55% decrease in the age-adjusted incidence in men, and a 57% decrease in the age-adjusted incidence in women, although statistical significance was only reached for women. The data for women were controlled for oral contraceptive/oestrogen use, and only 17% of the participants were taking disease-modifying anti-rheumatic drugs (DMARDs), which was far less than the observed drop in incidence. Prospective studies avoid the biases in retrospective or comparative studies of different cohorts. If the same disease definitions are used, any ascertainment bias would be systematic; and although absolute incidence rates may be debated, the trends over time should be meaningful.

A cross-sectional study in the UK published in 1993 looked at prevalence rate of RA [58]. In all women aged 45–64 in an 11 000-person general practice, the investigators found a prevalence rate of 1.2%. This was lower than the 2.5% rate found in a previous British study done between 1958 and 1960 [59]. Prevalence studies are difficult to interpret in a disease like RA where disease course waxes and wanes over time. A decreased prevalence can be caused by a shortening of the average disease duration: treatment rendering the disease so mild it is not 'captured' by the study criteria or by a true decrease in incidence. However, this study also supports the trend of a decreasing incidence.

Only two studies do not show a decline in RA incidence. Chan and colleagues found no secular change in the age-adjusted rate of RA in the population of Worcester County, Massachusetts, from 1987 to 1990, using ARA 1958 criteria [60]. This was a retrospective study based on chart review covering a short period of time. The incidence of RA was 60/100 000 in women and 22/100 000 in men. Gran and colleagues, in a published abstract, also found no change in the incidence rate of 21.1/100 000 among a Norwegian population from 1969 to 1981, also using 1958 ARA criteria [61].

Other factors could give the appearance of a decreasing RA incidence over time where none existed [63]. Earlier studies may have included patients who did not have RA, but had other inflammatory polyarthritides and spondyloarthropathies. There have also been changes in how RA is defined in studies over time [65–68]. When standard criteria are used, a patient who does not meet the definition cannot be counted even if they are felt to be a case. Kellgren and colleagues [62] and Valkenburg [63] estimated, respectively, that 25% of arthritis patients in urban England and the rural Netherlands never consult a physician. With systems of health care using primary care physicians as gatekeepers, RA patients may not see specialists or go to referral centres where studies tend to be done. Lastly, if RA is indeed becoming less severe—either 'naturally' or through more effective treatment strategies—fewer patients with the disease may be meeting the diagnostic threshold of criteria which were designed to identify the disease in its more classic and severe form.

In addition, we also note that incidence or prevalence rates that are not age adjusted, or alternatively ascertained within an age group, over time, cannot truly be compared, as the age distribution of the populations may be different or different over time. In populations where an increasing proportion is elderly, RA may be underestimated. In the elderly, synovitis can be subtle and symptoms mistakenly attributed to ageing, which could lead to under-ascertainment.

When one looks at studies which cover at least a decade of observation and use comparable case definitions, there are only the Mayo Clinic study, the Pima Indian study, possibly the study by Gran and colleagues and the study by Hannaford and colleagues which observe a population over a prolonged period of time. The Mayo study provides information only for the 1950s and 1960s. Each of these studies involves a relatively stable and homogenous population, although each is looking at a genetically dissimilar group.

If there has been a true decline in the incidence of RA what might be responsible? Investigators have looked at the effects of oral contraceptives (OCs) and oestrogen replacement on RA, and the data are conflicting. Some studies suggest that the use of oral contraceptives is protective against developing RA [69–72]. Other studies fail to find a correlation [73–77]. Two separate meta-analyses came to opposite conclusions [74,75]. These same discrepancies exist for oestrogen replacement therapy, with studies both supporting and not supporting its protective effects [78,79]. Earlier studies of OCs did not account for the lower pregnancy and breast-feeding rates in OC users. When that is done, and also adjusted for age of the mother when giving birth, the odds ratio (OR) for developing RA in women who had used OCs for < 5 years or > 5 years compared with never-users were 0.713 and 0.76, respectively [80]. Most European studies have been hospital-based, and most US studies population-based [69]. The data show a protective effect in Europe but not in the USA [81]. There may be protection in a selected population, but the difficulty in avoiding bias in observational studies of cause and effect relationships, especially related to oral contraceptives, has been discussed [82–85]. Nevertheless, a decrease in RA incidence has also been documented in women not using OCs and in data controlled for OC use, so it is clearly not the only factor [49,55]. Generally improved living conditions have been associated with improvements in other diseases such as bronchitis, peptic ulcer disease and coronary artery disease, but how this impacts on RA is as yet undetermined [64]. Finally, the possibility that the disease has 'burned itself out', and is now in its 'postepidemic phase' is a speculation based on the assumption of this being an infectious disease whose organism is still a mystery.

Secular trends in disease severity

In addition to a declining incidence there is also an impression that RA has become less severe [39,85]. The conclusion requires that we somehow quantify severity between populations and over time. This has been approached in three ways [64]. First, case fatality rates can be measured. Secondly, disability from the disease can be examined. Thirdly, trends in clinical and radiological features have been studied. A true decrease in severity is difficult to document, as study designs, definitions of RA and inclusion criteria vary tremendously in studies across time and populations.

These different definitions have important conceptual differences. Impairments such as erosive disease are anatomical damage, a 'physiological state'. Disabilities are functional limitations preventing the patient from performing desired activities. Function is the person's ability, usually self-reported, to navigate their world and is the result of a complex interplay of anatomy, motivation and social supports [86]. Clearly, functional status has dramatically improved, but these may be markers of more effective treatment rather than biological differences. Mortality may be considered to denote the most severe disease, but death rates may not reflect changes in morbidity or could be the result of treatment. Evidence of impairment, such as erosive disease, is comparable, but erosive disease does not correlate well with functional disability. In some studies those with more severe erosive disease may report less disability [87]. Looking at erosive disease at presentation may help delineate changes in RA epidemiology, but looking retrospectively at erosions in established disease could be confusing. These changes may reflect effective therapy or duration of treatment, rather than indicate true differences in biology. The same is probably true for rheumatoid factor, as this also appears to be an independent variable both for disease incidence and severity. A true decrease in incidence could also imply a decrease in severity, the decreased number of new cases reflecting a milder disease not captured by disease criteria.

Mortality

The majority of studies show that RA significantly reduces life expectancy. The standardized mortality ratio (SMR) in RA (the death rates in RA patients compared with the population as a whole) is 1.28–2.98 [88–90], which does not differ significantly from historical rates of 1.13–2.48 [90–92]. However, data from Australia show a significant fall in mortality in women with RA over the past 25 years, with the rate in men remaining stable [94]. Gabriel and colleagues examined mortality in three cohorts in Olmsted County and did not find convincing evidence of decreased RA mortality over time [95]. In fact, given the increase in life expectancy over this century, the lack of improvement in RA SMRs suggest that treatment of RA has been less effective than that of other diseases [94]. Major causes of excess deaths include infection, cardiovascular disease, renal disease and treatment-related deaths. Ulcer disease due to non-steroidal anti-inflammatory drugs (NSAIDs) makes up the largest proportion of treatment-related deaths. It is estimated that annually 7600 deaths in the USA are due to NSAIDs, one-third being RA patients [96]. There are estimates that 10% of deaths to RA are directly related to drug side-effects [97,98].

Functional severity

In the past, it is estimated that about 10% of patients with 10–15 years of RA would be in Steinbrocker's functional grade IV (wheelchair bound) [99–101]. A Canadian study looking at RA patients presenting between 1966 and 1974 found 16% were functional grade IV 16 years later [102]. A Finnish study showed a clear decrease in the number of people disabled due to RA between 1965 and 1985 [103]. Comparisons of two similar Finnish cohorts, one assembled in 1959 and one in 1982, shows 38% of patients in Steinbrocker's class IV at 9 years follow-up in the first cohort, compared with 2% in the later cohort [104,105]. In 1994 Hakala and colleagues published a study looking at 103 patients with RA of a mean duration of 16 years and found only 0.9% were Steinbrocker's grade IV [106]. Another study found that the percentage of patients with Steinbrocker' grade III and IV disability decreased from 32% to 19% when comparing cohorts from 1945–69 and 1980–89. However, these results were heavily influenced by one large study [107]. A Japanese study found no decline in severity over a 30-year period from 1960 to 1990 [108].

As mentioned above, improved functional status in RA may not be from differences in the biology of the disease but from improved management with more effective agents, physical therapy, occupational therapy, social work, orthopaedic surgery, etc. [109,110]. Total joint arthroplasty, in particular, has probably made a major contribution to improved functional status. Hakala and colleagues studied 103 RA patients in a catchment area of 13 000 adults and found an average of two orthopaedic operations per patient, and that 20% of their patients had had total joint replacements [106]. It is more difficult to evaluate the impact of drug therapy on improved outcomes. In the Canadian study cited above, a striking difference was the timing of initiation of DMARDs: on average 12.8 years after the first appearance of symptoms, as compared with 2.4 years into the disease in Hakala's study. Short-term studies show that DMARDs can slow the progression of joint erosions and thus improve function and this effect continues for at least 3 years [111–113]. The decreasing RA rates among Pima Indians could be in part due to the increasing use of DMARDs throughout the study, causing mild disease which was not 'captured' by the study. However, only 17% were using DMARDs by the last year of the study, far less than the observed drop in incidence [55]. In 132 women with RA followed for 6 years, only half had progressive disabling disease and 57% were treated with DMARDs during the follow-up period [114]. This contrasts with previous studies, which looked at disease progression prior to hospital admission in the pre-DMARD era. These showed 60–73% of patients had progressively severe disease [115,116]. However, different inclusion criteria again makes comparisons difficult.

Impairment (i.e. objective disease)

Severe erosive disease also appears to be on the decline. Silman and colleagues studied at 2000 patients with RA seen at the same institution since 1948 [117] taking into account indicators of severity such as seropositivity, subcutaneous nodules and radiological erosions. The patients were analysed in birth cohorts. Although there was an initial increase in the numbers of patients with severe disease, there was an ensuing decline over time. At age 50, those born from 1895 to 1904 had worse outcomes in all three measured outcomes compared with the other cohorts. Heikkila and colleagues studied joint radiographs in four cohorts, each with 50 seropositive female patients admitted to their hospital, who fulfilled their criteria in the years 1962, 1972, 1982 and 1992 and found a highly significant decrease in the number of damaged joints over time [118]. This is impressive since one would suspect that only the more severely affected patients are admitted. Silman found a similar decrease in erosive disease among English patients [85]. While Silman found a decrease in the frequency of rheumatoid nodules over time, a Japanese study saw no change in rates of nodules over a 30-year period [119]. Some investigators have linked nodules with increased mortality, while others have found no correlation [88,94]. Extra-articular disease such as vasculitis and rheumatoid nodules are linked to disease severity [120,121], and there is a prevailing impression that extra-articular manifestations are less frequent [58]. However, firm data are unavailable.

High titres of rheumatoid factor are linked to a higher risk of developing RA, and have been likened to a preclinical stage of the disease [122]. They are also linked to a worse prognosis and a higher mortality rate [89,123] up to six times higher than seronegative patients [124]. This has been found in both population- [91,92] and institution- [89,124] based studies. Studies have shown a decrease in the prevalence of rheumatoid factor since the 1950s, paralleling the decrease in disease severity [89]. Silman, studying RF status according to date of birth, found that younger patients with RA were less likely to be seropositive, suggesting a decrease in incidence as well as prevalence [85].

Conclusion

The difficulties in studying historical trends in incidence of a disease with a variable onset and evolution over decades are legion. The similarity of RA with other polyarthritidies such as viral polyarthritis, reactive arthritis and even spondylitic variants requires explicit inclusion and exclusion criteria and, more importantly, follow-up to ensure that one is studying RA. However, strict criteria may omit milder or atypical cases, or those modified by earlier use of DMARDs, NSAIDs or possibly exposure to exogenous oestrogens. Evolving case definitions for RA have attempted to address these issues (see Table 19.1). The most compelling studies are those which follow the same population over time, using consistent study criteria to define disease incidence. The studies of Linos et al., Hochberg, and Jacobssen et al. [40,50,55] all show significant decreasing trends in RA among women, although absolute incidence rates differed from 1150/100 000 to 39.7/100 000 person-years. Recent studies, such as Symmons et al. and Dugowsan et al. [53,54], show lower absolute incidence rates. These would be appropriate cohorts to be re-studied and compared with other cohorts in the same population 10 and 20 years hence. Whether they can be compared outright with studies of other populations is less clear. Chan and colleagues showed no change in incidence in their cohort from 1987 to 1990, but the time course may have been too short to pick up a change, or alternatively the study may indicate a plateau after the major decrease in incidence in the 1960s and 1970s. Changes in biological severity, best

Table 19.1 Evolving case definitions for rheumatoid arthritis (RA).

American Rheumatism Association (ARA) 1958 criteria [124]	Rome 1961 criteria for active RA [125]	New York criteria 1966 [126]	American College of Rheumatology 1987 revised criteria for RA [127]
1 Morning stiffness	1 Morning stiffness	1 History of an episode of three painful limb joints. Each group of joints (e.g. PIP joint) is counted as one joint, scoring each side separately	1 Morning stiffness
2 Pain on motion or tenderness in at least one joint	2 Pain or tenderness in ≥ 1 joint		
3 Pain of one joint, representing soft tissue or fluid			
4 Swelling of at least one other joint, with an internal free of symptoms no longer than 3 months	3 Swelling of ≥ 1 joint	2 Swelling, limitation of motion, subluxation and/or anklyosing of three limb joints. Necessary inclusion: (1) at least one hand, wrist or foot; (2) symmetry of one joint pair Exclusions: (1) distal interphalangeal joints; (2) fifth PIP joints; (3) first metatarsophalangeal joints; (4) hips	2 Swelling of ≥ 3 joint groups
5 Symmetrical joint swelling	4 Swelling of ≥ 2 joints		3 Swelling of MCP, PIP or wrist joints
	5 Symmetrical joint swelling		4 Symmetrical joint swelling
6 Subcutaneous nodules over boney prominences, extensor surfaces or near joints	6 Rheumatoid nodules		5 Rheumatoid nodules
7 Typical X-ray changes which must include demineralization in periarticular bone as an index of inflammation; degenerative changes do not exclude diagnosis of RA	7 Radiological abnormalities of RA	3 Radiographic changes (erosions)	6 Radiological abnormalities of RA

8 Positive test for rheumatoid factor	8 Rheumatoid factor positivity	4 Serum positive for rheumatoid factor	7 Rheumatoid factor positivity
9 Synovial fluid; poor mucin of clot formation on adding synovial fluid to dilute acetic acid 10 Synovial histopathology consistent with RA: (a) marked villous hypertrophy (b) proliferation of synovial cells (c) lymphocyte/plasma cell infiltration in subsynovium (d) fibrin deposition within or upon microvilli 11 Characteristic histopathology of rheumatoid nodules biopsied from any site	Exclusion diagnosis: SLE, histologically proven PAN, dermatomyositis, scleroderma, rheumatic fever, gout, infectious arthritis, joint tuberculosis, Reiter's syndrome, shoulder–hand syndrome, hypertrophic osteoarthropathy, neuroarthropathy, ochronosis, histological evidence of sarcoid, multiple myeloma, erythema nodosum, lymphoma or leukaemia, agammaglobulinaemia, or ankylosing spondylitis		
Classic, RA-7 criteria; definite, RA-5 criteria; probable, RA-3 criteria	*Classic, RA≥7 criteria; definite, RA≥5 criteria; probable, RA>3 criteria*	*RA is present if criteria 1 and 2 PLUS either 3 or 4 are met*	*Diagnosis: ≥4/7 criteria* *Criteria 1–4 must be present at least 6 weeks*
For criteria 1–5, symptoms or signs must be present for at least 6 weeks	*Criteria 1–5 must be present at least 6 weeks*		

SLE, systemic lupus erythematosus; PAN, polyarteritis nodosa. MCP, metacarpophalangeal; PIP, proximal interphalangeal.

evidenced by decreases in erosive disease and decreasing rheumatoid factor positivity, support the hypothesis that the disease has changed and is milder, but if true confounds the investigation of incidence, since mild cases may not meet inclusion criteria. Despite clear improvements in outcome and morbidity, mortality remains unchanged, suggesting all our efforts have done little to help the very worst off.

RA has not disappeared as predicted but the data suggest a diminution in incidence, impairment and functional severity. Whether this is due primarily to better treatment or to the natural history of a disease is unresolved. However, mortality remains fixed. Preventing deaths from RA will continue to challenge us as we enter the 21st century.

References

1 Buchanan WW, Murdoch R. That rheumatoid arthritis will disappear. *J Rheum* 1997; 96: 324–9.

2 Silman AJ. Is rheumatoid arthritis an infective disease? *Br Med J* 1991; 303: 200–1.

3 Fox DA. Rheumatoid arthritis —heresies and speculations. *Perspectives in Biology and Medicine* 1997; 40(4): 479–91.

4 Gregersen PK, Silver J, Winchester RJ The Shared epitope hypothesis: an approach to understanding the molecular genetics of susceptibility to rheumatoid arthritis. *Arthritis Rheum* 1987; 30: 1205–13.

5 Short CL. The antiquity of rheumatoid arthritis. *Arthritis Rheum* 1974; 17(3): 193–205.

6 Soranus of Ephesus. *On Acute Diseases and on Chronic Diseases*. Translated into Latin by Cmlius Aurelianus (fifth century AD), English translation by IE Drabkin. Chicago: University of Chicago Press, 1950: 923–39.

7 Sturrock RD, Sharma JN, Buchanan WW. Rheumatoid arthritis in Ancient India. *Arthritis Rheum* 1977; 20: 42–4.

8 Caughey DE. The arthritis of Constantine IX. *Ann Rheum Dis* 1974; 33: 77–8.

9 Sydenham T. *Medical Observations Concerning the History and the Cause of Acute Diseases*, translated by R.G. Latham. London: The Sydenham Society, 1848: 254–9.

10 Snorrason E. Landre-Beauvais and his Goutte Asthenique Primitive. *Acta Med Scand* 1952; 142 (Suppl. 266): 115–18.

11 Hartung EF. In: Bett W.R. ed. *The History and Conquest of Common Diseases* Norman, Oklahoma: University of Oklahoma Press, 1954: 136.

12 Garrod AB. *The Nature and Treatment of Gout and Rheumatic Gout*. London: Walton and Maberly, 1859.

13 Garrod AE. *A treatise on Rheumatism and Rheumatoid Arthritis*. London: Charles and Griffen, 1890.

14 Charcot JM. *Ètudes pour Servier a l'Histoire de l'Affection Decrite sous les Noms de Goutte Asthenique Primitive* .... Paris, Baillière, 1853: 38.

15 Adam RA. *Treatise on Rheumatic Gout or Chronic Rheumatic Arthritis of all the Joints*. London, Churchill, 1857.

16 Fraser KJ. Anglo-French contributions to the recognition of rheumatoid arthritis Ann. *Rheum Dis* 1982; 41: 335–43.

17 Buchanan WW. Rheumatoid arthritis: another New World disease? *Arthritis Rheum* 1994; 23(5): 289–94.

18 Ehrlich GE. Shakespeare's rheumatology. *Ann Rheum Dis* 1994; 26: 562–3.

19 Sharma P. Medicine, Durer and the praying hands. *Lancet* 1997; 349: 1470–1.

20 Dequeker J, Rico H. Rheumatoid arthritis-like deformities in an early 16th century painting of the Flemish-Dutch school. *JAMA* 1992; 268: 249–51.

21 Dequeker J. Siebrandus Sixtius: evidence of rheumatoid arthritis of the robust reaction type in a seventeenth century Dutch priest. *Ann Rheum Dis* 1992; 51: 561–2.

22 Dequeker J. The antiquity and origins of rheumatoid arthritis [Letter]. *JAMA* 1992; 268(19): 2649.

23 Appelboom T. *Art, History and Antiquity of Rheumatic Diseases*. Brussels: Elsevier, 1987.

24 Bridgeman GB. *The Book of a Hundred Hands*. New York: Dover, 1971.

25 Ruffer MA, Rietti A. On osseous lesions in ancient Egyptians. *J Pathol Bacteriol* 1912; 16: 439–65.

26 Bourke JBA. Review of the paleopathology of arthritic diseases. In: Brothweil D, Sandison AT, eds. *Diseases in Antiquity*. Springfield, IL: Thomas, 1967: 352–69.

27 Zorab PA. Historical and prehistorical background of ankylosing spondylitis. *Proc R Soc Med* 1961; 54: 415–20.

28 Wells C. Joint pathology in ancient Anglo-Saxons. *J Bone Joint Surg Br* 1962; 44B: 948–9.

29 Palmer DG, Marshall AJ, Buchanan WW *et al*. Eighteenth-century bone and joint disease: William Hunter's collection, Pathology Department, Royal Infirmary Glasgow. *Rheumatology* 1977; 4: 34–8.

30 Rogers J, Watt I, Dieppe P *et al*. Paleopathology of joint disorders: Evidence of erosive arthropathies in skeletal material. *Clin Rheum* 1985; 5: 15.

31 Rothschild BM, Woods RJ, Rothschild C, Sebes JI. Geographic distribution of rheumatoid arthritis in ancient North America: implications for pathogenesis. *Semin Arthritis Rheum* 1992; 22 (3): 181–7.

32 Rothschild BM, Turner KR, De Luca MA *et al*. Symmetrical erosive peripheral polyarthritis in the late archaic period of Alabama. *Science* 1988; 241: 1498–501.

33 Gilbert M. *Atlas of American History*. London, England: Dorset, 1985.

34 *Atlas of United States History*. Maplewood, NJ, Hammond, 1884.

35 Waidman C. *Atlas of the North American Indian*. New York, Facts on File, 1985.

36 Wolfe AM. The epidemiology of rheumatoid arthritis: a review. *Survs Bull Rheum Dis* 1968; 19: 518–23.

37 Naider SJ, Scharosch LL, Foto F, Howard EJ. Rheumatologic manifestations of human parvovirus B 12 infection in adults. Initial 2-year clinical experience. *Arthritis Rheum* 1990; 33(9): 1297–30.

38 Buchanan WW, Laurent RM. Rheumatoid arthritis: an example of ecologic succession. *Can Bull Med Hist* 1990; 7: 77–91.

39 Laurent R, Beller EM, Buchanan WW. Incidence and severity of rheumatoid arthritis: The view from Australasia. *Br J Rheum* 1989; 28: 360–1.

40 Linos A, Worthington JW, O'Fallan WM, Kurland LT. The epidemiology of rheumatoid arthritis in Rochester Minnesota: a study of incidence, prevalence and mortality. *Am J Epidemiol* 1980; III(1): 87–98.

41 Ropes MW. Proposed diagnostic criteria for rheumatoid arthritis. *Ann Rheum Dis* 1957; 16: 118–23.

42 Kellgren JH, Jeffrey MR, Ball J. *The Epidemiology of Chronic Rheumatism*, Vol. I. Oxford: Blackwell Scientific Publications, 1963: 324–7.

43 Wingrave SJ. Reduction in incidence of rheumatoid arthritis associated with oral contraceptives. *Lancet* 1978; 1: 569–71.

44 den Oudsten SA *et al*. *Longitudinal Survey of RA in an Urban District of Rotterdam*. Exerpta Medica International Congress Series No. 148, 1968: 99–105.

45 Wood JW, Kato H, Johnson KG *et al*. Rheumatoid arthritis in Hiroshima and Nagasaki Japan. Prevalence, incidence and clinical characteristic. *Arthritis Rheum* 1967; 10: 21–31.

46 Kato H, Duff IF, Russell WJ *et al*. Rheumatoid arthritis and gout in Hiroshima and Nagasaki Japan: a prevalence and incidence study. *J Chronic Dis* 1971; 23: 659–79.

47 Gabriel S, Crowson CS, O'Fallon M. The Epidemiology of Rheumatoid

Arthritis (RA) in Rochester, MN
1955–85. *Arthritis Rheum* 1998; 41
(Suppl.) Abstract 1950, S357.

48 O'Sullivan JB, Cathcart ES, Bolzan JA.
Diagnostic Criteria and the incidence
of Rheumatoid Arthritis in Sudbury,
Massachusetts. In: Bennett PH, Wood
PHN (eds) *Population Studies of the
Rheumatic Diseases.* Amsterdam:
Excerpta Medica Foundation, 1968:
109–15.

49 Bachman DM. Survey of rheumatoid
arthritis in Oregon. *Arthritis Rheum*
1963; 6: 761.

50 Hochberg MC. Changes in the
incidence and prevalence of rheumatoid arthritis in England and Wales
1970–82. *Semin Arthritis Rheum*
1990; 19 (5): 294–302.

51 Silman AJ. Has the incidence of
rheumatoid arthritis declined in the
United Kingdom? *Br J Rheumatol*
1988; 27: 77–9.

52 Hannaford PC. Oral contraceptives
and rheumatoid arthritis: new data
from the Royal College of General
Practitioners' oral contraceptive
study. *Ann Rheum Dis* 1990; 49:
744–6.

53 Dugowson CE, Kuepsell TD, Voigt LF.
Rheumatoid arthritis in women:
incidence rates in Group Health
Cooperative, Seattle Washington
1987–89. *Arthritis Rheum* 1991;
34: 1502–7.

54 Symmons DP, Barrett EM, Bankhead
CR, Scott DG, Silman AJ. The
incidence of rheumatoid arthritis in
the United Kingdom: Results from the
Norfold Arthritis Register. *Br J
Rheumatol* 1994; 33: 735–9.

55 Jacobsson LT Hanson RL, Knowler
WC *et al.* Decreasing incidence and
prevalence of rheumatoid arthritis in
Pima Indians over a twenty-five-year
period. *Arthritis Rheum* 1994; 37(8):
1158–65.

56 Del Puente A, Knowler WC, Pettitt DJ,
Bennett PH. High rate of incidence
and prevalence of rheumatoid arthritis
in Pima Indians. *Am J Epidemiol*
1989; 129: 1170–8.

57 Dewire P, Dugowson CE, Koepsell TP,
Voigt LF, Nelson JL. Incidence and
relative risk of rheumatoid arthritis by
race; a population based study.

Arthritis Rheum 1992; 35 (Suppl. 9)
S.101 (Abstract).

58 Spector TD, Hart DJ, Powell RJ.
Prevalence of rheumatoid arthritis and
rheumatoid factor in women: evidence
for a secular decline. *Ann Rheum Dis*
1993; 52: 254–7.

59 Lawrence JS. Prevalence of rheumatoid
arthritis. *Ann Rheum Dis* 1961; 20:
11–17.

60 Chan KW, Felson DT, Yood RA,
Walker AM. Incidence of rheumatoid
arthritis in Central Massachusetts:
Arthritis Rheum 1993; 36(12):
1691–6.

61 Gran JT, Magnus J, Mikkelsen K *et al.*
The incidence of classical and definite
rheumatoid arthritis in Lillehammer,
Norway. *Scand J Rheumatol* 1986; 15
(Suppl.): 7 (Abstract).

62 Kellgren JH, Lawrence JS, Aitken-
Swan J *et al.* Rheumatic complaints in
an urban population. *Ann Rheum Dis*
1953; 12: 515.

63 Valkenburg HA. Epidemiologic
consideration of the geriatric
population. *Gerontol* 1988; 34
(Suppl.): 2–10.

64 Silman AJ. Trends in the incidence
and severity of rheumatoid arthritis.
J Rheumatol 1992; 19 (Suppl. 32):
71–3.

65 Ropes MW, Bennett GA, Copp S *et al.*
1958 revision of diagnostic criteria for
rheumatoid arthritis. *Arthritis Rheum*
1959; 2: 16–20.

66 Kellgren JH, Jeffrey MR, Ball J *et al.*
*Proposed Diagnostic Studies for Use in
Population Studies, the Epidemiology
of Chronic Rheumatism.* Oxford:
Blackwell Scientific Publications, 1963:
324–27.

67 Bennet PH, Burch TA. New York
symposium on population studies in
the rheumatic diseases: new diagnostic
criteria. *Bull Rheum Dis* 1967; 17:
453–8.

68 Arnett FC, Edworthy SM, Bloch DA
et al. The American Rheumatism
Association 1987 revised criteria
for the classification of rheumatoid
arthritis. *Arthritis Rheum* 1988;
31: 315–24.

69 van Zeben D, Hazes JM,
Vandenbroucke JP, Dijkmans BA,
Cats A. Diminished incidence of severe

rheumatoid arthritis associated with oral contraceptive use. *Arthritis Rheum* 1990; 33: 1462–5.

70 Hazes JM, Dijkmans BC, Vandenbroucke JP, de Vries RR, Cats A. Reduction of the risk of rheumatoid arthritis among women who take oral contraceptives. *Arthritis Rheum* 1990; 33: 173–9.

71 Royal College of General Practitioners' Oral Contraception Study. Reduction in incidence of rheumatoid arthritis associated with oral contraceptives. *Lancet* 1978; i: 569–71.

72 Vandenbroucke JP, Valkenburg HA, Boersma JW *et al.* Oral contraceptives hormones and rheumatoid arthritis: Further evidence for a preventive effect. *Lancet* 1982; ii: 839–42.

73 Linos A, Worthington JW, O'Fallon WM, Kurland LT. Case control study of rheumatoid arthritis and prior use of oral contraceptives. *Lancet* 1983; i: 1299–300.

74 Spector TD, Hochberg MC. The protective effect of the oral contraceptive pill on rheumatoid arthritis: an overview of the analytic epidemiological studies using meta-analysis. *J Clin Epidemiology* 1990; 43: 1221–30.

75 Romieu I, Hernandez-Avila M, Liang M. Oral contraceptives and the risk of rheumatoid arthritis: a meta-analysis of a conflicting literature. *Br J Rheum* 1989; 28 (Suppl. 1): 13–17.

76 Hernandez-Avila M, Liang MH, Willet WC *et al.* Exogenous sex hormones and the risk of rheumatoid arthritis. *Arthritis Rheum* 1990; 33: 947–53.

77 Del Junco DJ, Annegers JF, Luthra HS, Coulam CB, Kurland LT. Do oral contraceptives prevent rheumatoid arthritis? *JAMA* 1985; 254: 1938–41.

78 Vandenbroucke JP, Witteman JC, Valkenburg HA *et al.* Non-contraceptive hormones and rheumatoid arthritis in perimenopausal and postmenopausal women. *JAMA* 1986; 225: 1299–303.

79 Spector TD, Brennan P, Harris P, Studd JW, Silman AJ. Does estrogen replacement therapy protect against rheumatoid arthritis? *J Rheum* 1991; 18: 1473–6.

80 Jorgensen, Picot MC, Bologna C, Sany J. Oral contraception, parity, breast feeding and severity of rheumatoid arthritis. *Ann Rheum Dis* 1996; 55: 94–8.

81 Vandenbroucke JP, Hazes JM, Dijkmans BA, Cats A. Oral contraceptives and the risk of rheumatoid arthritis. The great transatlantic divide? *Br J Rheumatol* 1889; 79 (Suppl.): 31–2.

82 Esdaile JM, Horwitz RI. Observational studies of cause–effect relationships: an analysis of methodological problems as illustrated by the conflicting data for the role of oral contraceptives in the etiology of rheumatoid arthritis. *J Chron Dis* 1986; 10: 841–52.

83 Spector TD, Silman AJ. Oral contraceptives and rheumatoid arthritis [Letter]. *J Chron Dis* 1987; 40(11): 1063–4.

84 Esdaile J. Response. *J Chronic Dis* 1987; 40(1): 1065–8.

85 Silman AJ *et al.* Is rheumatoid arthritis becoming less severe? *J Chron Dis* 1983; 36: 891–7.

86 Karlson E, Katz JN, Liang MH. In: Spilker B., ed. *Chronic Rheumatic Disorders, Quality of Life and Pharmacoeconomics in Clinical Trials*, 2nd edn. Philadelphia: Lippincott-Raven Publishers, 1996: 1029.

87 Hameed K, Gibson T. A comparison of the clinical features of hospital out-patients with rheumatoid disease and osteoarthritis in Pakistan and England. *Br J Rheum* 1996; 35(10): 994–9.

88 Myllykangas-Luosujarvi R, Aho K, Isomaki HA. Mortality in rheumatoid arthritis. *Semin Arthritis Rheum* 1995; 25(3): 193–202.

89 Wolfe F, Mitchell DM, Sibley JT *et al.* The mortality of rheumatoid arthritis. *Arthritis Rheum* 1994; 37(4): 482–94.

90 Jacobsson L, Knowler WC, Pillemer S *et al.* Rheumatoid arthritis and mortality: a longitudinal study in Pima Indians. *Arthritis Rheum* 1993; 36: 1045–53.

91 Allebeck P, Ahlbom A, Allander E. Increased mortality among persons with rheumatoid arthritis, but where RA does not appear on death certificate: eleven year follow-up of

an epidemiological study. *Scand J Rheumatol* 1981; 10: 301–6.

92 Prior P, Symmons DP, Scott DL, Brown R, Hawkins CF. Cause of death in rheumatoid arthritis. *Br J Rheum* 1984; 23: 92–9.

93 Cobb S, Anderson F, Bauer W *et al.* Length of life and cause of death in rheumatoid arthritis. *New Engl J Med* 1953; 249: 553–6.

94 Wicks IP, Moore J, Fleming A. Australian mortality statistics for rheumatoid arthritis. 1950–81: analysis of death certificate data. *Ann Rheum Dis* 1988; 47: 563–9.

95 Gabriel S, Crowson C, O'Fallon WM *et al.* Mortality in rheumatoid arthritis (RA): Have we made an impact in three decades? Abstract 1770, American College of Rheumatology National Meeting, Washington DC, 8–12 November 1997.

96 Fries JF. NSAID gastropathy: the second most deadly rheumatic disease? Epidemiology and risk appraisal. *J Rheumatol* 1991; 8 (Suppl. 28): 6–10.

97 Mitchell DM. Survival, prognosis and causes of death in rheumatoid arthritis. *Arthritis Rheum* 1986; 29: 706–14.

98 Myllykangas-Luosujarvi R, Aho K, Lehtinen K, Kautiainen H, Hakala M. Deaths attributed to antirheumatic medication in a nationwide series of 1666 patients with rheumatoid arthritis who had died. *J Rheum* 1995; 22(12): 2214–17.

99 Steinbrocker, Traeger CH, Batterman RC. Therapeutic criteria for rheumatoid arthritis. *JAMA* 1949; 140(659–62): 99.

100 Duthie JJR, Brown PE, Truelove LH, Baragar FD, Lawrie AJ. Course and prognosis in rheumatoid arthritis: a further report. *Ann Rheum Dis* 1964; 23: 193–202.

101 Jacoby RK, Jayson MI, Cosh JA. Onset, early stages and prognosis of rheumatoid arthritis: a clinical study of 100 patients with 11 year follow up. *Br Med J* 1973; ii: 96–100.

102 Sherrer YS, Bloch DA, Mitchell DM, Young DY, Fries JF. The development of disability in rheumatoid arthritis. *Arthritis Rheum* 1986; 29(4): 494–500.

103 Isomaki HA *et al.* Rheumatoid arthritis as seen from official data registers. Experience in Finland. *Scand J Rheum* 1989; 79: 21–4.

104 Aho K, Kirpila J, Wager O. The persistence of the agglutination activation factor (AAF) in the circulation. A nine-year study of twenty-seven patients. *Ann Med Exp Fenn* 1959; 37: 377–81.

105 Aho K, Tuomi T, Palosuo T *et al.* Is rheumatoid arthritis becoming less severe? *Clin Exp Rheumatol* 1989; 7: 287–90.

106 Hakala M, Nieminen P, Koivisto O. More evidence from a community series of better outcome in rheumatoid arthritis. Data on the effect of multidisciplinary care on the retention of functional ability. *J Rheumatol.* 1994; 21(8): 1432–7.

107 Anderson JJ, Felson DT, Meenan RF. Secular changes in published clinical trials of second-line agents in rheumatoid arthritis. *Arthritis Rheum* 1991; 34(10): 1304–9.

108 Imanaka T, Skichikawa K, Inoue K *et al.* Increase in age at onset of rheumatoid arthritis in Japan over a 30 year period. *Ann Rheum Dis* 1997; 56: 313–16.

109 Williams MH, Bowie C. Evidence of unmet need in the care of severely disabled adults. *Brit Med J* 1993; 306: 95–8.

110 Brooks PM. Clinical management of rheumatoid arthritis. *Lancet* 1993; 341: 286–90.

111 Fuchs HA, Pincus T. Analysis of progression of radiographic damage in hands and wrists of patients with rheumatoid arthritis. *Arthritis Rheum* 1990; 33 (Suppl. 9): 69 (Abstract): 521.

112 van der Heijde DM, van Riel PL, Nuver-Zwart IH, van de Putte LB. Sulphasalazine versus hydroxy-chloroquine in rheumatoid arthritis. 3-year follow up. *Lancet* 1990; 335: 539.

113 Borg G, Allander E, Birger L. Auranofin improves outcome in early rheumatoid arthritis, results from a 2-year, double blind, placebo controlled study. *J Rheumatol* 1988; 15: 1747–54.

114 van Zeben D, Hazes JM, Zwinderman AH, Vandenbroucke JP, Breedveld FC. The severity of rheumatoid arthritis: a 6 year follow-up study of younger women with symptoms of recent onset. *J Rheumatol* 1994; 21: 1620–5.

115 Short CL. Rheumatoid arthritis: types of course and prognosis. *Med Clin North Am* 1968; 3: 549–57.

116 Duthie JJ, Thompson M, Weir MM, Fletcher WB. Medical and social aspects of the treatment of rheumatoid arthritis with special reference to factors affecting prognosis. *Ann Rheum Dis* 1955; 14: 133–48.

117 Silman AJ, Davies P, Currey HLF, Evans SJW. Is rheumatoid arthritis becoming less severe? *J Chron Dis* 1983; 36: 891–4.

118 Heikkila S, Isomaki H. Long-term outcome of rheumatoid arthritis has improved. *Scand J Rheumatol* 1994; 23: 13–15.

119 Imanaka T, Shichikawa K, Inoue K *et al.* Increase in age at onset of rheumatoid arthritis in Japan over a thirty year period. *Ann Rheum Dis* 1997; 56: 313–16.

120 Geirsson AJ, Sturfelt G, Truedsson L. Clinical and serologic features of severe vasculitis in rheumatoid arthritis; prognostic implications. *Ann Rheum Dis* 1987; 46: 727–33.

121 Vollertse RS, Conn DL, Ballard DJ *et al.* Rheumatoid vasculitis: survival and associated risk factors. *Medicine* 1986; 65: 365–75.

122 MacGregor AJ, Silman AJ. Rheumatoid factors as predictors of rheumatoid arthritis. *J Rheumatol* 1991; 18: 1280–1.

123 Spector TD, Hart DJ, Powell RJ *et al.* Prevalence of rheumatoid arthritis and rheumatoid factor in women: evidence for a secular decline. *Ann Rheum Dis* 1993; 52: 254–7.

124 van Schaardenburg D, Hazes JM, de Boer A *et al.* Outcome of rheumatoid arthritis in relation to age and rheumatoid factor at diagnosis. *J Rheumatol* 1993; 20: 45–52.

125 Ropes MW, Bennett EA, Cobb S *et al.* 1958 revision of diagnostic criteria for rheumatoid arthritis. *Bull Rheum Dis* 1958; 9: 175–6.

126 Kellgren JH, Jeffrey MR, Ball JF. eds. *The Epidemiology of Chronic Rheumatism*, Vol. 1. Philadelphia: FA Davis Co., 1963.

127 Bennett PH, Burch TP. New York Symposium on Population Studies in the Rheumatic Diseases: New Diagnostic Criteria. *Bull Rheum Dis* 1967; 17: 453.

128 Arnett FC, Edworthy SM, Bloch DA *et al.* The American Rheumatism Association 1987 revised criteria for the classification of rheumatoid arthritis. *Arthritis Rheum* 1988; 31: 315–24.

20: Should limited funds be directed at patient care or research?

F.A. Wollheim

Introduction

The theme of this book is to question old and new dogma. This is basic-ally a useful exercise, because so much of what we teach does not qualify as evidence-based medicine. We live in a time when technological advances and many investigators' hard labour have resulted in an explosion of knowl-edge regarding health and disease mechanisms. We are able to transplant organs, and gene transfer experiments in humans have started. Products of recombinant technology can be used to interfere with physiological and patho-logical processes with increasing accuracy and power. Yet we also live at a time when increasing numbers of patients turn to so-called alternative medicine, to shamans and religious sects. Book titles like 'We kill ourselves with cures' appear in paperback [1]. The paradox is that despite advances in knowledge and new technical possibilities the position and usefulness of basic science is being questioned by the public. At a time when more and more heroic medical intervention becomes feasible, economic restrictions constitute a growing limit to growth and indeed result in often drastic shrink-ing of healthcare resources. In times of decreasing resources one is forced to reconsider priorities, which may actually be a healthy thing to do. It is my task to address this problem and in particular examine whether prior-ity should be given to more research or better implementation of current knowledge to patient care.

Cortisone and rheumatoid arthritis

Modern rheumatology was born 50 years ago at the Mayo Clinic when Drs Slocumb and Polley, while their chief Philip Hench was touring Europe as the Heberden orator, treated 14 patients with crippling rheumatoid arthritis (RA) with the first available pure cortisone [2]. The isolation of 17-hydroxy-11-dehydro-corticosterine by the biochemist Harold L. Mason in Dr Ed Kendall's laboratory, as well as other chemical characterization of adrenal mineral corticoids by Dr Tadeus Reichstein in Switzerland, was the result of years of labour-intensive research. The wisdom of the brothers Mayo in the 19th century enabled practising physicians to live and work side by side with investigators and still close to patients. Finally Dr Hench had an idea that RA perhaps was a disease that could be controlled by a substance X produced in stimulated adrenals in such conditions as jaundice and pregnancy. He had the perseverance not to give up despite a series of failed attempts to support his idea. He also had a superb partner in the research laboratory funded by the Mayo Foundation. In the end, success was dependent on the devoted unprecedented synthetic work in the Merck laboratory, resulting in the production of a few grams of pure substance. This was the time before ethical committees and extensive safety studies in animals: the adrenalectomized dog was the animal model used to isolate cortisone and other adrenocortical hormones.

Fifty years later, millions of patients worldwide are given oral gluco corticoids by physicians who *believe*, but do not really know, that this will benefit their patients. A recent study in the UK highlights the problem. A protocol of adding 7.5 mg prednisolone or placebo to conventional non-steroidal anti-inflammatory drugs (NSAIDs) and disease-modifying anti-rheumatic drugs (DMARDs) seemed to show that this regimen resulted in a reduced occurrence of new erosions in the prednisolone arm after 2 years [3]. Some senior rheumatologists in my part of the world hailed this as a big breakthrough. Practising rheumatologists who perhaps had not read the paper critically, or even had only heard about it, changed their routines and are now giving 'low-dose' prednisolone to every new patient. Yet what the study really showed was only that after 2 years the patients in both groups were symptomatically and functionally indistinguishable. Also the radiological changes 1 year after the study were similar. It is *possible* but not certain that continued prednisolone after the 2 years would have been beneficial. There is also concern of long-term vascular injury and increased mortality. Another effect of this and other recent work is apparent in a Swedish health authority document which will provide firm guidelines regarding pharmacotherapy in RA. It will state that the decision to start glucocorticoid therapy should only be made by or in consultation with a rheumatologist. If the rheumatologist is to be able to make this decision on a rational basis it is mandatory at this time to give priority to patient-orientated research. We need long-term placebo-controlled trials looking at both benefit and its opposite, in well-balanced patient groups. Eventually we will perhaps know whether current enthusiasm among some colleagues is warranted or not.

Intra-articular administration of microcrystalline glucocorticoid preparations has a well-documented beneficial effect when given at the right stage.

In a paper published in 1994 it was shown that 24 h of bed rest, following injection of inflammatory knee joints, prolonged the effect from weeks
to several months [4]. The economic impact of implementing this important finding should be enormous. Yet it can be considered unethical or at
least suboptimal care not to admit such patients to hospital. This is a
simple example where a straightforward comparison of no vs. 3–4 h of post-
injection rest could pay off handsomely. This shows how great a knowledge gap exists for how to best use a drug that has been available for half
a century.

DMARD research

A classical example of physician–drug company interaction in rheumatology is Nanna Svartz' idea of combining an antibacterial with aspirin into
one pill, to treat both the aetiological agent and disease symptoms simultaneously. We all know that nobody is acknowledged in his own country,
but Nanna was highly respected and feared in Sweden. She 'knew' that
her sulphasalazine worked in RA [5], and this was not a fact that one
questioned if one wanted to be or remain in her favour. When she retired,
sulphasalazine popularity decreased dramatically and one further study performed in Scotland showed no effect. This study [6] gave such a large starting dose of sulphasalazine (in comparison to gold) in a small number of
patients that severe side effects precluded adequate assessment of efficacy.
The flawed study did not encourage further investigation at the time. Then
in 1980 Brian McConkey achieved the rediscovery which in essence was
to produce scientific evidence in a controlled study for its efficacy [7]. By
that time the producer had just managed to terminate the licensing for RA.
Thus, failure on the part of Swedish rheumatologists (I was one of them)
delayed wider use of sulphasalazine in RA for some decades. Therapeutic
trials had low status in those days, there was a shortage of rheumatologists and other drugs, such as d-penicillamine, interested us more.

  DMARD research is often funded by the industry, which favours
research on new drugs. Increasingly we are ignorant of the long-term features of older drugs, should they not be used in combinations with a 'new'
one. Industry funding will always depend on market projections, and academic funding is notoriously difficult to get for this type of research. Yet
it is so important for optimal patient care. One example of how relatively
simple but controlled clinical investigations can generate information useful in the practice of rheumatology is the placebo-controlled withdrawal
study [8], addressing the question of whether to withdraw DMARDs from
a patient when stable remission has been achieved. This trial showed that
the risk of disease flare doubled over the next year. A later study looked
at effects of resuming therapy and showed that although some benefit

occurred, the patient's condition did not improve to the level it had before the initial stopping [9]. A lesson that world rheumatology could learn from this is how much patient care can gain from organizing it in a way that facilitates controlled studies. In the Netherlands, hospital-based and private rheumatologists cooperate in a network allowing implementation of structured protocols and collection of outcome measures. This does require additional funding but in the end is probably cost effective, providing better quality and lower costs to society. In Sweden a cooperation between rheumatology units has been started and given the name RAMONA (Rheumatoid Arthritis MONitor Activities). Its goal is to register all new cases of RA in a uniform way, and monitor therapy so that pooling results and long-term assessments will be possible. This system should also facilitate large-scale formal trials in the future. The goal must be to find a balance between service provision and clinical research and development. In most countries and environments I believe the balance is heavily tilted toward providing suboptimal care. Several factors favour imbalance. The media, in their pursuit of scoops, produce premature and unproved solutions to clinical problems, giving politicians and consumers of care the false impression that research is superfluous. Routine workload is often overwhelming, and few have the mental and physical strength to plan and take part in research. The reward of possible but uncertain scientific progress in the distant future competes with family life, hobbies and inertia.

Losec—a success story in the end

Few drugs have in recent times helped more patients from both incapacitating symptoms of disease and from the surgeon's operating knives. The pharmaceutical chemist Ivan Östholm was chief of research for more than 25 years at Hässle, a subsidiary of Astra, and has told the story of omeprazole and other drug developments in a book that to my knowledge is only available in Swedish [10]. Its subtitle is '50 years of success and failure in the world of drugs'. The story of what has been called the greatest Swedish invention in modern times goes back to 1956, when Hässle was gathering some local doctors in a restaurant to tap them for ideas, to develop new drugs. The best suggestion was made by a young haematologist, who during the walk home stressed the need for a good liquid antacid. This proposal was turned down by the marketing division who estimated the potential market to be too small. However, the following year, Östholm hired a pharmacologist who worked on such a project, and after 3 years a product was launched with some success. This generated enough income to motivate more innovative research around 1965. In 1966 a focused effort was started to find new substances able to inhibit secretion of gastrin, the hormone responsible for acid secretion. In 1967 the first new substance H68/51 was ready for animal testing. Ignoring external academic advice, rats were chosen. The results looked promising and experiments in human volunteers were planned when dogs given the substance developed liver toxicity. In 1968 the next compound H81/58 was given to healthy individuals. However, even before effects on acid secretion began, liver toxicity stopped development. Two years later the new H81/75 was well tolerated but sadly completely lacked effect on acid secretion in the volunteers. Again strong voices within the company wanted to terminate the project. The budget was reduced. It was realized that the rat model was no good. External support was obtained by signing a contract of collaboration with Abbott. This company was to supply new substances from their large pool of candidate companies.

In 1972 a new strategy was started, aiming at finding cellular inhibitors of acid secretion rather than inhibitors of gastrin production. A toxic substance owned by a French company was found to be effective in the Pavlov dog model. Now the news of the H2 blocking agent Tagamet as well as the failures with Hässle's own endeavour generated strong support for switching efforts towards finding new H2 blockers. Also company goals were adapted to the new competitor, into searching for a drug that was to be better than Tagamet. The task seemed more impossible than before, but the decision was made to continue the search for a new type of substance.

In June of 1973 a new agent, H124/26, was tested at Abbott. Its structure had similarities to the later omeprazole (Losec). It was toxic to the liver. However, a metabolite was found, H83/69, and this turned out to be far more potent than some 200 previously tested agents. In 1974 Abbott lost interest and terminated the cooperation with Hässle. The project was again close to failure when it was discovered that H83/69, unexpectedly, was toxic in the thymus and thyroid gland. Now a grant of 1.5 million Swedish crowns from a new Swedish State agency to help developing new products for the export industry allowed work to continue. A new substance, H149/94, was not toxic to thymus or thyroid gland. It was called picoprazole.

In 1977 at one of the symposia arranged to celebrate the 500th birthday of Uppsala University, George Sachs from the USA presented data on a new enzyme, hydrogen–potassium adenosine triphosphatase (ATPase), present in parietal cells of the stomach and involved in 'pumping' out acid by these cells. It turned out that this enzyme only occurred in three locations, the other two being thymus and thyroid. This information led to the assumption which was soon confirmed, that the compounds under development were inhibitors of this enzyme.

However, more problems turned up. In 1978 dogs given picoprazole developed vasculitis. This serious adverse effect could have stopped development, but thanks to a senior professor of pharmacology a closer look was taken when he discovered what had not been noticed by others, that one puppy in the control group also developed vasculitis. This revealed that all puppies that had developed vasculitis were fathered by one dog, Fabian, and further testing confirmed the innocence of the drug.

In 1979 a new compound, H168/68 (omeprazole), was synthesized and found to be even more potent as a proton pump inhibitor. A year later clinical programmes started and results looked excellent. Then in 1984 oncogenicity tests in a research laboratory in the USA seemed to show occurrence of gastric carcinomas in rodents. All development was immediately stopped. The pathologist Havu was sent by the company to the laboratory, and soon he found out that the tumours were carcinoids of enterochromaffin-like cells [11]. In 1985 the clinical trials were resumed and in 1988 Losec was licensed in Sweden.

What can one learn from this? I think several conclusions can be drawn. It is perseverance that is a prerequisite for success in research. Experts are more often wrong than right, not least when predicting potential markets for new drugs. Animal models are often misleading and there is no substitute for careful clinical trials. Perhaps most important in the context of this chapter: we, the clinicians, must provide the industrial or basic scientist the problems to work on.

Biologicals—waste of money or sound investment?

In recent years a considerable amount of excitement has been created by reports of dramatic improvements in RA induced by administration of monoclonal anti-tumour necrosis factor (TNF) [12,13] or a construct of human IgG and two p75 soluble TNF receptors [14]. This is understandable, since these are the first controlled studies with confirmed and significant clinical effects of biologically engineered products in RA, and since they followed a number of disappointing trials of anti-T-lymphocyte reagents reactive with CD4, CD5 and CD7 (reviewed in [15]). The optimistic interpretation of the work is that we now know better how to manage aggressive RA and should use any funding in the widespread implementation of TNF inhibition. If the compounds indeed are licensed, continued rigorous trials of combination therapy, dosing and duration and timing of therapy must follow. TNF inhibition may be a powerful way to diminish inflammation and acute-phase reaction, but will it alter the course of RA? There is anecdotal evidence that radiological deterioration continues despite effective anti-TNF therapy. Will it cause severe toxicity? Ten per cent or more of patients develop antibodies against native DNA. Perhaps inhibition of interleukin 1 beta (IL-1β) would be a better treatment over time? Better still would be a low molecular product that could be administered orally. Clearly we need to address these and other queries by carefully planned clinical investigation in prospective trials. This will not be cheap and the industry may not pay the whole price. In the end it will result in better and safer therapy for a disease that is still crippling in a proportion of victims. There is no ethically proper alternative to further research and the end result is likely to be more cost-effective management.

Haemophilia—the cost for a normal life

Haemophilia is a rare disorder which, if untreated, results in crippling joint disease. In the 1950s three young academic physicians, the Blombäck couple in Stockholm and Inga Marie Nilsson in Malmö, started an all-out effort to improve the lives of the ≈ 200 patients from 200 families in Sweden. Having trained in both biochemistry and medicine and expending a great amount of enthusiasm, they managed to combine basic patient care and the persuasion of industry to improve factor VIII and factor IX production. They also talked their respective chiefs and hospital administrations into making modest investments in infrastructure. The efficacy of intravenous therapy of fresh plasma and later purified fractions was proved. An ambitious and centralized programme for orthopaedic reconstructive surgery was organized [16]. The various efforts over the decades has prolonged the life expectancy and increased the chances to live a normal life dramatically. In 1991 recombinant factor VIII was marketed and in 1997 factor IX followed. Today replacement therapy usually starts at the age of 1 year in severe cases. Life expectancy is normal and new joint damage rarely or never occurs [17]. The reverse side of the coin is cost. Abortion of all affected male fetuses would not solve the problem, since 50% of cases have unaffected parents. Further research is needed. At present intravenous administration, usually performed by the mother, is given three times a week. Lower total amounts of factor could, however, be effective if the frequency of administration were increased [18]. Preparations with prolonged half-life could be engineered. Such developments will substantially decrease costs for maintenance therapy. In the end gene therapy may be achieved, although the involved genes are rather large.

Lyme disease—what does it really teach us?

The discovery of Lyme arthritis [19], hailed as one of the most important rheumatological contributions of its decade, was the result of an unusual number of children in a small town taken ill with what observant mothers reported to their listening doctors as tick bites, followed by skin and joint manifestations. For 5 years Lyme disease was described and treated like a new form of juvenile chronic arthritis, occasionally giving rise to erosions and treated with such drugs as antimalarials and glucocorticoids. The efficacy of penicillin was rediscovered and in 1982 the spirochaete that caused the problem was isolated [20]. By then cases had been identified from several places in the USA and other countries. Serological diagnosis was soon developed and the widespread occurrence of Lyme borreliosis confirmed. For unknown reasons arthritis was considered a rare manifestation in Europe. The condition was unknown to a young MD (Dr Johan Berglund) taking up primary care practice in a rural district in southern Sweden in the early 1990s. He was confronted with three cases of what was diagnosed as Lyme arthritis within less than a month and decided to take a closer look at the problem. He established contact with the nearest rheumatologist, with a university hospital-based infectious disease department and with a department of primary care, and within a few years he had completed the largest epidemiological study outside the USA [21] and produced evidence that arthritis was not less prevalent among infected individuals than in the USA [22]. Ongoing studies investigate the transmission of other infectious agents by tick bites. This project has already resulted in earlier diagnosis and better management of a treatable disease. The costs have been modest and partly covered by the local health authorities.

Oral vaccination—dream or reality?

In early years of training we learnt that RA was unusual in rural areas in Africa, just like poliomyelitis, and the idea that in primitive societies, as with poliomyelitis, was associated with early exposure to an environmental organism causing RA seemed basically sound. Consequently the idea of looking for a protective vaccine against RA was rather attractive. Causative agents remain elusive but autoimmunity stays with us. Oral tolerance can be induced by administering antigens in low dose. Oral tolerance in animals can be induced to antigens other than the one that is administered, and this approach is particularly interesting in RA. Animal experiments show some efficacy of collagen II in both collagen-induced arthritis and adjuvant arthritis [23].

Human trials were first published in 1993 [24] but were inconclusive. Later, larger studies were negative or inconclusive [25]. Many sceptics may think little of the idea to continue along this line of research. But perhaps we are facing a 'Losec' problem again. One recent and very intriguing development is coupling of antigens to cholera toxin B, which is inert but has a strong affinity for gut mucosa [26]. It therefore can be considered as a powerful biologic delivery device to the gut membrane. Encouraging animal results have been published where administration of conjugated human insulin prevented spontaneous autoimmune diabetes in mice [27]. The mechanism may be modulation of T-cell function from Th1 to Th2, changing cytokine patterns [28]. The same principle has also been used successfully in the treatment of experimental autoimmune encephalitis (EAE) by administration of conjugated myelin basic protein [29]. Similar experiments giving conjugated collagen II to animals with latent or manifest collagen-induced arthritis are very encouraging (A. Tarkowski, personal communication, 1997). Since RA shows several features suggestive of a Th1-induced disease it is indeed tempting to start trials in humans with antigens like collagen II conjugated to cholera toxin B.

Optimizing quality in patient care and research

The ultimate goal of our profession must be to move towards a balance between management of patients as we understand it today and research directed at improving the management of tomorrow. By definition this will obtain the most benefit out of limited resources. One can see this process as travelling by car from one place to another. There will be stretches of highway with adequate traffic flow, there will be terrible bottlenecks and there may be wastefully oversized parts of the road. Basic science is producing results at an ever-increasing speed thanks to technological advances. Many of these results could be of fundamental interest to investigators of disease mechanisms and further down the road to investigators involved in patient-orientated disease. Unfortunately, the different categories of people do not always communicate well enough.

Measures to implement delivery of patient care will differ much between countries and whereas needs are well satisfied in some countries they are not at all met in others. When the good data to support a rationale for better resources are available, it is the duty of the profession to fight for their implementation. Patient organizations will gladly use their influence, to which politicians are sensitive, to do the same.

Optimizing research is a more complex matter. In a recent editorial the Nobel laureates Goldstein and Brown [30] examine this problem. They make a distinction between basic research, disease-orientated research and patient-orientated research. The last is research where the investigator shakes hands with the patient. This is also called clinical research, and whereas basic and disease-orientated research are flourishing, clinical is not. In the past the clinical investigator could spend part of the time on the wards and the rest in the research laboratory. Patient problems were always the inspiration for the work in the laboratory. Today this type of academic double life is more difficult and both laboratory and other research work are increasingly performed by PhDs. It becomes more important to build bridges between bedside medicine and disease-orientated research. Goldstein and Brown give examples of fruitful twin teams, such as their own and that of Hench and Kendall [2]. I could add several more, one being that between my teachers Jan Waldenström, the great clinician, and Carl-Bertil Laurell, the chemical pathologist, and another between the rheumatologist Tore Saxne and the biochemist Dick Heinegård. In such teams each partner understands and has some knowledge of the other's work but also some unique skills that are not shared. They have to be good enough friends to be able to criticize each other briskly.

In order to facilitate application of new basic knowledge, we must try to stimulate bright young doctors to embark on a career in clinical research, and help them to build bridges to basic science laboratories.

Looking out of the window at the department of rheumatology makes me hopeful. I can watch the digging of a big hole for the new biomedical centre, which when completed will bring all so-called preclinical and clinical research within spitting range of the emergency room, clinics and patient wards. Several bridges will connect the buildings. If things go well this will result in more interaction between doctors caring for patients and those working in the laboratory, and stimulate faster patient-orientated applications of progress in basic science.

References

1 Krämer W. *Wir Kurieren uns zu Tode.* Berlin: Ullstein Taschenbuch 1997.

2 Hench PS, Kendall EC, Slocumb CH, Polley HF. The effect of a hormone of the adrenocortical cortex (17-hydroxy-11-dehydrocorticosterone: compound E) and of pituitary adrenocorticotropic hormone on rheumatoid arthritis: Preliminary report. *Proc Staff Meet Mayo Clin* 1949; 24: 181–97.

3 Kirwan JR. The effect of glucocorticoids on joint destruction in rheumatoid arthritis. *N Engl J Med* 1995; 333: 142–6.

4 Chakravarty K, Pharoah PDP, Scott DGI. A randomized controlled study of post-injection rest following intra-articular steroid therapy for knee synovitis. *Br J Rheumatol* 1994; 33: 464–8.

5 Svartz N. Salazopyrin, a new sulfanilamide preparation. *Acta Med Scand* 1942; 110: 577–98.

6 Sinclair RJG, Duthie JJR. Salazopyrin in the treatment of rheumatoid arthritis. *Ann Rheum Dis* 1948; 8: 226–31.

7 McConkey B, Amos RS, Durham S *et al*. Sulphasalazine in rheumatoid arthritis. *Br Med J* 1980; 280: 442–4.

8 ten Wolde S, Breedveld FC, Hermans J *et al*. Randomised placebo-controlled study of stopping second-line drugs in rheumatoid arthritis. *Lancet* 1996; 347: 347–52.

9 ten Wolde S, Hermans J, Breedveld FC, Dijkmans BA. Effect of resumption of second line drugs in patients with rheumatoid arthritis that flared up after treatment discontinuation. *Ann Rheum Dis* 1997; 56: 235–9.

10 Östholm I. *Från örtavkok till läkemedel*. Stockholm:

Apotekarsocietetens förlag, 1991: 5–295.

11 Havu N. Enterochromaffin-like cell carcinoids of gastric mucosa in rats after life-long inhibiton of gastric secretion. *Digestion* 1986; 35 (Suppl. 1): 42–55.

12 Elliott MJ, Maini RN, Feldmann M *et al.* Randomised double-blind comparison of chimeric monoclonal antibody to tumour necrosis factor alpha (cA2) versus placebo in rheumatoid arthritis. *Lancet* 1994; 344: 1105–10.

13 Rankin EC, Choy EH, Kassimos D *et al.* The therapeutic effects of an engineered human anti-tumour necrosis factor alpha antibody (CDP571) in rheumatoid arthritis. *Br J Rheumatol* 1995; 34: 334–42.

14 Moreland LW, Baumgartner SW, Schiff MH *et al.* Treatment of rheumatoid arthritis with recombinant tumor necrosis factor receptor (p75) -Fc fusion protein. *N Engl J Med* 1997; 337: 141–7.

15 Moreland LW, Heck LW Jr, Koopman WJ. Biologic agents for treating rheumatoid arthritis. Concepts and progress. *Arthritis Rheum* 1997; 40: 397–409.

16 Ahlbeck Å. Haemophilia in Sweden. VII. Incidence, treatment prophylaxis arthropathy other musculoskeletal manifestations of haemophilia A and B. *Acta Orthop Scand* 1965; (Suppl. 77): 3–132.

17 Nilsson IM, Berntorp E, Lethagen S, Ljung R, Petersson C. *Haemophilia*. Uppsala, Sweden: Pharmacy Plasma Products, 1944: 1–100.

18 Carlsson M. *Pharmacokinetic dosing of factor VIII and factor IX in prophylactic treatment*. Thesis, Lund University, 1997.

19 Steere AC, Malawista SE, Syndman DR *et al.* Lyme arthritis. An epidemic of oligoarticular arthritis in children and adults in three Connecticut communities. *Arthritis Rheum* 1977; 20: 7–17.

20 Burgdorfer W, Barbour AG, Hayes SF *et al.* Lyme disease—a tick-borne spirochetosis? *Science* 1982; 216: 1317–19.

21 Berglund J, Eitrem R, Ornstein K *et al.* An epidemiologic study of Lyme disease in southern Sweden. *N Engl J Med* 1995; 333: 1319–27.

22 Berglund J, Blomberg I, Hansen BU. Lyme borreliosis in rheumatological practice: identification of Lyme arthritis and diagnostic aspects in a Swedish county with high endemity. *Br J Rheumatol* 1996; 35: 853–60.

23 Weiner HL. Oral tolerance: immune mechanisms and treatment of autoimmune diseases. *Immunol Today* 1997; 18: 335–43.

24 Trentham DE, Dynesius-Trentham RA, Orav EJ *et al.* Effects of oral administration of type II collagen on rheumatoid arthritis. *Science* 1993; 261: 1727–30.

25 Sieper J, Kary S, Sorensen H *et al.* Oral type II collagen treatment in early rheumatoid arthritis. A double-blind, placebo-controlled, randomized trial. *Arthritis Rheum* 1996; 39: 41–51.

26 Holmgren J, Lycke N, Czerkinsky C. Cholera toxin and cholera B subunit as oral-mucosa adjuvant and antigen vector. *Vaccine* 1993; 11: 1179–84.

27 Bergerot I, Ploix C, Petersen J *et al.* A cholera toxoid-insulin conjugate as an oral vaccine against spontaneous autoimmune diabetes. *Proc Natl Acad Sci USA* 1997; 94: 4610–14.

28 Ploix C, Bergerot I, Fabien N, Perche S, Moulin V, Thivolet C. Protection against autoimmune diabetes with oral insulin is associated with the presence of IL-4 type 2 T-cells in the pancreas and pancreatic lymph nodes. *Diabetes* 1998; 47: 39–44.

29 Sun JB, Rask C, Olsson T, Holmgren J, Czerkinsky C. Treatment of experimental autoimmune encephalomyelitis by feeding myelin basic protein conjugated to cholera toxin B subunit. *Proc Natl Acad Sci USA* 1996; 93: 7196–201.

30 Goldstein JL, Brown MS. The clinical investigator: Bewitched, bothered, and bewildered—but still beloved. *J Clin Invest* 1997; 99: 2803–12.

Index